The Insiders' Guide to UK Medical Schools 2(

The Insiders' Guide to UK Medical Schools 2007/2008

The Alternative Prospectus compiled by the BMA Medical Students Committee

Edited by

**Sally Girgis,
Leigh Bissett and
David Burke**

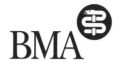

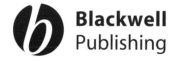

Published by Blackwell Publishing Ltd

Blackwell Publishing, Inc., 350 Main Street, Malden, Massachusetts 02148-5020, USA
Blackwell Publishing Ltd, 9600 Garsington Road, Oxford OX4 2DQ, UK
Blackwell Publishing Asia Pty Ltd, 550 Swanston Street, Carlton, Victoria 3053, Australia
The right of the Author to be identified as the Author of this Work has been asserted in accordance with the Copyright, Designs and Patents Act 1988.

First published 1998
Second edition 1999
Third edition 2000
Fourth edition 2001
Fifth edition 2002
Second impression 2002
Sixth edition 2003
Seventh edition 2004
Eight edition 2005
Reprint 2006
Ninth edition 2007

ISBN: 978-1-4051-5748-3

A catalogue record for this title is available from the British Library

Set in 9/11 Helvetica by Sparks, Oxford – www.sparks.co.uk

Printed and bound in the United Kingdom by TJ International Ltd, Padstow, Cornwall

Commissioning Editor: Mary Banks
Editorial Assistant: Victoria Pittman
Development Editor: Simone Dudziak
Production Controller: Rachel Edwards

Cartoons © Clive Featherstone
For further information on Blackwell Publishing, visit our website:
http://www.blackwellpublishing.com

The publisher's policy is to use permanent paper from mills that operate a sustainable forestry policy, and which has been manufactured from pulp processed using acid-free and elementary chlorine-free practices. Furthermore, the publisher ensures that the text paper and cover board used have met acceptable environmental accreditation standards.

Contents

Foreword   ix

Preface   xi

Acknowledgements
and contributors   xiii

Meet Mikey and Michelle   xv

Part 1: Insiders' information   1

    1.   Is medicine right for you?   3
    2.   Life as a medical student   7
    3.   Applying to medical school   20
    4.   Graduate and premedical courses   39
    5.   Funding your way through   46
    6.   Life beyond graduation …   55

Part 2: The A–Z of UK medical schools   61

    How to use Part 2   61

    Aberdeen   65
    Barts and The London   73
    Belfast   82
    Birmingham   90
    Brighton and Sussex Medical School   98
    Bristol   107
    Cambridge   115
    Cardiff   125
    Derby   134
    Dundee   141
    East Anglia   150

Edinburgh	159
Glasgow	167
Guy's, King's and St Thomas'	175
Hull and York	183
Imperial College London	192
Leeds	200
Leicester	208
Liverpool	217
Manchester and Keele	224
Newcastle and Durham	234
Nottingham	244
Oxford	252
Peninsula	261
Royal Free and University College London	270
St Andrews	279
St George's	286
Sheffield	294
Southampton	302
Warwick	310
Appendices	317
Mikey and Michelle's quick compare table	318
Glossary	321
Further information	325

Leigh Bissett is a final-year medical student at the University of East Anglia in Norwich. He qualified in law before going on to medicine and he thought this was an excellent career choice. Leigh joined the BMA Medical Students Committee in 2002 and rose in the ranks to become the Chair of the MSC between 2003 and 2005. He worked passionately on welfare issues and continues to take an interest in such issues. He has been involved with the development of the BMA/CHMS School Charter and the MSC document on minimum standards in undergraduate medical education *Medicine in the 21st Century*. He has had experience on various committees including the Modernising Medical Careers board as well as chairing local groups such as the UEA Student's Union Council.

David Burke is in his final year of studying medicine at The University of Nottingham. He entered the course as a graduate, with a first class honours degree in Medical Biochemistry, from The University of Birmingham. He was formerly a member of the BMA Medical Students Committee, and is joint editor of the BMA document *Medicine in the 21st Century*. He is also a trustee of the British Medical and Dental Students Trust. At Birmingham he was chairman of the Guild Council and held a seat on the University Senate.

Sally Girgis has worked for the British Medical Association for the past five years. She has worked for the General Practitioners Committee, Medical Students Committee and currently works for the Medical Academic Staff Committee. This is the fourth and final edition of the *Insiders' Guide to Medical Schools* that she has co-edited.

Foreword

Let's face it, we don't expect to choose which medical school we go to – most of us go to the one we get in to. Just one offer is all we need. Bearing that in mind, it makes sense to spend some time thinking through what we really want from our medical school and university. Where do we want to spend the next 5 or 6 years of our lives and – potentially – the few years after medical school when we start our first job?

Five or six years may seem like a long time now, but, before you know it, you have nearly finished your course and are considering where you would like to live and work. A few years ago a BMA survey indicated that over 75% of final-year medical students wanted to work where they had studied medicine. This never occurred to us when applying to medical school! What did occur to us was that, as only one of four schools is likely to offer us a place, we should be sure that we would be happy there.

The Insiders' Guide to Medical Schools is a guide to all the things that might make your experience of medical school better or worse. Do you think that a problem-based learning course would suit you, or would you prefer regular examinations? Are you desperate to do anatomical dissection? Would you like the option of undertaking an intercalated degree during your time at medical school? These things are covered in this book too. It may seem now that putting four schools on an application form is an easy decision, but if you are using this book, you have already realised that there are many choices to be made. What is the city like? What facilities does the university have that you may be interested in using? Is an Olympic-size swimming pool important? Or do you desire to be a short drive from the sea?

Researched by current medical students, *The Insiders' Guide* gives the student perspective on each medical course in the country. Of course, medical education is not static, and universities and medical schools have to respond to new evidence about training, changing demands from the General Medical Council and students' evaluations of their own courses. This means that not everything in this book can be completely up-to-date with regard to the specifics of each medical course. What *The Insiders' Guide* does is help you access relevant information about each medical course, as viewed by current students, that may help narrow down your options.

An important consideration for students, and their families, is the cost of funding ourselves throughout our studies. The arrangements can seem complicated and overwhelming, but this book gives an idea of the costs of living in different cities, along with the distances travelled to peripheral hospital placements, and points to several useful websites. These could be important considerations for you when weighing up which school gets a place on your UCAS form.

We didn't know about this book before we applied to medical school, but we wish that we had. We did realise that taking the huge step into medical training would need us to be happy where we lived and studied, and we both feel we would have been happy at any of our four choices. Our own research paid off, but would have been made much easier and less time-consuming if we had known about *The Insiders' Guide.*

Medical education in the UK is known to be world class: we can expect that wherever we study we will access excellent teaching and gain the necessary skills and experience to become excellent doctors.

Studying medicine is challenging but it is an immensely rewarding experience. There is a breadth of opportunities available to you throughout your medical career: a degree in medicine opens many doors, not just into clinical practice. We wish you the best of luck in your application to medical school and subsequent medical education and career.

Kirsty Lloyd
Chair
BMA Medical Students Committee 2005–06

Emily Rigby
Chair
BMA Medical Students Committee 2006–07

Preface

Obstacles cannot crush me
Every obstacle yields to stern resolve
He who is fixed to a star does not change his mind.

Leonardo da Vinci

Why we dream for the things we do often eludes us, but the realisation of ambition should not. Preparation paves the way to success; leaving your future to chance leads to ambiguity at best. Entry to the medical profession is fiercely competitive, but if you are well informed, and truly understand what you are undertaking, you will maximise your chances of success.

Being a doctor offers the chance to alleviate sickness, heal the wounded, deliver babies, comfort the dying and even avert death. In which other profession could you see the human brain, hold a heart, work as part of a close multidisciplinary team to save lives, help children to grow up safely and yet watch people slowly demise despite your best efforts? It requires a lot from the individual too: you will have to break bad news, announce good news, listen, examine, investigate and diagnose, and apply a thorough understanding of the human being in order to treat. Don't ask yourself *can I do this?* but rather, *after training, do I want to do this?* If your answer is a well-considered *yes*, then with the proper work experience and knowledge you should be able to convince others at interview.

The medical course is longer than most other degrees, but the clinical years deliver a welcome boost with an apprenticeship-style feel that smoothes the transition to doctor. Occasionally you will have to work hard into the late hours of the night, and yet at other times you will have the odd day off – you and your life need to be flexible. With tuition fees, accommodation costs, exorbitant social life, clinical clothes, and the long duration of the course, your costs are going to be high. However, after qualification medics are fairly paid and the expense should not deter the genuine applicant.

There are more medical school places available in the UK than ever before, and the decision of where to apply should not be taken lightly. Benefiting from nearly a decade of contributors, our book is written by preclinical and clinical medical students from every UK medical school – truly making it *The Insiders' Guide*. From course structure and teaching methods, to application statistics and tips, placement distances, accommodation prices, opportunities to travel, assessment methods, and much, much more: this book has it all!

We wish you the best of luck with your application.

Leigh Bissett, David Burke, and Sally Girgis
BMA House, London 2007

Acknowledgements and contributors

We would like to thank all the many individuals and institutions that have provided the information and views contained in this book. This book would not be possible without their help. We would also like to thank the numerous BMA and Blackwells staff who have contributed at various stages in the preparation of this book. Their support and efforts on our behalf have been invaluable and are very much appreciated.

The need for an *Insiders' Guide* and the vision for its production were first dreamt up many years ago by members of the Medical Students Committee who have long since graduated and are busy working as doctors. Each edition has built upon the hard work and ideas of the editions that preceded it and to these past pioneers we are truly grateful. Finally, we would like to thank all the members of the BMA's Medical Students Committee, both past and present, who have contributed to *The Insiders' Guide*. We believe it is a fantastic resource and hope it will continue to go from strength to strength in the years to come.

If you have any suggestions for ways in which *The Insiders' Guide* could be improved we would very much like to hear them. Please email: info.students@bma.org.uk

Student contributors in the 2007–08 edition
Ashraf Abbas, Mobeen Ahmed, Clare Aitchison, Lucy Alego, Ferras Alwan, Harnaik Bajwa, Alison Barbour, Laura Barnfield, Rosalind Benson, Tom Berry, Delphine Boury, Emma Brandon, Rebecca Bright, Megan Broomfield, Nicola Browne, David Connell, Lucy-Jane Davis, Laura Davison, Angela Deeley, Melissa Evans, Jane Farrow, Helen Gordon, Sharon Hadley, Jason Holdcroft, Gurjiven Hothi, Hardeep Hunjan, Bala Karunakaran, Fionla Lynch, Ian MacCormick, Swetha Maddula, Matt Mak, Nigel Mendes, Vasantha Muthu, Brendan O'Brien, Gemma Owens, James Piper, Jerry Raju, Helen Reilly, Clare Russell, Indira Sabanathan, Carolyn Scott, Louise Shinn, Ross Spackman, Leo Smith, Sabrina Talukdar, Joannis Vamvakopolous, Helen Wagstaff, Siobhan Wilson, Noamaan Wilson-Baig, Rebecca Wells, Andrew Wickham, Paul Young and Anthi Zeniou.

Previous editors
Alex Almourdaris, Jo Burgess, Simon Calvert, Jennie Ceichan, Deborah Cohen, Lizz Corps, Chris Ferguson, Sally Girgis, Karen Hebert, Kristian Mears, Richard Partridge, Kinesh Patel, Philip Smith, Jill Spencer and Ian Urmstrong.

Special thanks
Ann-Marie Aleppo, Mary Banks, Natalie Breeze, Kevin Hand, Andrew Pearson and Kirsty Lloyd.

Cartoons created by:
Clive Featherstone

Editorial assistance:
Helen Paddock and Jason Penn

David's personal acknowledgements:
To my mum, dad and sister, and for my granddad.

Leigh's personal acknowledgements:
Most importantly thank you mum, dad, Craig, and the rest of the Bissett/Small family, who have allowed me to pursue all my dreams, and set me up for life – I know I could not have done it without you. Thanks also to the other special people in my life – Ed, Sarah, the Chrises, and Karen.

Sally's personal acknowledgements:
A big thanks to Richard Cashman, the inspiration for me agreeing to edit my first IGMS four years ago. To mum and dad for letting me loose on the other side of the world – promise I'll come home soon.

Meet Mikey and Michelle

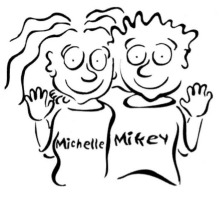

If you are reading this book, congratulations – you are certainly doing your research! This book hopes to give you a view of medical schools from a student perspective, and it is the only one that can boast insider information. Michelle and Mikey, the two characters on this page, are here to help you around the book and point out interesting issues for students applying to medical school. On occasion you will come across a word, phrase or abbreviation that you may be unaware of – we have tried to pick these out and put them in a list which you can find on the pages that follow.

So, how do you use this book? This book has had a huge number of contributors, all with specialist insight into the medical schools. The book cannot claim to be totally impartial as the contributors have written about their own medical schools and if you have any doubts we recommend that you contact the school directly.

The book has been divided into two parts:

Part 1

Part 1 contains general information designed to help you decide whether medicine is right for you as a potential career or study subject. It also makes suggestions about your personal statement, interviews, and considerations you must take when making an application through UCAS. The new examinations and processes that you must undergo to gain a place at medical school in the United Kingdom are also described. We recommend that you read the finance section, as this has changed quite considerably since the introduction of top-up fees. The BMA's student finance guru has spent a great deal of time giving you the detail you need when you attend medical school.

All chapters in Part 1 have been written by individuals with specialist insight into finance, welfare systems, and future careers for doctors, so it is well worth reading them in order to give yourself a good insight into studying medicine, and it will be very helpful for your interviews.

Part 2

This is the section that makes this book unique. No other book has access to medical students from *every* medical school in the United Kingdom. Every medical school has a chapter that aims to give you as much insider information as possible to you the applicant. The chapters formally cover key facts about the school, the educational structure, the placements, opportunities to travel, information on sports and societies, and a short list of the good and the not so good things about each school.

We have used the symbols below to make skim-reading easier when looking up specific topics:

 Education

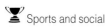 Welfare

Sports and social

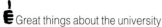 Great things about the university

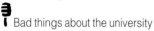 Bad things about the university

At the end of the day, you need to choose a medical school which offers the right social and educational set up for you. It is therefore advisable to have your own list of ideals and then see which of the medical schools match them. This might be the need for early patient contact or the presence of a Duke of Edinburgh Society. This will allow you to really pinpoint schools which will suit your needs, and ultimately make your time there far more enjoyable. For students with disabilities or any other special requirements, it is advisable that you make contact with the schools directly to discuss any reasonable adjustments that you may require when you attend medical school.

Whilst this book does attempt to provide all the information you need, it is impossible to cover everything. We therefore advise that you read the other information that is out there.

Remember:

- Access websites run by medical schools (the school will often have a medical society)
- Talk to the medical students at the school
- Attend the open days
- Read the school's prospectus
- Look around the town and surrounding area
- Look at transport links for travel to and from home
- If you have any other needs, enquire about them with the support structures at the school.

A book like this could never claim to be totally objective or definitive about all the differences and similarities, or strengths and weaknesses between the medical schools. Every effort has been made to ensure that the opinions of the medical students who contributed to the book are based on factual information. Take the opinions offered here into account and we strongly recommend this book alongside other material you will have collected (from prospectuses to the opinions of others) as you draw up your shortlist of where to apply.

Part 1
Insiders' information

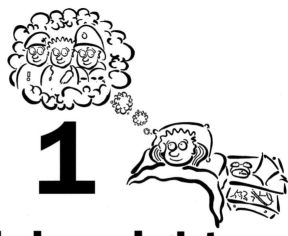

1

Is medicine right for you?

Guido the plumber and Michelangelo obtained their marble from the same quarry, but what each saw in the marble made the difference between a nobleman's sink and a brilliant sculpture

Bob Kall

If you were to ask the average student why they chose to put medicine on their UCAS form, the responses would vary wildly. At interview the answers fall in to three major categories:

'I enjoy science.'

'I want to help people.'

'I know I would get job satisfaction from a career in medicine.'

The medical school is going to delve a little deeper when deciding who to give their oversubscribed places to, and will want to know the other reasons for choosing medicine over other career options. Some people may have chosen medicine because of parental pressure, job security in the future, steady income, because family members are doctors or they have the grades, or for the raw sex appeal and kudos that goes with the job! Whatever your reasons, you should certainly discuss the career options with your friends, family, and careers advisors, and reflect upon any experiences you may have had with the medical profession to focus your motivations for such a big leap. Do not let anybody else make the decision for you.

Doctors continue to be held in high regard by the general public. The 2005 MORI public opinion poll reported that doctors continue to be the most trusted profession in the UK. But, with this trust comes a great deal of responsibility which must be borne out in high professional standards, personal integrity, and a willingness to constantly evaluate the work you undertake, in order to improve care for the patients you and your colleagues treat. You need to have these values both at medical school and upon qualification.

Medicine, like nursing and other vocational courses, makes greater demands of your time whilst at university. There is plenty of time for partying and play, but, unlike other courses, time management and commitment to clinical attachments is a core aspect of study. Turning up to clinical practice worse for wear is not an option when you consider important issues such as patient safety and comfort; the last thing you want as a patient in hospital is a recovering medical student trying to examine your lungs or take a history about your shortness of breath.

Every day, medicine poses unique ethical, emotional, clinical, and cultural challenges – some of which can be stressful and unpleasant. Important ones to consider include breaking bad news, dealing with abusive patients, dealing with uncertainty, feeling frustration at the lack of time or resources available to you, long days and long nights, and your beliefs about abortion, euthanasia, and other controversial topics. Some medical school interviews may even discuss these things with you in an attempt to glean information from you – it is OK to have an opinion but try and remain measured and balanced.

We seem to have painted a pretty negative picture about medicine, but actually everything mentioned above makes it a diverse and stimulating environment in which to work, with fresh challenges every single day of your working life. Treating patients and their relatives can be a huge buzz, especially when you improve their quality of life. At times your ability to intervene will be limited and patients get progressively worse or may suffer pain, but very often it is the care and compassion you can offer the patient that will make the big difference, not the medical intervention.

Every year, large numbers of students apply to enter medical school. There has been a steady expansion of medical school numbers in an attempt to train more doctors, and most importantly to encourage greater diversity in the medical profession. This ease of access is being slowly improved through innovative and intensive fast-track degree courses and access/foundation courses. However, this massive step forward faces a significant challenge with the introduction of top-up tuition fees and the ever-increasing costs of living as a student.

Salaries for junior doctors have increased significantly over the last few years and are set to continue rising, so whilst you can expect high levels of debt, the salary at the other end will enable you to enter the black within a few years of qualification. Indeed, some junior doctors can be paid an annual salary of around £34,000 (before tax). The workload can be very demanding and salaries do reflect the need to do night shifts, work long hours, and face significant time away from family and friends. Saying this, the introduction of the European Working Time Directive (EWTD) has improved the working conditions for doctors.

If your aim is to make huge piles of cash, to run around in a white coat looking like a star from television's *Casualty*, or to demonstrate your academic prowess, you are not likely to enjoy your time at medical school, so make sure you have considered all careers. There are easier ways to make money and the work is not glamorous: 400 blood samples later you'll be cursing those late night *ER* sessions! Your major influence should be dedication to patient care and continual learning, as this is the reality of a career as a doctor. Whilst many of your friends in other professions will be able to relax at the end of a working day or even be earning money, you may finish a long shift only to have to begin your study for the evening, and young doctors frequently spend their weekends working. Whatever combination of reasons has made you consider medicine, remember it is a vocation. Those who enter medical school with a strong commitment to work hard, learn, and serve patients to the best of their ability are the people most likely to find life as a doctor richly rewarding and stimulating.

As mentioned previously, widening participation has been a key agenda for the government, professional bodies, and medical schools, and the Human Rights Act introduced in 2001 offers greater protection than ever before to people who are not treated equally in society. To this end, the General Medical Council (GMC) states that all applicants who have the potential to meet the learning outcomes set by the GMC should be considered for admission to medical school without prejudice. There has been progress over the last few years and medical schools and professional bodies have been trying hard to ensure that students from all backgrounds have fair access. As the medical student population becomes increasingly diverse, it is much easier for mature students and students with dependents, disabilities, and ill health to study medicine than in the past. The enactment of the Disability Discrimination Act in 2004 has ensured that disabled applicants have a fairer chance when applying to study medicine. The Council of Heads of Medical Schools (CHMS) have also joined the GMC in acknowledging that students with a blood-borne virus (HIV, hepatitis B, hepatitis C) should be allowed to study and qualify as doctors with suitable career plans that do not pose a risk to patients. In addition, the Age Discrimination Act came into force in 2006 and may make it unlawful to impose age limits for entry to medicine.

All this said, students with particular needs should consider the medical schools carefully and should liaise with the individual school (contacts at the back of each chapter) to ensure that additional support is provided and that you yourself are happy with arrangements and facilities available.

Medical schools have also made huge steps over the last decade, with ethnic minorities comprising 30% of the intake and 60% of the population are now female. Discrimination does still occur in medical schools and the health service, often in subtle ways, but the BMA, the Department of Health, and all medical schools are committed to equal opportunities for all.

Gay, lesbian and bisexual applicants are often concerned about the implications their sexuality will have upon their career progression and work environment. Whilst some members of the medical profession do have intolerant attitudes towards an individual's sexuality or gender, they are a dwindling breed and all employers should protect you from any form of discrimination you may face. Groups do exist to support doctors and students (see Further Information) and gay and lesbian doctors can be found across all grades and specialties.

Some people know before they start medical school what medical career they want, but it is probably better to remain open-minded as you will have an opportunity to experience a whole range of specialties whilst at medical school and during your first job. Whatever you do, it is vital that you continue your medical education throughout your entire career to keep your skills and knowledge up to date.

It is worth remembering that the decision to study medicine could change your life and many students in your position will be toying with the idea of studying pharmacy, law, veterinary science, and other courses. How then can you be sure medicine is for you?

- Speak to doctors – your own GP might give you some good pointers.

- Get some work experience at your local hospital if they allow students to.

- Look at the internet, read books, go to the local library and order other books on the subject – volumes and volumes of information are available.

- First-hand experience in a medical environment is beneficial but if you can't access this, involve yourself in the community, for example by offering to be a helper with charitable organizations.

- Whatever you do, make sure you understand that medicine involves a huge service commitment to other people, and if this is a driver for you then being a doctor may be an ideal job for you.

Finally, and most importantly, the decision to study medicine is yours, and yours alone! The hours will be long, whether it is revising for that clinical exam or writing up another patient log book. You will be at university for longer than the majority of your friends, and whilst the financial rewards are significant in medicine, there is always room for earning more in other professions. Studying medicine will truly be the first step toward a future in which people will rely upon your integrity, your passion for the job and your compassion for serving others. It is a fantastic career, with the potential for tremendous job satisfaction that is worth all the associated stress, study, and pressure.

Key Points

- Try and get as much information about the medical profession as possible. This will benefit you for your interview and will help you decide whether medicine is actually for you.

- Speak to as many doctors as you can and arrange a placement in a hospital or general practice surgery if possible.

- Ensure that the medical school can facilitate learning if you have any special requirements.

- Discuss the full career options with your friends, parents, and careers advisor, and consider important features such as salary, job demands, and career progression.

- Make the decision based on your own feelings, not what others tell you.

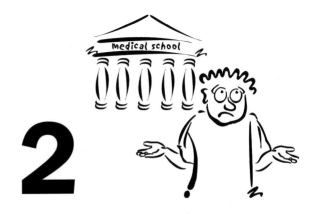

2

Life as a medical student

Medical education is not completed at the medical school, it is only begun.

William H. Welch (1850–1934)

How unfair! Only one health, and so many diseases.

Victor Schlichter, attributed by his son Dr. Andres J. Schlichter,
Children's Hospital, Buenos Aires, Argentina

How am I going to be taught?

In the past, there was a view that medical students spent their first couple of years cramming a vast amount of knowledge without ever seeing a patient, and then emerged brainwashed, unable to think and unable to communicate.

If this ever was the case, it is now very much a thing of the past. Recommendations in the General Medical Council (GMC) report *Tomorrow's Doctors* encouraged medical schools to reduce the emphasis on learning factual information and concentrate much more on developing the skills and attitudes needed to become a doctor. The foundations of factual knowledge established at medical school would then be built on whilst practising as a doctor. The report also recommended the introduction of special study modules (SSMs) to give students the chance to undertake projects of their own choosing. Alongside this, the GMC encouraged schools to adopt a more 'problem-based learning' (PBL) approach to teaching, where facts are taught within a framework of real-life clinical scenarios.

Developing research skills and encouraging intellectual curiosity and enthusiasm for learning are now as important as knowledge. The emphasis is placed very firmly on producing graduates who will be life-long learners – preparing students for the necessity of continuing professional development once qualified. The majority of medical schools have already changed their curricula so that older courses, in which science and clinical practice were taught separately, have given way to more integrated curricula. In other words, instead of learning subjects separately – for example, anatomy, biochemistry and physiology (subject-based teaching) – students learn about respiration, reproduction, diet and metabolism in a more systems-based approach.

Mikey's view: a day in the life of a preclinical student

Just another Tuesday. My alarm clock sounds and I realise I have 20 minutes to make the bed-to-medschool journey. Suffering slightly from a cold, I head with the feeling of impending doom towards the dissection room. Anatomy is tough to learn and requires more than rote learning alone. I'm hoping that the anatomy tutor isn't going to pick me today to demonstrate the route of some obscure vessel or nerve. We start by reviewing the liver and gastrointestinal (GI) system. Unfortunately, the air conditioning system seems to be on the blink as I am quite sure that the smell from the cadaver really isn't meant to be quite so pungent. Despite feeling distinctly nauseous all morning I seem to be ravenous by the time our coffee break arrives and treat myself to a chocolate muffin.

The anatomy session overruns and, after the 10-minute break, I arrive slightly late for my 2-hour lecture block consisting of physiology of the liver followed by pathology of the GI system. I arrive at the back of the lecture theatre only to realise that the only spare seats are at the front! Clutching my anatomy tomes I try to slip in unnoticed – but fail miserably.

We learn about the release of digestive enzymes from the pancreas and the role of the liver in the absorption of nutrients from the gut into the blood. I furiously scribble notes only to find, at the end of the lecture, that the professor has kindly printed off all of his PowerPoint slides. In the pathology lecture we are shown pictures of removed and dissected specimens. 'If I have a picture of it,' says the pathologist, 'they didn't survive it.' Hmm ... what an interesting thought before lunch.

A well-deserved hour-long lunch break is followed with my favourite lecturer in the clinical skills lab. We're learning the basics of urinalysis and how the presence of certain molecules in the urine indicates particular diseases. They used to taste for glucose in the urine, once upon a time, to check for diabetes mellitus: I'm sure grateful for medical research! At the end of the session, we are asked to read up on good communication skills in preparation for next week when we will role-play different clinical scenarios.

It always amazes me how the end of the day makes me feel so energised. My housemate and I start planning the night ahead on our walk home. Feeling very self-righteous I decide that I will be sensible and stay in, as I have a hospital visit tomorrow and must be in for 8:30 AM. Hospital visits are a real highlight, and one of the few opportunities we preclinical students get to experience clinical life as a doctor. I get home, dust down the stethoscope, and start re-reading my notes. After some revision I feel I've definitely earned some time to myself, so I head down to the rugby ground for a rather intense training session. Our team's doing really well this year, and there's an important tournament on the horizon. It's late when I get back, so a big group of us order takeaway and stay up for hours talking shop. I am sure I had to be up for something in the morning but can't quite remember what …

In the past, medical courses were very much split into preclinical (academic-led) and clinical (clinician-led) phases. The divide is far less dramatic these days and, in most schools, students will have regular contact with clinicians and patients from the outset. The early years still have less clinical content and more lecture and laboratory teaching, but the traditional preclinical/clinical divide is dying. An important effect of these changes is that students need to be much more responsible for their own studies, and self-motivation and self-discipline are essential. Clinical skills laboratories have been introduced in most schools so that students can practise procedures and take examinations on dummies; this helps to build confidence before going on the wards and carrying out the same examinations on patients. The balance between lectures, PBL, SSMs, and clinical exposure will vary between schools and is worth considering carefully in order to help you choose the medical school which best suits your preferred style of learning. You need to decide what type of learner you are: some people prefer more structured timetables, and so prefer the lecture-based curricula; others prefer more independence and flexibility, and are likely to enjoy problem-based learning more.

Clinical work takes place in local teaching hospitals and district general hospitals (DGHs), which can be many miles away from the medical school. These attachments take you out of town, but getting away from the big city hospitals often provides the opportunity to be more involved in a team, gain more hands-on experience, and, ultimately, to learn more. The group of healthcare professionals and other students you are attached to are known as your 'firm'. Most schools provide free accommodation within the hospitals if commuting is not practical. Some schools will even allow overseas attachments in addition to the elective. Due to the increasing number of students studying medicine, most universities have to send their students further afield for a longer period of time. It is important that you fully understand the implications of this, as it is almost certain that you will be spending significant time away from your main university address.

But I'm squeamish!

As you would imagine, there is a fair amount of blood and gore in medicine at various stages: for example, physiology practicals, post-mortems, dissection, and taking blood. Many students become used to this remarkably quickly. For others, it may take longer. It may surprise you to know that some doctors are still squeamish after many years of practice. If you are very concerned about how you might react, try to arrange some appropriate work experience at your local hospital.

I've heard it's really hard work!

Now that the emphasis is placed more on learning appropriate skills and attitudes, rather than cramming vast amounts of facts, the ability to be able to list reams of detailed biochemistry or pathology is less important. Nonetheless there are still exams and the amount that a medical student is expected to know on graduation is still considerable. More importantly, the amount that you learn during your time at medical school will have a direct impact on your ability to perform as a new doctor, and the thought that the wellbeing of patients will shortly be in your hands is an incredible motivation to work hard.

Medicine remains a very demanding course and friends studying for other degrees may have as many hours timetabled per week as you will have in one day. Attendance at lectures and practicals can last from 9 AM until 5 PM every day, and regular evening and weekend study is essential. During the clinical years the hours spent in hospital are frequently much longer and additional time is still needed for personal study and revision. There is no doubt that if you want an easy option at university, medicine is not the right subject for you.

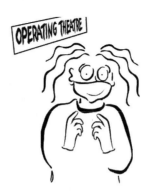

Michelle's view: a day in the life of a clinical student

The day starts with the rather unwelcome sound of the alarm clock at the comical hour of 6:30 AM. It's still pitch black outside. After showering, dressing, making my lunch, and managing only half of my measly slice of toast, I'm already running late. I jump into the car at 7:45 AM, only to end up in a traffic jam! Typical!

After the 20-mile journey, which has taken 45 minutes, I manage to make it to the outpatients department where the urology clinic starts at 9 AM. Actually, I'm on take today which means I need to help receive the surgical emergency patients into hospital. However, normally nothing really happens until after lunch when the GPs have had a chance to send some patients in, which is why I'm attending the clinic in the meantime. At the clinic, one patient has a hydrocoele (a collection of fluid in the scrotum) which is a condition I have never seen before. At 11:30 AM I have to leave, as radiology teaching is about to start.

Together with the fellow students of my firm, we await the arrival of the consultant. Twenty minutes after the session was due to begin, a message is sent to say that our teaching has been cancelled as the consultant is too busy with an ultrasound list to teach us this morning. It is a nuisance, as the clinic I had been at was really interesting, but cancelled teaching is something we have to accept as part of the course.

It's midday and things are quiet at the surgical admission unit, except for one patient who needs a cannula inserted (a cannula is a needle to give medication and fluid through). As I'm the only person who has turned up to the unit in the last 4 hours, the nurses jump on me as though I'm their oasis of hope and ask me to do it. My blood pressure's rising as I've only done one before, but it's a good chance to practise my clinical skills and hey, they do say 'see one, do one, teach the rest.' I have to look in three different places for a vein that I can use, as there doesn't seem to be a decent one (they're not the greatest I've ever seen). However, I finally decide on the best. Confidence is definitely not oozing from me, and I'm half expecting the vein to disappear, but despite shaking I manage to get it in. I am filled with pride and really feel quite useful for a change!

The on-call registrar arrives on the ward, so I let him know the cannula is in and find out an emergency appendicectomy (removal of the appendix) is about to take place. As a result I rush to eat my sandwiches whilst walking to theatres; it's 2:15 PM and I'm hungry. Having changed into scrubs, the surgeon asks me to 'scrub up' – that is, wash and put on gown and mask – and assist. Unfortunately, the appendix has ruptured so laparoscopy (a minimally invasive surgical technique commonly called 'keyhole surgery') can't be used. He lets me hold things out of the way and cut a few stitches as he talks me through the anatomy of something called Calot's triangle.

After completing the operation in 3 hours (it was complicated), a vascular surgeon informs me that there is a patient who is coming in with an abdominal aortic aneurysm which is suspected to be leaking. An aortic aneurysm is when the main artery in the body is dangerously dilated. As he is currently on the CT scanner having images to identify any problems, I head towards the radiology department again. However, there is hoard of people running in that direction too and when I arrive I find that the patient has had a cardiac arrest. As medical students, we're advised to observe such situations if we can for learning purposes. However, I feel awkward standing in the corner watching the patient being resuscitated. A nurse spots me and asks me to count how long they've been resuscitating for. Although for once I'm being useful, the scuffle in front of me is a distraction. I don't want to be seen as a gawking spectator. This isn't *ER* or *Casualty* – and it's certainly not *Holby City* – this is a real person dying in front of me. After 20 minutes, the patient is pronounced dead. People gradually exit one by one and I'm left not quite knowing what to do. I wonder how my feelings may change when I've been to many more crash calls as a qualified doctor …

A junior doctor comes over: 'Is that the first person you've seen die?' 'Yes,' I say still trying to take the situation in. 'If you need to talk about what you've just witnessed, then I'm happy to listen.' 'Thanks, but I'll be okay.' At 9.00 PM (how time flies …) I make the decision to leave for home, recounting the events of the day. I'm exhausted and feel quite drained. After walking what seems like 20 miles through the hospital back to the car, driving home in the dark is not fun – I've barely seen the light today!

(*Continued*)

(Continued)

It's been a very busy day and I've been running on only some toast and a sandwich. Time for food! But before bed, preparation of some material must be done for a presentation tomorrow to one of the consultants. Sleep finally calls to me at midnight, but I must be up early again for the post-take ward round to review all the patients admitted today …

In recent years, many medical schools have placed a greater emphasis on continuous assessment and a number have rearranged final exams so that they are taken over a longer period rather than all at once. Many students have found this to be a sensible development which has reduced a lot of the episodic pressure. Some, however, argue that this has only spread the pressure throughout the year: the increased number of exams can lead to exam fatigue and at schools with more traditional courses, *finals* are still dreaded. Although medical degrees are not classified in the way that other degrees are (1st, 2:1, 2:2, 3rd), some schools offer a distinction grade for those aficionados who perform exceptionally highly in exams.

Is it fun?

Absolutely! Despite all these pressures, medical students have no trouble being sporty and socia-ble. In fact, we often excel at both. There is a wide mixture of students at every medical school and every group will contain a range of public school and state school, working class and middle class, medical family and non-medical family type backgrounds. You will be able to pursue your non-course interests as well as your studies. 'Work hard and play hard' is the maxim that unites medical students, and the medical profession has an enviable community spirit – a 'we're all in it together' attitude. Year groups vary in size but are often large (200+). Nonetheless, because everyone is doing the same course, you get to know your colleagues very quickly and very well. The downside of this is that medical students sometimes have a reputation for not mixing with students on other courses. It is also why we have the enviable reputation for the best social life! The common purpose among those studying medicine results in a closeness, which is one of the best aspects of life as a medical student.

Getting the balance right …

Maintaining a healthy balance between academic and extra-curricular activities whilst at medical school is very important. One of the greatest benefits of university life is in enabling students to develop as people as well as train as doctors. A healthy interest in sport, music, theatre, or even in just spending time relaxing with friends will be important to your development as a well-balanced person, in addition to influencing your success as a doctor. Medicine is a demanding course and learning how to manage a healthy work-to-life balance early on will enable you to maintain it through the pressures of life as a doctor and increase your ability to cope with stress.

If you find that you have no time at all for socialising or pursuing a hobby, then something is wrong. Either you are working too hard and need to relax, possibly with the help of university pastoral care systems, or you are living and/or studying in an inefficient way and would benefit from some coach-

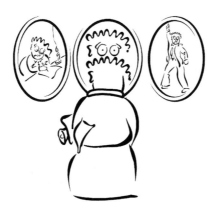

ing on organisation and study techniques. This is available at most universities, in addition to a range of written resources including *How to Study Medicine* produced by the BMA. The importance of developing a well-balanced life during medical school cannot be over emphasised. Doctors are particularly vulnerable to stress-related conditions, depression, divorce, and alcohol dependence, and developing good practices as a student will help safeguard your health and happiness in the future.

It is also important to note that with the seemingly endless range of opportunities available at university, and the active social life, it is easy to become involved in too much and find yourself pulled in too many directions. This situation can prove equally stressful and may cause academic difficulties. Most medical schools provide so-called formative exams during the early terms, which should help you to gauge your academic progress, without contributing to your final degree mark. Use these as the excellent tool they are to check that you have an appropriate balance between study and play, and adjust your activities as necessary.

Finally, it is worth bearing in mind that at the end of your time at medical school you will be applying for Foundation Programme (see Chapter 6) positions alongside a great number of other medical students with almost identical qualifications. Whilst there are enough jobs for everyone, if you have your heart set on a particular job it is helpful to have something that makes your CV stand out from the crowd.

Can I combine medicine with pursuing another degree subject?

You can interrupt most courses to study for an extra intercalated degree, normally a medical science degree (BSc, BMedSci) undertaken during an extra year of study. This is particularly worthwhile if you are considering a career in research or academic medicine. For sheer pleasure, you may wish to enrich your knowledge with a non-related subject such as art history or music, but disappointingly only a few medical schools now allow this. Intercalated degrees are commonly taken after the second or third year, and entry policies vary between schools. They are compulsory in some, e.g. Oxford, Imperial, and Cambridge, actively encouraged in others, while some allow students to intercalate by invitation only. In some schools, where it is voluntary, as many as 50% of each year group intercalate at some stage in their studies. Students on the 5-year programme at the University of Nottingham undertake a research project in their third year and, if satisfactory performance is achieved, graduate with a BMedSci degree in addition to their medical degree in just 5 years. It is ordinarily not possible to intercalate on the 4-year graduate-entry courses, at Nottingham or elsewhere. The main consideration to extending an already long course is the issue of financing an extra 12 months. At some schools tuition fees for the intercalated degree year are paid for, but you will still need to finance your living costs for an extra year. There are a number of significant bursaries available for intercalating students, both via the university and via external bodies, and it is definitely worth finding out about these.

Is it possible to travel abroad for any part of the course?

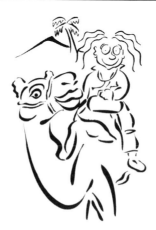

People say the world is your oyster, and there is really no other profession that this applies to more aptly. Medicine truly is your passport to the world and doctors are trusted and welcomed in every corner, culture, and society. Medical schools have embraced this fact for many years now, and have incorporated a period within the medical curriculum dedicated to the students' self-arranged and self-directed learning, termed an *elective*. The elective is usually over a period of between 8 and 12 weeks, depending on which medical school you attend. To many students this means the chance to study overseas for a prolonged period. The elective is viewed as one of the major highlights of the undergraduate curriculum. Not only is it a fantastic learning experience but it is also a chance to escape the NHS and see part of the world you have never seen before. Medicine is practised in diverse environments and settings, many of which are very different to the healthcare system students will eventually enter. The elective allows the opportunity to experience how different healthcare systems contrast to our own. This may be the ultra-sophisticated and technologically advanced system that exists in the USA or the humble resource-stricken system that exists in much of the developing world. Many students choose to place themselves in the latter environment because they are likely to gain a level of hands-on experience unavailable in more developed and regulated health services.

The timing of the elective varies between medical schools, but usually takes place during the clinical years so that students have a broad base of clinical knowledge before embarking on the elective period, to maximise learning. All schools encourage the elective period to be used primarily as an invaluable learning resource and not just a holiday, although a holiday certainly can be incorporated.

A number of schools require either clinical or academic research to be undertaken as part of the elective. Students decide to go on a particular elective depending on their interests and what they intend to achieve. For example, the adventurous may choose trauma in Johannesburg, whilst a student keen for a more relaxed experience may prefer to spend their elective in the Seychelles. With enough time and motivation, the opportunities are endless. For example, previous students have benefited from electives with NASA in the USA, The Flying Doctors in Australia and the mountain rescuers in Nepal.

You do not have to go abroad for your elective and many students choose instead to organise an equally rewarding experience in the UK: perhaps delving into medical politics, carrying out a project at an academic or pharmaceutical research centre, or working with the team doctor at a football club. The elective really is what you make it. Generally, students organise their own elective with the assistance of the medical school, reports from previous students, and relevant elective literature. There really is no limit to what you can get out of your elective if you are prepared to put the effort into organising it.

It can be expensive, depending on what you choose to do, but numerous grants and prizes are available which allocate money especially to medical student electives: if you are well-organised it is often possible to obtain considerable financial support. Generally it is easier to obtain sponsorship and grants if your elective incorporates research. Many organisations award money on a means-tested basis, but the British Medical and Dental Students Trust (BMDST) award considerable sums based on how well-organised and beneficial, to you, your project is. In addition, the BMA produces a guide to funding your elective that you may wish to consult.

Whatever you choose to do as part of your elective, the memories and experience you will gain will be something you will never forget throughout your future career as a doctor.

In addition to electives, a few medical schools allow students to take one or more special study modules (shorter periods designed to allow students to study an area of particular interest) abroad. Furthermore, a small number of universities allow medical students to take part in exchange programmes with other European nations for part of the course, and even to study a foreign language. This is called *Erasmus*, and the ability to undertake these at each medical school is outlined in the second half of the book. If these opportunities interest you then it is important to read the information for each medical school carefully as practices vary considerably and medical schools facilitating such opportunities are currently in the minority.

Is it wise to study medicine with a chronic illness or disability?

Medical school is tough. It is tough for everyone – even those who are totally healthy. It places pressures on students academically, financially, and emotionally. The decision to study medicine should not be taken lightly or without prior knowledge of these facts, particularly if you are chronically unwell or have a disability to contend with in addition to studying, and even more so if your health status fluctuates. This all sounds very daunting and may make you wonder whether you should even consider doing medicine. However, in many respects you are well-equipped to tackle this vocational subject. The challenges and obstacles that you may have faced are the same ones that the patients you will eventually serve experience. Your deeper understanding of illness is something that is invaluable to you and the profession.

Medical schools are endeavouring to widen access to all potential students, whatever their circumstances, and all medical schools are obliged to provide some form of pastoral care and support. However, the approach of different medical schools to students with health problems and disabilities varies, as does the quality of the pastoral support available. Unfortunately, the 'caring profession' isn't always as caring to its own. It is well worth considering these factors carefully when choosing which medical schools to apply to. This is explained in more detail in Chapter 3.

As mentioned in Chapter 1, the Disability Discrimination Act is now in force and requires universities and medical schools to take into account the needs of disabled students. They must provide statements about the facilities available for such students, which should include details about access, the specialist equipment and counselling available, admission arrangements, and complaints and appeals procedures for disabled students. The Act applies in Northern Ireland with exceptions.

Depending on the disability or health problem, medical schools may require the applicant to have a skills assessment to ensure that they are fit to perform the tasks involved in becoming a doctor. This will focus on what the student can do, rather than what they can't do. Medical school faculties and occupational health services may be able to offer skills assessment and deans of medical schools should be able to offer further information and advice. Students may be eligible for financial help, such as the disabled students' allowance. Following a publication by its Disabled Doctors Working Party – *Meeting the Needs of Doctors with Disabilities* – the BMA launched a service for disabled medical students and doctors. This aims to provide information about aids, facilities, equipment, and financial help. It also puts disabled medical students and doctors in touch with each other. Further information may be obtained from the Medical Education Department of the BMA (see the Further Information section at the end of the book).

Despite the efforts of good medical faculties and the best intentions of the majority of students within a year, it is very easy to feel isolated when you are struggling with health problems. In order to reduce the impact of this on both your studies and your health, it is helpful to:

- investigate which specialties are, and which are not, realistic options: once you know what the options are, consider these in light of any limitations you may have;
- keep the relevant people informed at all times, particularly when you feel there may be a problem around the corner – medical faculties are able to help and to take circumstances into consideration if they know in advance;
- don't be afraid to ask for help – you are only human;
- always remember your health is the most important thing – you don't want to end up next to the patients you are treating.

Medicine should be for everyone so do not be put off. The old mentality of 'if it's too hot, get out of the kitchen' is gradually fading. Indeed, the editors personally know of examples where people have been aided tremendously by their medical school. As more people with illnesses and disabilities enter the profession, the negative attitudes will hopefully disappear completely.

What about studying medicine as a mature student?

For the sake of clarity when we say 'mature students' we mean individuals who are over 21 when they commence the course, irrespective of whether they hold a degree. 'Graduate students' are clearly those who hold a degree, and if over the age of 21 they are also mature. In recent years there has been a dramatic increase in the number of applications from both graduate and mature students wanting to study medicine. Much of this has resulted from the introduction of 4-year fast-track medical degrees for students who meet certain criteria (see Chapter 4 for more information), but mature and graduate applications to traditional 5- and 6-year courses have also increased. Previous experience and maturity are becoming increasingly valued, and medical schools often view mature students as reliable and likely to stay the course. These applicants have often achieved another degree or worked in professions allied to medicine, such as nursing, and many argue that they have spent more time assessing whether they really want to be a doctor before taking the plunge into medicine.

When considering applying as a mature or graduate student it is important to realise that attitudes towards mature students, and the support systems in place to help with their needs, vary across UK medical schools. The majority thoroughly enjoy their training, but you must choose a university carefully. Indeed, until relatively recently there were a significant number of medical schools that would not even accept applications from those aged over 25, 30, or 40. In general, the graduate-entry courses are better placed to deal with the needs of older students, and you might wish to contact admissions officers about the schools' demographics.

The BMA's graduate and mature students' group has identified specific issues that cause additional concern for those who are planning to change their lifestyle to study medicine. As a mature applicant you will need to consider:

- *Finance* – can you afford it? What about your tuition fees/mortgage repayments?
- *Partners and family matters* – what will this mean for them and for your relationship(s)?
- *Children, childcare, and future pregnancies* – how will you fit them in?
- *Lifestyle changes* – e.g. loss of regular income, working unsociable hours. How will you cope if you are expected to live in a shared student flat? (This is usually only necessary on distant clinical placements, but most schools take your placement needs into account if you have dependants.)
- *Work/study mix* – due to the demands of the course, most students are not able to work enough part-time hours to fund their courses.
- *Attitudinal challenges* – both your own and from teachers and fellow students.

A large proportion of mature students will be self-funding if they have previously completed undergraduate degrees, and consequently are likely to incur higher levels of debt than their younger colleagues. However, finances should not put you off applying to medical school if you are motivated and have a true desire to study medicine and become a doctor. Before applying however it is worth listing honestly the pros and cons of returning to or continuing education for at least another 4 years. This is not a useless exercise as you can be sure that those interviewing you will want to be very sure of your motives and future plans.

Chapter 4 covers mature and graduate entry to medicine in some detail. This chapter also includes the routes available to A level leavers who did not take chemistry, as it covers premedical courses.

Do many students manage to study medicine and care for dependants?

As if studying for one of the longest degrees, arguably involving some of the most mind-numbing

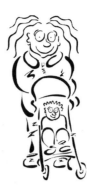

memory work, was not enough, some students like to liven things up a bit by choosing to start their studies with a ready-made family of their own in tow. Others add the challenge of a pregnancy or two, to the otherwise all-too-quiet time we have as medical students.

In fact medical students have always done this. It's just that with more mature students these days, and greater choices for women in the workplace, it has become talked about, and rightly so. Scan the website of any of the university medical schools in the UK for their maternity policy for students and you'll be hard-pressed to find one. The sad fact is that when you approach your tutor to say:

- you need to take time off because your child has chicken pox;
- your child-care has fallen through and you'll be late for lectures;
- you want 6 months off because you're pregnant …

you are not likely to get the sort of treatment you would get if you were at work. For example, we are aware of a case of a student whose daughter died but whose university tried to give her a fail mark for missing the OSCE she should have sat rather than being at her daughter's bedside in paediatric intensive care. Another university offered such scant support to one pregnant student that she felt forced to leave and transferred to another medical school.

Nevertheless, there are success stories and the graduate-entry courses have so far shown greater flexibility and compassion to parents. An increasing number of students manage to give birth and pick up on their studies by timing matters to fit in with holiday periods (especially in the preclinical years when the holidays are longer). Others take a full year out and slot back in the next year. Indeed, some think having a baby as a student is the best way to do it. After all, it's not going to be any easier when you are a stressed-out junior doctor, or when you're 15 years older and a consultant.

As more and more students with children or other dependants enter medicine, the provision of sup-port and understanding will improve in the same way that flexible working patterns for doctors have had to radically improve as a result of the large number of both male and female practitioners who have demanded a better work-to-life balance. In the meantime enjoy your family and your time as a student. Remember many people are already doing just that. And the more students that do it, the more we can one day look forward to persuading universities to offer flexible degrees in the same way as there are flexible working arrangements.

Studying as a European Union or international student

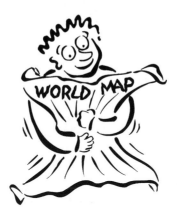

Medical students come from all over the world to study in the United Kingdom, with the majority coming from the Republic of Ireland and former Commonwealth nations in East Asia, South Asia, the Middle East and Africa. Students come from a wide variety of backgrounds and experiences, and find it to be a great opportunity to meet people and learn about cultures that they would never be able to in their own country. Universities are generally very keen to receive such students as diversity enriches the profession.

Coming to the UK can be an overwhelming experience, as things can be quite unlike what you are accustomed to at home. From the type of food and entertainment, to the cultural values and way of life, you may find it very different from what you are used to – but this can be a good thing. The UK is a very multicultural society, and it is generally easy to fit in and feel comfortable with your surroundings. It also means that you are likely to find at least one restaurant that serves a dish from your country, as there is more to British food than fish and chips!

It is generally a good idea to live on campus for the first year, so you can get to know other students at your university and make new friends. It also gives you time to adapt to the culture and way of life, before you move out into the *real* world. Some universities allow international students to live on campus for up to 2 years. When students do move out, they tend to share accommodation with friends and colleagues they have met during their first year, which is the norm in the UK.

Funding for EU and international students is rather different from domestic UK nationals. For international students in particular, tuition fees can be substantial. Bursaries may have to be applied for from your home country. Consult Chapter 3 and Chapter 5 for more information.

If you can get over the weather and the funny accents, the United Kingdom is an excellent place to undertake your undergraduate training. Most people involved in your training are keen to teach, the nurses and staff are helpful, and the patients are very friendly and willing for medical students to practice their clinical skills on them – all in the name of learning.

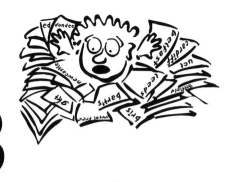

3

Applying to medical school

The most revolutionary act you can commit in our society today is to be happy, that if you really want to change the world, then you be your own focus for celebration of life and let it be known, whatever it is that gives you that happiness. Then, pursue your dreams.

Patch Adams

Introduction

Most will have heard Bob Dylan's dulcet tones exclaiming, 'the times they are a changing,' and the same is true of admission to medical schools. This year we see the introduction of a new form of admissions test called the *United Kingdom Clinical Aptitude Test* (UKCAT) in many, but not all, of the UK medical schools. Not only this, we have also witnessed a further rise in applications to medical schools, an increase in medical school places, a potential age limit for applications to medical school being introduced, and much more. The Universities and Colleges Admissions Service (UCAS) have also announced that a major reform of the application process is to be undertaken in the next 5 years; fortunately, this is unlikely to have any impact on the applications process during the lifetime of this edition of *The Insiders' Guide*.

In this chapter we outline many of the key methods of accessing medical school, although this is not an exhaustive list by any means. At the end of this section we have included some flow diagrams which we hope will act as quick reference guides for you.

Entrance requirements

School leavers

Most medical schools require students to get A and B grades in at least three full A level subjects, or five Scottish Highers (one sitting), which equates to 360 points in England, Wales, and Northern Ireland and 336 points in Scotland (according to the UCAS tariff system). Some schools prefer Scottish students to have attained a Scottish Certificate of Sixth Year Studies in a science subject, although this seems to be a reversing trend.

The entry requirements have continued to rise even though there has been a downward trend in the applicants-to-places ratio. In 2005, there were 15,635 applicants fighting for 7100 medical school places, which translates to about 2.2 people fighting for every medical school place in the UK. Many schools require the student to be predicted AAB (A level) and AAABB (Scottish Highers) at the time of application. Some schools demand that you have an A or B in a science subject but this varies from school to school (some demand it in biology and others in chemistry). Whilst some schools do not make any demand for particular subjects at A level or Higher Grade, it is reasonable that some of your choices in the final year of school include subjects related to medicine. More importantly, if you have a particular medical school in mind, check their entry requirements: if they require chemistry, and you do not have it, yours may be a wasted application.

Medical schools also vary in their attitude towards other subjects selected. For example, if you were considering making an application to one of the more traditional universities, you may struggle to gain a place if you have chosen biology, drama, and art as A level subjects. However, substitute drama with maths or chemistry and you may well have a good chance to get in.

At other medical schools, admissions personnel look for a broad range of knowledge, communication skills, and interests outside of science; and it may well be desirable to have an arts or humanities subject on your application. The editors of the *Insiders' Guide* cannot encourage you enough to make note of the requirements laid down by each school in Part 2 of this book. Be aware of what schools expect of applicants.

Many medical schools now require students to sit the UKCAT, which is explained in more detail below. This test has been added to the application process in order to make it easier for medical schools to discern before interview between students with maximum UCAS points. Some courses use similar, but more established, access tests, which include GAMSAT and BMAT. These are also explained briefly below.

Conversion into medicine from related degrees

Some medical schools will permit a few top students in certain subjects to transfer internally into medicine in the early stages of the degree. If you have missed the grades and are determined to get into medicine, undertaking a degree in a related field (e.g. biochemistry or physiology) can offer you this opportunity but you would need to check with the individual schools concerned. Should you fail to come top of your class it is not the end of the world – there is always the graduate-entry route.

Few medical schools offer such opportunities to medical students, however, and it really should not be considered as a typical entry route if you want to change medical schools.

Graduate entry

More and more applications are being considered from graduates, so much so that there has even been talk of having an American-style model in which all medical students have degrees in other fields before attending medical school (this is unlikely to happen any time soon).

The UK has witnessed a number of new graduate courses being established in England and Wales. These courses are 4 years in length and are aimed at a variety of different graduates, often those with scientific backgrounds. There has been talk about establishing a graduate course in Scotland, although at the time of writing this had not been confirmed. Competition for places at graduate institutions remains very high due to the high standard of candidates, the small number of places available and the significant financial incentives accompanying the shortened courses.

In response to the proliferation and success of graduate-entry courses, Chapter 4 of this book has been dedicated to such programmes along with other non-school leaver entry routes. Graduates can also apply to undergraduate medical courses, and a number of medical schools now welcome applications to the undergraduate 5-year course. It is worthwhile checking which schools welcome graduate students, as some are more accepting than others. The BMA Medical Students Committee may be able to offer some advice about graduate friendly courses. Also, contacting the school itself may give you some idea about the attitudes held by the school – what was the warmth of the response you received? Most schools ask for a minimum 2:1 and you will also have to go through the formal processes as with any other undergraduate applicant (UKCAT or equivalent).

Access, foundation, and premedical courses

Access, foundation, and premedical courses are for those students who did not study relevant subjects at school. Such courses are usually undertaken the year before starting the medical course and have been traditionally aimed at students who have not taken the correct A levels or Scottish Highers to access medicine. They are open to other students but are still predominantly aimed at younger applicants. Many schools continue to run these – see Chapter 4 for details. Premedical courses generally demand that you undertake the UKCAT or equivalent.

Access courses are for those students who have chosen a non-traditional route. A number of these courses have opened at various colleges in the last few years and they often have a link with a specific medical school. For example, Kings Lynn has a link with Norwich (UEA) and any student who passes the course at Kings Lynn is offered an automatic interview at UEA, although not an automatic place. These courses are usually intensive 1-year programmes. Again, UKCAT will likely be a requirement as part of the application process for many schools. Consult Chapter 4 for more information.

How do I get into medical school?

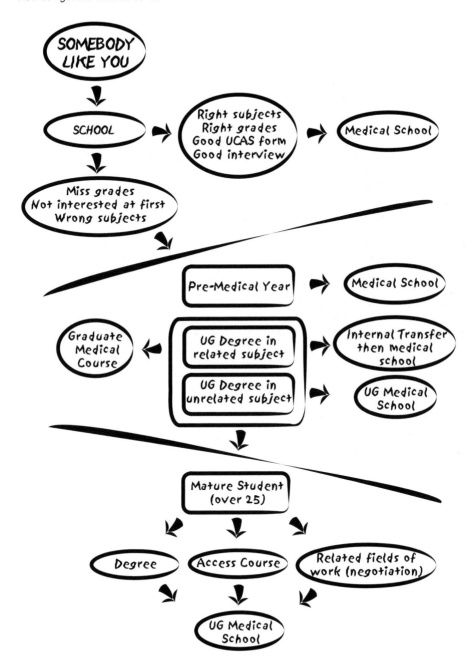

Mature applicants

As with graduate students, talk to the admissions tutor to get an idea of the medical school's attitudes toward mature applicants. There are an increasing number of schools welcoming such applicants, but at the time of writing some schools were attempting to cap the application age at 41.

As a mature applicant, you can send supporting material to the admissions teams in addition to your UCAS form – do not just limit this to a CV. If you decide to do this, discuss with the school the form that this material should take to determine what will make your case most effective. For example, you can use letters of support, details of relevant courses and work experience. You can quickly determine the schools that will be open to your application – one of the editors sent his CV and copies of certificates to all medical schools in the UK and had an overwhelming response.

The newer medical schools are reported to be much more welcoming to those who have had a career elsewhere or who do not fit the typical school-leaver applicant's profile. Some older establishments, however, are also keen to recruit more mature students. Contact the schools directly and read the prospectuses carefully.

Above all, be sure that medicine is what you want to do. At interview, prepare to be grilled as to the reasons why you want to change your life at this point in time. Remember, nothing sounds as good or as convincing as the truth!

UK Clinical Admissions Test (UKCAT)

The official website (http://www.ukcat.ac.uk) describes the test as something to 'help universities make a more informed choice from amongst the many highly qualified applicants who apply for the medical degree programmes'. UKCAT is a computer-based assessment and does not aim to test candidates on their scientific or general knowledge; it specifically aims to assess the cognitive ability needed to be a new doctor – and we weren't sure what that meant either!

Those that designed UKCAT state that you cannot practise for the assessment, although having undertaken the practice questions online, the editors suggest that this may not be the case. Many similar problem-solving and analytical books are sold in good bookshops in the UK. Although UKCAT do not publicise any particular practice books, they do give some good ideas about what kind of books you could use. It is worth taking a look. For those people who cannot access such books, the internet may be of some use. Get online: do the practice questions. If you cannot get online, or cannot afford any books, do not panic: the problems do not seem to be overly onerous. There is a charge for sitting UKCAT although bursaries are offered to those people from poorer backgrounds.

At the time of going to print, applicants to the following universities and courses will need to undertake the UKCAT to gain access to the course:

- University of Aberdeen
- Brighton and Sussex Medical School
- Cardiff University
- University of Dundee
- University of Durham

- University of East Anglia
- University of Edinburgh
- University of Glasgow
- Hull York Medical School
- Keele University
- King's College London
- University of Leeds
- University of Leicester
- University of Manchester
- University of Newcastle
- University of Nottingham
- University of Oxford Graduate Entry Medical Degree
- Peninsula Medical School
- Queen Mary, University of London
- University of Sheffield
- University of Southampton
- University of St Andrews
- St George's, University of London.

Consult the annually published *UCAS Handbook* for information about course codes and institutions. Application dates, bursary details, international students application information, and key dates are all on the UKCAT website.

BioMedical Admissions Test (BMAT)

Some universities are not taking part in the UKCAT but require applicants to complete the BMAT. This examination does look more at your scientific understanding and analytical skills. This test has information online and the medical schools clearly state where this is a requirement. More information can be found at http://www.bmat.org.uk/index.html

The BMAT is a biomedical entrance examination undertaken by students who want to get in to specific universities. It is really an aptitude test which enables the universities to differentiate between students who generally all come with high educational standards.

Heinemann have published a book called *Preparing for the BMAT: The official guide to the BioMedical Admissions Test.*

Graduate Australian Medical School Admissions Test (GAMSAT)

One or two universities continue to use this test for graduate entrants, although many have opted to move from this form of testing to the UKCAT. The GAMSAT is very much like the UKCAT and some books exist to help you through this examination, which has elements of psychometric testing and analytical reasoning. Contact UCAS for more information about it. GAMSAT results remain valid for 2 years, and some universities who do not formally demand it will informally take results into account. GAMSAT is described on the websites as a multiple-choice question exam which tests reasoning and analytical skills. A small minority of the universities in the UK continue to use this process to select students for university.

A number of preparatory books exist and many self-help websites can be found free of charge online which you can use to research for your exams.

Health and disability issues

Introduction

It is important to remember that, if you feel that you have a medical condition that may put patients at risk, it is your responsibility to disclose this to occupational health and to modify your medical practice accordingly. The reality is that there are very few cases in which reasonable adjustments cannot be made, and medical schools are obliged to make every reasonable attempt to accommodate students with disabilities (including blood-borne viruses, or BBVs).

There has been a push towards testing students for a whole range of conditions but this has been avoided so far, on the basis that there is a lack of uniformity on testing throughout the medical profession. The BMA Medical Students Committee believes that it is pointless testing a medical student for HIV if surgeons and other health professions do not get similar screening. That said, as health professionals we may need to lead the way in breaking the stigma associated with HIV and other BBVs.

Medical schools themselves have made big steps forward and have categorically stated that BBVs and disability are not a bar to studying and practising in certain areas of medicine.

Disability

Medical schools do not generally accept students unless they are convinced that they have the potential to meet the requirements of the Foundation Year 1 (the F1 is your first year as a junior doctor). The learning outcomes required by an F1 doctor can be obtained from the General Medical Council, either online, by email or by telephone. Where an applicant has a disability or chronic health problem which may impact on their study, good admissions practice suggests that medical schools should assess an applicant on their merits and without reference to their illness or disability. If the school is happy to offer that student a place, but feels that clarification of the health challenge is necessary, the applicant should undergo a separate occupational health assessment to determine whether they would be physically and mentally capable of meeting the learning outcomes of the preregistration year.

As with everything, some schools are better equipped and have better attitudes towards students with disabilities and it is important that you make every effort to find this out. Speak to the medical faculties prior to applying in order to gain an impression of their attitudes. The good medical schools will have past or present students with health problems or disabilities whom they can put you in touch with, and the medical faculty personnel will be encouraging and keen to help. It can be beneficial to arrange a meeting with the admissions officer before applying to give yourself as much information as possible when it comes to making an application.

Organisations to contact include SKILL – the National Bureau for Students with Disabilities (see Further Information). If you feel at any point you have been treated unfairly, we would encourage you to seek assistance and ensure that medical schools are challenged for poor practice. The road may be paved with obstacles but attitudes are changing.

Immunisations and testing

Certain health-related requirements need to be fulfilled, although in future occupational health checks will be conducted after admission to medical school. Individual schools will outline their requirements in the prospectus but, in general, you will need the following:

- rubella immunity
- meningitis C vaccination
- hepatitis B antibody confirmation
- BCG required

Some schools are considering testing for hepatitis C and HIV but it is important to note that it is not compulsory at the moment.

As with any medical condition, ensure that you have had the correct information and counselling. It may be useful to speak to the school's own occupational health team if you require specific guidance, as your own GP may not have all the information available.

Applicants with dependants

Before selecting where to apply, talk to the universities on your short list. Find out:

- whether it has any medical students with dependants that you can talk to;
- its policy on maternity leave for students;
- whether childcare is provided, and whether it is subsidised for students;
- whether there is specific support available for mature students or students with dependants;
- whether there are any special hardship grants for students with dependants.

Apply to universities that are encouraging and positive towards you. The admissions tutor's response to your initial enquiries will speak volumes about the university's potential attitude towards you in the future. Remember, mature women students with young children are more likely than any other group to abandon their course and it doesn't take many brain cells to work out why.

International applicants

The first step for a prospective international student considering studying in the UK is to determine the cost of education in its entirety (including tuition fees, equipment, books, and living expenses) as this can be extremely high. The second step is to find out if your country of origin offers any loans, scholarships, or grants to study abroad, as some governments do offer financial relief for their citizens to experience medical training in another country. It is also worth finding out if the university you are considering offers any scholarships to international students. The best way to find this out is to contact the university directly. The British Embassy or High Commission, or your own country's education authority, may be able to advise you about grants and scholarships.

It is important to note that the rules for working in the UK are changing for international students who graduate in medicine. Whilst you are guaranteed a job in the UK until you complete the first 2 years of work, there is no guarantee you will have a job after this time. It is essential that you understand the new arrangements and any implication this may have on your employment status if you want to work in the UK for any length of time upon qualification. Check the English Department of Health (http://www.dh.gov.uk) and the Immigration and Nationality directorate (http://www.ind.homeoffice. gov.uk/) for the most up-to-date information.

After reading the university prospectus, it is a good idea to contact the school and clarify any information, as situations can change rapidly: this may influence your decision to attend a particular school. The British Council (http://www.britishcouncil.org/home.htm) has information about UK universities and medical schools and may be able to guide you on whether your qualifications are recognised in the UK. If you are not studying UK-examined A levels, then contact the admissions office at the medical school to check whether your subject choices and qualifications are acceptable. There are growing links between overseas medical schools and UK medical schools, and you may be able to do some of your studies in the UK even if you don't get a full-time place on the course. If you are applying to medical schools in other countries you might want to enquire about this.

Applicants from outside the UK must also apply via UCAS and should follow the instructions in the *UCAS Handbook*. You can get copies of UCAS information from British Council offices or by writing to UCAS. Many schools and colleges will order supplies for you.

Finally, but most importantly, a number of private medical schools have opened in the UK in the last 5 years: these schools are not recognised by the UK regulatory body (the GMC) so it is important that you establish that the medical school does qualify you to work in the UK (all medical schools registered with the GMC grant degrees which permit medical practice in the UK).

Gap years

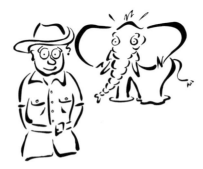

Most colleges and universities look on gap years favourably. The majority, however, expect you to use the time in a constructive way by working and/or travelling. It is important that you check the medical school's attitude before you apply if you intend to defer entry. Time out between school and university is not just for those who have the money for a 'round-the-world' air ticket: a well-planned gap year will give you time to think about how to get through university. Use the time to boost your confidence by gaining new and challenging experiences – which will be of benefit to you at medical school.

Student debt is at an all-time high. You could try to save some money in a gap year and be in better financial shape for your eventual university career. A gap year may also be used to gain some more work experience in healthcare, although do not overdo it – you'll have a lifetime of it ahead of you.

Note: A minority of colleges at Oxford and Cambridge do not approve of gap years, so do check up beforehand if you are desperate to do one. Schools cannot retract an offer but you must give plenty of notice if you intend to take a gap year as they can stop you taking up a place the year after if you do not inform them of your intentions.

Work experience

Work experience is a fantastic way to gain exposure to medicine and can be incredibly enjoyable and rewarding. It is also a good opportunity to test whether life as a healthcare professional is the right choice for you.

Although not a stated prerequisite for entry to all medical schools, some exposure to the healthcare setting is regarded by many medical schools as evidence that you are seriously interested in a medical career. It is helpful, therefore, if your personal statement shows that you have tried to understand what a medical career will entail. You don't need to shadow a doctor for a few days – it is accepted that this is difficult enough given the busy nature of doctors' lives, but even harder if you do not know any doctors to contact. There are many opportunities to undertake work experience in caring roles, and working as a nursing auxiliary or volunteer within a hospital will enable you to experience the broader healthcare environment. It will also give you invaluable insight into the role of other healthcare professionals in the overall system. Think laterally about the range of opportunities open to you, including contacting current medical students to ask what they did. Why not ask if your local GP can take you on for a while – a taster to medicine in the community?

If you do contact a doctor for work experience, remember to adhere to patient confidentiality rules and observe your own limitations. It is particularly important that you do not agree to do anything for which you are not qualified, or that you would not want someone of equivalent experience to do to you or a member of your family. The BMA has produced a set of work experience guidelines, available on the BMA website, and the Department of Health also provides guidance for NHS managers to which you can refer.

Several universities offer opportunities to participate in summer schools or medical student shadowing schemes to give a taster of medical student life; use the contact details later in the book to find out what is available – universities local to you may have specific programmes for those attending local schools, and remember to apply early!

Open days and further information

It is very important that you find out as much as possible about the medical schools that you are considering applying to. In Part 2 of this book we give you admission information, and views and opinions for you to consider. Only by visiting the school and reading the prospectus, and any alternative guides, will you be able to assess the atmosphere and whether you will enjoy studying there. Remember, no one knows what life at medical school is like better than those already there. Don't be afraid to approach current medical students: we are generally a friendly bunch and would be more than happy to chat over a coffee about *any* aspect of medical school life.

Open days will help you decide whether you would prefer a medical school that is part of a larger university, on a campus, spread across a town, in a big city, or near the countryside, and give you an idea of where you'd like to live should you accept a place there. It will also allow you to talk to the medics who are already there. Starting university can be a daunting – even scary – experience, but if you know what to expect, you will be much more at ease. If you can't afford the cost of travelling, get a group together and ask if your school or college will sponsor a minibus or take a coach to an open day. Many open days take place in the summer after students have had their exams and before applications are due. It is better to go early, before students go on vacation, although there are clinical students milling around all year. Well-organised open days have a welcoming team to escort visitors from the station, and organise events, talks, tours, displays, and demonstrations. However, organisation varies greatly from school to school.

Some medical schools run intensive open days during which you may sample lectures, and some operate summer schools – extended periods of experience of life as a medical student – with opportunities to work alongside students and others interested in applying to medicine. There are commercially run courses giving application advice as well as an insight into life as a medical student. These can be expensive but may be a good way of helping you decide whether medicine is the right choice for you. Your careers tutor might be able to help you find out about these courses and open days.

If you can't attend an open day, or decided to apply too late, there are a number of people you could write to. The students' union can deal with enquiries and may have promotional material to send you. The medical faculty office should also be able to supply you with the name of the president of the medical society (MedSoc: the student group responsible for representing medics and organising sports and social events) so you can contact the students directly. BMA student representatives are always happy to answer questions, and they may be contacted through the medical school or via the BMA Medical Students Committee (see Further Information).

The application process

UCAS forms

Medical schools only accept applications made through UCAS. There is detailed information in the *UCAS Handbook*, which you should consult to ensure that you understand what you need to do. Make several drafts of your UCAS form, using photocopies (the quota of forms for each school is limited) before finalising your application. Your careers tutor at school or college will be able to help you fill in the form. If you do not have a careers tutor, try and find someone else to read through a draft version for you before you write it up – perhaps a family friend or your work experience supervisor. It has been said that only critical advice is useful – those who tell you 'yeah, it's good,' and that's all, may not be the best people to consult. Give them a red pen and tell them to be brutal. Choose your critics wisely! When you do write it up, remember to make it accurate and legible.

Personal statement

The most important part of the form is the personal statement. This is your chance to stand out from the crowd and make the admissions tutors want to interview you. What you write will go a long way towards determining how many medical schools offer you an interview or a place. The comments below apply equally to electronic and paper applications.

You can expect – not surprisingly – that the medical school will want to know why you want to study medicine and, as there is so much competition, you must use this opportunity to demonstrate your commitment to joining the profession. For example, you may want to try to describe what drives you to pursue a career in medicine. Medical schools will want to be sure that you know what you are getting yourself into and so it is very important to demonstrate how you have gone about trying to understand what a medical career will entail. However, don't take too much space to do this, as it will be at the expense of other important information. The challenge is to do this effectively with supporting evidence of a well-balanced character; for example, a healthcare assistant job or regularly visiting a local old people's home – along with captaining the school netball team or editing the school magazine. These examples will prove to them that you are a good candidate and that you are well rounded in your interests. Make sure you outline your strengths – if you play an instrument with proficiency, dance, act or paint, then say so.

In addition, it should be clear from the information supplied by your school or college whether you have the potential to get the grades, so the personal statement must show you as a potential asset to the medical school and, later, the medical profession.

They will be looking for:

- signs of good interpersonal skills;
- evidence of a social life;
- details of your interests/hobbies;
- any notable achievements;
- an understanding of what being a doctor may entail.

You should mention:

- sports achievements;
- academic prizes;
- organizational or supervisory positions of responsibility;
- voluntary work, part-time work, or work experience;
- musical or travel interests;
- projects you have particularly enjoyed, or unusual hobbies.

If you are deferring entry for a year, you should explain how you are going to use your time.

There is no need to defend your choice of A levels/Highers unless you have something interesting to comment on, for example: 'I am studying computing as an A level as I think it may lie at the heart of medicine in the future.' Don't be afraid of making bold statements but prepare to be questioned on them. Ultimately, you want to offer signposts for interviewers that will allow them to interview you and find out more about what makes you tick.

If you are called for an interview, the panel will question you on the contents of this section. You may be asked to talk about any of the things you mention in the personal statement, so be truthful – it will probably show very quickly if you have embellished a little too much! Do not lie.

Remember, admissions staff read hundreds of UCAS forms, and yours should stand out – if it does, it will give you a better chance of being called for interview. The admissions tutor will want to know that you are prepared for a career in medicine, and that you have realistic expectations of what the future holds. So do your research early on: it will stand you in good stead throughout the application process.

This book will hopefully give you a good indication of the medical school you wish to attend; however, the personal statement should not give a personal preference. Another medical school may dismiss your application if they think that you will turn down their offer, and if you change your mind or your first-choice medical school does not offer you a place, you will have limited your options.

The best advice is to ask other people to read and comment on your personal statement: they may pick up errors and statements which do not adequately convey the message you intend to send. It is also worth remembering that medical schools are trying to determine if you will be happy at their institution, so your passions and ambitions should fit with the medical school on your forms. For example, if you express a passionate interest in Premiership football, an admissions tutor at Peninsula might think you would not enjoy being miles from any of the top clubs and so not offer you an interview. Equally, an application to a Scottish medical school might appear eminently sensible from a student interested in Ceilidh dancing.

WARNING! The examples below are for demonstration only – do not copy these …

Example of a bad personal statement

- John, aged 18, is applying to Cambridge, Bart's, St. George's and Guy's, King's and St Thomas'.

I have always wanted to be a doctor cause I care about people and have family members who have also been to medical school. I wanted to be a dentist at first but dentists need to work very long hours and don't really get to talk to their patients. I like football and rugby and support Manchester United – I would like to join the football team when I come to university.

I think I would be a good doctor as I am top of my class in A-Levels for General Studies, Art, Drama and Chemistry. I have done loads of work experience in general practice, hospital departments, etc. I am keen to stay close to home and would prefer to study in medical schools close to London.

I speak Spanish which I think would be useful for studying medicine and I am very good with computers.

Example of a good personal statement

- Parveen, aged 24, is applying to Peninsula Medical School, University of East Anglia, Brighton and Sussex, and Edinburgh.

For many years I have had a serious determination to enter the medical profession. Although it is difficult to gain extensive work experience, I believe I have gained sufficient experience to know what the vocation truly involves, and that I would be suitably challenged if I had the opportunity to become a doctor – diagnosing and problem solving. I think I have developed many of the skills required to be a good doctor and have worked hard to improve my abilities to work in a team, to lead, to communicate effectively and to get the job done. I have been the Vice-Chair of the Federation of Islamic Women at my university and played netball for the local team. These were occasions which I developed some of these skills referred to above, although I have a long way to go ...

A good personal statement would then continue to give details of work experience, including things witnessed and what you learned. Give details of voluntary work and how it has benefited you, etc.

When to apply

Apply as early as possible, but do not rush your application form. Importantly, remember to submit it well before the appropriate deadlines, bearing in mind that applications to certain universities, such as Cambridge and Oxford, may need to be earlier than others. The *UCAS Handbook* and website will give you all the details. You can submit your application electronically. You may receive replies from medical schools virtually as soon as you apply or you may be kept waiting until the last week that offers can be made, as other interviews are ongoing. Either way, do not read too much into delays and be patient – phoning the medical school on a daily basis will not speed up the process but may make you more anxious.

By the end of the process you may have been given a selection of the following offers:

- *Unconditional offer* (unusual for medicine) – offered a place with no conditions attached.
- *Conditional offer* – offered a place with conditions (e.g. you must get 2 As and a B in your A levels). If you fail to meet these conditions by a few marks, the medical school may be willing to give you some leeway; so always contact a school when you get your results.
- *Rejection* – remember, it is not the end of the world: there are other medical schools and there is an opportunity to get in to medicine via other means.

It is unlikely that schools will forget about your application, but it has happened. As deadlines approach, contact the admissions office to enquire about any possible delays. You can arrange for UCAS to acknowledge receipt of your form, and you will be given an application number so you can check progress if you feel it is taking too long. Admissions offices will be very busy during this time, but a telephone call may put your mind at ease even if they can't give you a decision on your application. Do not be afraid to make the occasional call.

The interview

If you are called to an interview, remember that it is a great opportunity to really sell yourself. The

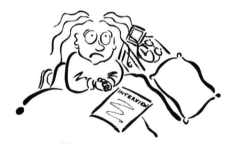

keys to a good interview are preparation and lots of practice. Prepare draft answers to questions you are likely to be asked. Don't learn things by heart, as you will sound rehearsed; but thinking ideas through before the interview will prepare you for possible pitfalls and you will have thought about the most important information to include. Practise interviews with anyone who is willing to spare 10 minutes. Ask them to suggest ways of improving your answers or style. This will help you to be more relaxed when it comes to the real thing.

Interviewers will look at your UCAS form for inspiration. They will be interested in the special and unusual (but not weird) about you: they would be fascinated to find out what drove you to do a llama herding course in South America during your gap year – so tell them! Reread your personal statement and anticipate the kinds of questions you might be asked. This is where your personal statement and your interview should mesh. As stated before, place signposts in your personal statement so that interviewers can pick up on and question you about them. Remember, they may be interviewing 40 people that day, and you can make it easier for them by doing this. You should also keep up to date with medical news stories and developments, as these may be the subject of some questioning.

Dress smartly and arrive in good time. If you are going to be shown around the medical school, remember that this is an opportunity to ask current students any questions you might have. Students will give you a good idea about the medical school – and proud students are often a good sign! In the interview, do not feel obliged to ask questions, and do not ask questions which are answered in the prospectus. In some ways an interview is a chance for the medical school to assess the potential it has recognised in your application form, but it is not an academic test. Treat it as an opportunity to show that you are serious about your career choice, and that you will be an asset to them and the medical profession.

If you do not think that the interviewers are asking you the questions that allow you to shine, it is possible to use an answer to one question to lead on to the subject that you would like to talk about. For example, if they have not asked you about your sporting activities then you can reply to a question about why you have applied to their university to talk about the excellent sporting opportunities available and how that would suit you well in your endeavours as a county junior athlete. Whilst it is not a good idea to start rambling off on a complete tangent, a skilful interviewee can heavily influence the direction of the interview.

Most importantly, enjoy your interview. You are more likely to excel and be well-regarded if you try to enjoy the experience. It is an opportunity for the panel to get a feel for the sort of person you are. Be polite and respectful, but try to be yourself – that is what the interviewers are there to see. If you don't agree with something then say so, as long as you can justify your disagreement logically and concisely.

It is difficult to predict the questions you will be asked, but below are some questions that you should be prepared to answer.

- Why do you want to be a doctor? Why a doctor and not a nurse?
- If you are so fascinated by the human body, why don't you do biology or physiology instead?
- Why do you want to come to *this* medical school?
- What can you offer the medical school?
- What are the most important characteristics of a doctor? What makes a good doctor?
- How would you go about researching a topic?
- Do you think you are suited to problem-based learning (if applicable to the course)?
- Do you know about the medical career structure?
- Do you know what sort of doctor you would like to be?
- What is the one thing you would like to change about the health service?
- Please give me three of your strengths and three of your weaknesses? (Be careful when selecting your weaknesses – you do not want to be so honest that it counts against you. An example would be 'I'm prone to being too much of a perfectionist at times. I think that I will have to work on this during my time at medical school so that I can manage the demands of being a doctor without getting too frustrated at the lack of time to do everything quite as well as I would like.')
- Please describe a situation when you worked well in a team.
- Please describe a time when you have had to make a difficult decision. What is the hardest decision you've ever had to make?
- Have you ever felt out of your depth? How did you handle that situation?

You may also be asked:

- questions that try to elicit whether you can think from a doctor's AND a patient's perspective.
- to work through an ethical situation. Here interviewers may be looking for characteristics such as teamwork and dealing with uncertainty.
- how you would go about researching medical information.
- to talk about a life-changing event.

What if I don't get in?

As mentioned earlier, medical schools are still oversubscribed. Only a small number of candidates will make it to interview and they will be selected on the basis of their UCAS forms and references. Surprisingly, medical schools like Oxford and Cambridge have fewer applicants per place but selecting medical schools on the basis of ratios is not advisable.

We must now emphasise something! Not getting a place to read medicine this year may not be a reflection on your personal abilities, but rather simply a reflection of the pressure for places. Even if you maximise your chances of being selected for interview, you may still be unsuccessful in your application. Don't be disheartened, but have a plan.

Firstly, think long and hard! Do you still want to study medicine? Medical schools try to select people who will make good doctors and who have the right ability and motivations for studying medicine, but even so some students choose to leave mid-course and others fail exams. The interview panel has a responsibility to make the right decision for the medical school, and you have a responsibility to yourself and your potential future patients to make sure you are making the correct choice. Examine your reasons for wanting to study medicine. If in doubt, or if you have felt pushed in a different direction, it might be a good idea to consider different courses or careers.

If you still want to study medicine, start by asking yourself why you weren't successful in your application. Did you get an interview? If you did, your school might be able to get some feedback from the medical school. This is unlikely to be in depth, but might give you some useful information. Discuss the prospect of your chances with teachers. Reflecting on your disappointment at this stage may prove difficult, but it is in your interests to be honest and realistic. Think about the possibility of following another course, whether in a related field – for example physiology, pharmacy, physiotherapy, biochemistry – or something totally unrelated. Most universities offer places on degree courses through *clearing*. If your grades are good then many other courses will be open to you. It is possible to reapply to read medicine, but some medical schools will only consider a second application if you applied there first time round. If you do reapply, your A level results should be at least as good as the estimates that your school originally made. There are some medical schools that will consider candidates who are re-sitting but others do not, and some medical schools actually give you extra points for persevering. Save your own time and energy by asking your preferred schools if they would accept an application from you. This could prevent you from wasting future UCAS choices. It is only advisable to re-sit exams if you are sure about getting A grades the second time around, or if there were extenuating circumstances, such as bereavement or serious illness, in the months preceding your A levels first time around.

There are a growing number of places available for graduates to read medicine, which means that you could do a degree and see after graduation whether you still want to become a doctor. Some students start university studying a parallel course, such as physiology, and then apply to switch to medicine at the end of the first or second year when the university has had a chance to measure their potential and character. These students would still have to start medicine from the first year though, and this method of entry is very rare and should not be relied on. Graduates usually follow the full undergraduate medical course unless they can be exempted from part of it because of the nature of their first degree (for example, biochemistry or dentistry). Graduates with a purely arts background at A level or as a degree could try to take a medical foundation year (premed year) before the medical course proper. This is not available at all institutions. Many schools don't normally consider applicants over 30 years of age. Graduate entry, however, is one of the ways into a career as a doctor. The BMA, and many other interested parties, have recognised the desirability of graduate entry and, as more places are being reserved for graduates, it is sensible to consider this route as an option.

I have been made an offer – what do I do now?

UCAS should explain this in more detail but if you have been offered a place at medical school you should accept it. If you have been lucky enough to be offered more than once place then you are required to give a first choice and a second choice. Some students are tempted to put the university asking for the highest grades first, then the lower of the two second due to the perception that the higher one is a better medical school. This is not necessarily the case. In fact, you may have performed less well in your interview at that school. Choose the medical school that is best suited to your personality and learning methods.

I have accepted a place at medical school – what next?

You are undoubtedly both nervous and excited about starting medical school. Most students are

The application process

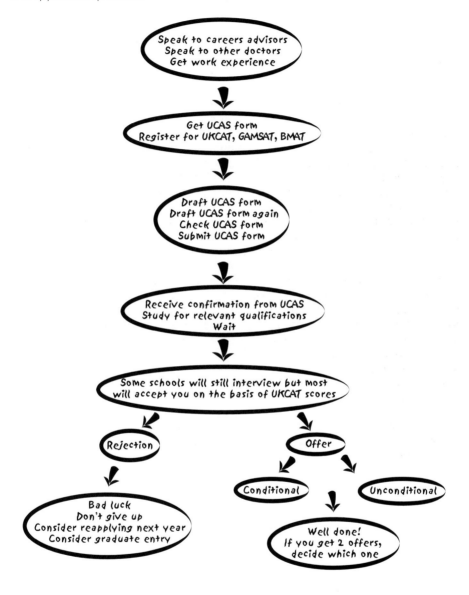

eager to get started and throw themselves into student life. Having been there already, here are a few pointers we thought might come in handy.

- Once you have accepted a place on a course, you are obliged to start it that year. If you wish to take a gap year you must seek permission to defer, or be released (and lose the offer) if you change your mind.

- Don't buy textbooks until you start the course. Freshers tend to buy an armful of books which they hardly use and could have easily borrowed from the library. Wait a while and make selective purchases.
- Make sure you read and are happy with everything you sign. Many medical schools will require you to sign a student contract. Most of these are reasonable and follow the GMC's requirements. However, it is important that you understand what you are signing so do ask a tutor for explanations and advice if you feel unhappy or unsure about the content. If you are a member of the BMA, you can also contact your local office.
- Get involved with the medic social scene. As a fresher it may seem daunting, but these people will be your colleagues for the next five years at least and it is amazing how many friendships stem from the very first week at medical school. Most medical schools will organise a specific medics' freshers' event and this is often well attended by the more senior medical students. Get to know them – their advice will be invaluable later on. It may seem cheesy but medics can provide a real family away from home and this support will prove essential.
- Come to medical school armed with some decent passport photos. You will be surprised at how many people want a photo of you!
- Make the most of the free offers available at freshers' events. Organisations like the BMA offer free membership to first-year medical students and can provide invaluable support and benefits to you, throughout the course and when you become a doctor.
- Don't feel pressured to drink or take drugs – standing up for your opinion from the start will make things an awful lot easier in the long run.
- Make the most of freshers' weeks and do sign up to be part of any medical school mentoring system.
- Make the most of your time at medical school: it really does fly by.

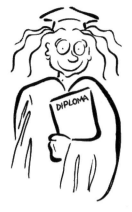

4

Graduate and premedical courses

The work of the doctor will, in the future, be ever more that of an educator, and ever less that of a man who treats ailments.

Lord Horder

If you want something done right, you have to do it yourself. This especially includes your healthcare.

Dr. Andrew Saul

Not everyone knows from an early age that medicine is the career for them. Many students have long possessed A levels or even degrees before deciding to pursue a career in medicine. Others may decide on a late career change with relatively few, or 'non-standard', qualifications. This section gives pragmatic advice for these applicants, along with details of application procedures. This chapter is a 'must read' for:

- graduates of any discipline;
- mature students who do not have A levels or do not have a degree;
- students with A levels but who did not take chemistry (or biology – relevant for some medical schools).

Graduate entry programmes (GEP)

In the USA, and more recently Australia, only graduate students may apply to study medicine. In the UK, more and more entrants to medical school have already completed an undergraduate degree, and some people even believe this should be the only way into the profession. In 2003, some 20% of applicants to medicine were over the age of 21, and in some undergraduate medical courses as many as 15% of students are mature (aged over 21).

As a graduate student you have two options – either apply for a 5 or 6 year course, or a graduate-entry course.

Since 1999 and the opening of the first graduate-entry 4-year course at St George's, an almost frenzied emergence of graduate-entry programmes has swept across the UK, and created a second possibility for graduates. This has been in response to the government's plan to increase the number of doctors in the NHS, and medical schools have been keen to absorb the extra funding for such courses. Graduate-entry programmes vary considerably in their entry requirements so it is worth investigating them thoroughly. Universities operating most of the new courses require graduates to hold a medically-related life science degree in, for example, biology, biochemistry, or genetics. Others require students to hold a healthcare-related degree in, amongst others, nursing, radiography, or midwifery. A 2:1 classification or higher is ordinarily required. A couple of courses, St George's (London) and The University of Nottingham at Derby, allow graduates with at least a 2:2 in any discipline to apply; however, applicants must pass the fiendish GAMSAT, described in Chapter 3, in order to secure an interview.

If you are still completing your first degree you can obtain a UCAS form from your university careers office. Universities are usually happy to make offers based on predicted degree class, but make sure you smooth-talk your personal tutor and express the importance of a good predicted grade and reference. Your careers department may also be able to provide you with a mock interview.

Details on the graduate-entry programmes offered by universities can be seen in the table below. However, students are encouraged to contact the relevant universities for more information.

University	Places	Course details
Birmingham	40	• Four-year medical course open to graduates of life science subjects with a first class degree. A sound knowledge in chemistry (equivalent to grade C at A level) required. • Students are taught in a separate stream for the first two years, before joining the specialty clinical rotations of years 4 and 5 of the 5-year MBChB degree.
Bristol	19	• Four-year medical course requiring at least a 2:1 degree in a life science subject. Healthcare degrees not accepted. • The first year of the course is a condensed and truncated version of the first 2 years of the 5-year course. The latter 3 years are identical.

University	Places	Course details
Cambridge	20	• Four-year medical course open to graduates of any discipline, with at least a 2:1. Various science GCSEs and A levels required too. • All candidates are required to take the BioMedical Admissions Test (BMAT – see Chapter 3), after application and before interview. • No elective period. • Graduate applicants may also apply to Oxford.
Derby (Nottingham University)	90	• Four-year medical course open to graduates of any discipline who have obtained, or are predicted to obtain, a minimum honours degree classified 2:2 or better. • Applicants have to complete the GAMSAT (see Chapter 3). Those who achieve the highest marks will be offered a structured interview for a place on the course.
GKT	40	• Four-year medical course open to graduates of any discipline with at least a 2:1 in their first degree. Other qualifications considered. • Applicants take a written aptitude test (MSAT). Interviews offered on the basis of the application form and MSAT results. • First year is unique, but years 2–4 are integrated with the final 3 years of the 5-year course.
Leicester	64	• Four-year medical course open to graduates with a least a 2:1 healthcare degree. • Applicants must sit the UKCAT examination (see Chapter 3).
Liverpool	40	• Four-year medical course open to graduates with at least a 2:1 in a biomedical or health science degree. BBB also required at A level, along with various GCSEs. • The programme covers the first 2 years of the 5-year course in one academic year.
Newcastle	95	• Four-year medical course open to graduates of any discipline, with at least a 2:1. Alternatively, postgraduate qualifications may be accepted. • Evidence of academic achievement in the last 3 years is also required: e.g. A levels, GAMSAT, Open University, etc. All applicants must sit UKCAT.
Oxford	30	• Four-year graduate entry course for applied and experimental sciences graduates (see their website for list; it is extensive) with at least a 2:1 honours degree. • Applicants must complete the UKCAT (not the BMAT). • Applicants may not apply to both the 4- and 5- year courses: only one. • Graduate applicants may also apply to Cambridge, unlike school leavers.

(Continued)

(*Continued*)

University	Places	Course details
Southampton	40	• Four-year medical course open to graduates of any discipline with at least a 2:1 in their first degree. A level requirements also. • The course has differences from the 5-year course throughout the whole 4 years.
Bart's and the London	40	• Four-year medical course open to graduates with at least a 2:1 degree in life sciences or healthcare. • Applicants must sit the Medical School Admission Test (MSAT) – those who score highest are interviewed.
St George's	70	• Four-year medical course open to graduates in any discipline. They must have or be predicted at least a 2:2 degree in any discipline. • Applicants have to complete the GAMSAT test. Those who perform well in the test are offered an interview. • No upper age limit at present!
Swansea	70	• Four-year medical course open to graduates of any discipline with at least a 2:1 in their first degree. • Applicants have to complete the GAMSAT test. Results of this test are not used for the purposes of selecting for interview and are, instead, a contributing factor to the final decision.
Warwick	164	• Four-year degree open to biological science graduates with at least a 2:1 in their first degree. • Applicants sit MSAT and complete a supplementary application form.

Whether leaving behind a well-paid career, supporting a family, or only recently having completed your previous degree, finances should not put you off applying to medical school if you have a true desire to become a doctor. UK nationals and those domiciled for a sufficient period on approved 4-year graduate-entry courses will have their tuition fees paid from year 2 onwards, and are means-tested for a yearly bursary. More information is contained in Chapter 5 and you should contact the NHS Student Grants Unit for more information (see Further Information).

It has been known for students in their late forties and fifties to be admitted to graduate-entry courses. Ideally, any capable candidate who wants to study medicine should be able to, and the Age Discrimination Act, enacted in 2006, prohibits discrimination on the basis of age. However, some medical schools have argued in the past that older students will generally not serve as long as younger ones and thus the cost to the public purse is significantly more. The current shortage of doctors in the NHS has been used to argue against this.

Access courses

Access courses are a relatively new invention and offer an alternative to A levels, typically with less stringent entry requirements. Most are run by further education colleges and provide a 1-year intensive course in the subjects required to study medicine. This can be a quicker option than taking 3 A levels, but be sure to investigate the acceptance of particular courses by the universities you might like to go to. Access courses too can provide useful preparation for GAMSAT. Obtain statistics regarding the successfulness of previous cohorts. Institutions providing Access courses are listed here (we apologise for any omissions):

- University of Bradford
- City and Islington College
- Lambeth College
- University of Lincoln
- Birkbeck College (University of London)
- Manchester College of Arts and Technology
- City College Norwich
- St Martin's College Lancaster
- Sussex Downs College
- College of West Anglia.

Some universities claim that it is possible to transfer to medicine partway through another course, e.g. biochemistry. If a formal mechanism is not in place, be very wary of such claims, since it rarely happens in practice. Some departments deliberately, and not inappropriately, recruit hopeful medics who do not make the grade, through the UCAS clearing process.

Premedical courses

While most medical degrees last 5 or 6 years some schools offer a premedical year. This year is intended as a foundation year in basic sciences and gives students with good non-science A level grades (and some non-science graduates, if you decide against the 4-year fast track option) a way into the medicine degree course.

There are significant variations in the way these courses are taught and organised, and the exact nature of the premedical course varies from school to school. At some schools, students who complete the year successfully can apply competitively to join the medical degree course, whereas at most there is automatic transfer to year 1 of the 5-year course.

Premedical courses may be taught within the medical faculty or in other university departments. Exemptions from parts of the course may be offered if that subject has already been studied to a sufficient level, and some schools offer a choice of subjects studied. Certain schools also specify that particular science subjects are needed at GCSE/Standard Grade level. Some institutions offer 1-year *widening access programmes* for applicants from disadvantaged backgrounds, or for people who have not demonstrated the usual acumen required of applicants but show great potential. Under the confusing guise of many different names, these courses are offered by GKT, Kingston (in association with St George's), Newcastle, and Southampton, amongst others. These courses are not included in the table overleaf.

Instead of a premedical year, some people choose to take evening courses in science A levels: usually biology and, more importantly, chemistry. This is obviously also an option if you currently have no A levels and, not being too put-off by the long haul, find yourself wanting a drastic career change.

This may also be a useful way of preparing for the GAMSAT (see Chapter 3) if you are a non-science graduate and want to commence a suitable graduate-entry course.

Medical schools offering premedical courses are listed below, along with some course details. However, students are encouraged to contact the relevant universities for more information.

University	Places	Course details
Bristol	10	• Students who studied non-science A levels or degree are admitted into a preliminary year where they can acquire the necessary science background before automatically commencing the 5-year programme. • The premedical year is spent studying the equivalent of A levels in chemistry, anatomical sciences and physics. • Entry requirement (any subject): AAB at A level or 2:1 degree.
Cardiff (Wales College of Medicine)	16	• The premedical course is restricted to applicants who do not meet the subject requirements for direct entry to the 5-year programme, but who have shown high academic achievement elsewhere. • It is a modular programme and studies centre on the chemical and biological sciences, or other subjects selected according to the student's prior qualifications.
Dundee	14	• The year is provided for applicants with good passes in non-science subjects and is not available for applicants whose passes in science subjects do not meet requirements for first year. • Premed students join with first-year BSc courses in chemistry, biology, and physics. • Entry guaranteed to medical course upon successful completion.
Edinburgh	No set number	• The premedical year is an extra year of study for applicants who do not have the subject entrance requirements for the 5-year programme. • It consists of selected courses from the first year of the biological sciences course. • Successful students continue on to the 5-year course.
GKT	40	• The premedical year is an extra year of study for applicants who do not have the subject entrance requirements for the 5-year programme, but achieve the academic requirements. • Applicants must sit the UKCAT. • The course covers biology, chemistry, physics, and maths. Students study alongside those taking BSc degrees. • An additional premedical course exists for people who have not demonstrated the usual academic acumen, but who show potential and live in inner London.

University	Places	Course details
Manchester	20	• This programme occupies a single year and is designed for students who do not have the required science qualifications for direct entry into 5-year programme but have achieved good grades, in mainly arts subjects or, in the case of mature students, have a good arts degree. • Students learn fundamentals of biology, physics, and chemistry at Xaverian college near the Manchester campus. This is achieved with problem-based learning cases, theatre events and skills sessions. • Entry to the next year of the medical course is automatic on satisfactory completion of this year. • Applicants must sit the UKCAT and pass an interview.
Newcastle	10–15	• The premedical year is open only to applicants without a science background. • Students study a combination of chemistry, biological sciences and medical data-handling.
Sheffield	15	• The premedical science foundation course is a modified 'Access to Science' course, tailored to give students with a non-scientific background the necessary knowledge to undertake the medical course. • The course is designed to prepare students for the first part of the medical degree, and is studied at Barnsley College. There are visits to the medical physics, clinical chemistry, and anaesthetic departments of a local hospital. • Additionally, students gain basic scientific knowledge through studying biology, chemistry, and physics.

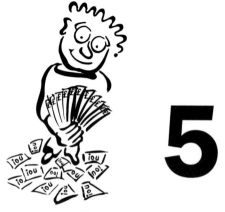

5

Funding your way through

The physician should not treat the disease but the patient who is suffering from it.

Maimonides

What to expect

Money is an issue close to most students' hearts, and medical students are no exception. For the past few years, graduating medical students had to pay tuition fees while studying; fees have now been increased with the introduction of 'top-up' fees for new students. As a result, the issue of money will be very different for students starting medicine today, even compared with those who have recently graduated.

A recent BMA report, *Annual Survey of Medical Students' Finances 2004/2005*, found that the average total debt among final-year students was over £20,000. The survey found that debt varied enormously: some students had no debt but a small number had debts of over £50,000. These students were under the old tuition-fee system, and those entering medicine now are likely to come out with much higher debts. The main reason for this is that, from September 2006, all new medical students are liable to pay £3000 per year in tuition fees. Although this does not have to be paid until you are earning over £15,000, the days of many doctors paying off their debts within a few years of qualifying are becoming, for many, a thing of the past. Many entering medical school now may well take over 10 years to pay off the debt after graduating. While this may be a heady concept to come to terms with, it is important to remember that, while this situation is far from ideal, few will regret their decision to study medicine. Don't let finances alone put you off studying medicine. Yes, you are likely to be in more debt after graduation than someone who takes a 3-year degree course, but you must balance this with the excellent future career prospects and good job security that medicine provides. Medical student intake reflects all sectors of society. If you are not supported by wealthy and generous parents, you won't be alone in being in debt.

Depending on where you choose to study medicine and the requirements of the course, it can take you between 4 years and 6 years to complete, and you will have to consider how you will support yourself for that time. The first 2 years are often the least financially demanding as you will probably have longer holidays, which allows time to earn cash if you want or need to; it is also more possible to work a few hours per week in term-time in the less demanding, earlier years. Working to support yourself gets a little trickier in your clinical years when you spend more time in hospital – a total annual holiday of 6 weeks is considered good by most students! Finding paid work when you have only 6 weeks off can be difficult, and it can be hard to fit in term-time work with a gradual increase in the intensity of the course.

There are many expenses involved in studying medicine and debt is likely to stare you in the face earlier than you might anticipate. Medicine is different from almost any degree course: for example, there are many expensive books to buy (you could spend at least £150 per year) and travel expenses to peripheral placements can really add up. Medical equipment, such as stethoscopes, can cost around £60. As always, however, the advice remains that you should shop around where possible as there are good deals out there! Don't get excited and buy every book and piece of equipment at the start of your first year. Speak to students in years above – do you really need that expensive piece of equipment? You can often pick up books secondhand. If you've got good library facilities which are convenient for you to study in, you may not need to buy that many books – but this will vary enormously from medical school to medical school. In addition, some organisations offer medical equipment – the BMA, for example, has run programmes where membership entitles you to a significant discount on a range of medical equipment. You will also need to spend money on some smart clothing once you're in hospitals regularly. This is to make you look and feel like part of the medical profession, and to help you gain the trust of your patients.

Top-up tuition fees

As mentioned above, the vast majority of medical students entering medical school will have to pay variable fees (or 'top-up' fees), up to a maximum of £3000 per year, although there are some exceptions. In reality, there's a high supply of medical school applicants and all medical schools charge £3000 per year. If you haven't done a previous degree in the UK then you will be entitled to a fee loan which allows you to defer payment of tuition fees until after you graduate, when you will pay back the fees gradually. At the time of writing, the Department of Health will pay the tuition fees of medical students in certain years of the course, depending on whether you are on a 6-year course or a graduate-entry course.

The obvious question is: 'How will I pay for all this?' One port of call for some people will be parents, guardians, or family, who may be able to give you something towards the cost of studying. The amount of government support that you are able to receive will, for most students, depend upon your parents' earnings. Some students with wealthy parents receive good support from them. Students with very low parental incomes will get good government support. Potentially, the most difficult financial situation a medical student could be in is having medium- to high-earning parents who can't or won't provide sufficient support. If you think that this may be your situation, it doesn't mean you can't go to medical school; it just means that financially it will be trickier. You'll have to rely more on commercial debt and possibly do a lot of paid employment.

Some students can be considered 'independent of their parents' and hence have their own income rather than their parents' subjected to means testing. Many find the strict criteria unfair, finding themselves not classed as independent even though in reality they haven't lived with or received money from their parents for many years. In the early years, the most common way to be classed as independent is to be over 25 years old at the start of the academic course.

At the time of writing, the rules around the age of independence, at least for support provided by the English Department of Health, were changing due to the introduction of the Age Discrimination Act, and the BMA was in discussion with the government about the implications of independent status for students studying medicine. At the time of going to print, future entitlement to support may depend on demonstrating that you have been financially self-sufficient for a set period of time. In view of this, it is well worth investigating your entitlements very early on.

Government support

The type of government funding you receive depends mainly on two factors:

- where you lived before entering medical school (which becomes more complex than that if you've recently done a first degree, been to boarding school or have moved about in the past three years);
- how much your parents earn (or, if you are deemed 'independent' from your parents, *your* earnings and your spouse's earnings).

With devolution, the involvement of different government departments, and EU rules, medical student finance has become incredibly complex for some students, and it isn't likely to simplify any time soon. The key is to plan well. To plan well you need to know what you are going to get from government sources and consider all other options available. It's important to remember that most government finance websites, guides, and helplines are primarily aimed at standard students on standard courses. Medical students are different: both the course and the length of terms are longer, and government support, such as the NHS bursary, isn't available to most other students. The hard facts are that you will have to fill in many forms and spend time investigating what you are entitled to, including reading the small print very carefully. It isn't fun, but nor is realising you're not eligible for a particular bursary or loan with only a few days to go before the start of a year and with no Plan B!

On top of this, some of you may have different circumstances which may make finding out your entitlements even trickier. Examples are if you haven't lived in the same part of the UK for the past few years or if you are studying medicine as a second degree. There are some good sources of information in the Further Information section of this book – our advice is to read through these carefully and be persistent in finding out what you're entitled to. But remember, try not to become too frustrated if the call-centre guy on the government helpline can't answer your question (even after you've spent 45 minutes in a queue listening to immensely annoying music!). Don't give up: there are people who can help – for example, the new www.money4medstudents.org website is superb.

If you've already completed a degree in the UK, funding is going to be more difficult. At the time of writing, you'll have to fund your tuition fees up front in year 1 if you're on a 4-year course and pay the full £3000 per year during years 1 to 4 of a 5-year course. This means ensuring you have access to money at the start of the course and probably means, for those on a 5-year course, a high reliance on commercial debt later on in the course.

Listed below are some of the key costs for most students. It doesn't cover every eventuality – so if you fall into a complex scenario, please refer elsewhere, being mindful at all times of which nation you are living in. Also, things change over time and the details below may not be up-to-date when you read this, so please check carefully. All figures quoted relate to 2006–07 rates and we have tried, where possible, to list differences in the devolved nations.

Sources of funding

Tuition fees

If you're studying medicine in England you'll have to pay top-up tuition fees, which were capped at £3000 per year. If it's your first UK degree, you are entitled to a fee loan to cover the entire fee. This is like a government loan which will only increase with inflation (i.e. you pay back in real terms what you borrowed). In 2007, the requirement was that the loan has to be repaid once you are earning over £15,000.

If you've already done a UK degree, you will have to pay tuition fees upfront to your university – most likely in instalments of £1000 per term.

Nobody will have to pay fees in their fifth and subsequent years of study. When tuition fees were originally introduced, the BMA's Medical Students Committee persuaded the government that special consideration needed to be given to medical students because of the length and expense of the course. The Department of Health subsequently agreed to pay tuition fees for medical students from their fifth year of study onwards. This arrangement also applies to students doing premedical or intercalated years, so you will only pay top-up tuition fees for your first four years of your course.

If you are on a 4-year accelerated graduate-entry medical course, you must pay the fee for the first year upfront. Then if you're from England or Wales, or most other places in Europe, you will pay no fees. If you're deemed to be from Scotland or Northern Ireland and you're studying in England you may have to full upfront fees throughout your degree!

If you're studying in Scotland and you're deemed to normally live in Scotland (or anywhere in the EU except England, Wales, or Northern Ireland) and you are studying medicine as your first UK degree, you won't have to pay fees. You will have to pay a small, deferred fee (or 'graduate endowment') when you graduate, but this can be covered with a student loan and paid off with the rest of your student loan. If you fit the above category but you've already got a UK degree, then you will have to pay around £1200 per year upfront. If you normally live in England, Wales, or Northern Ireland but are studying in Scotland, you'll have to pay fees of £2700 per year for years 1 to 4. If medicine is your first UK degree, you are entitled to a fee loan to cover this. If you're not, you'll have to pay the fees upfront.

If you're studying in Wales your fee will depend on where you're deemed to normally live – and the rules are as bizarre as for Scotland. If you're from anywhere in the EU (including Wales) except England, Scotland, or Northern Ireland, you will pay around £1200 per year (first UK degree students can defer payment of this fee with a fee loan). However, if you're deemed to be from England, Scotland, or Northern Ireland and you are studying in Wales you'll have to pay £3000 per year! (Fee loan is available if you are taking your first UK degree.) These complex absurdities may change in future …

The fee structure in Northern Ireland is similar to that in England for students from anywhere in the UK or Europe. We have not referred to arrangements for graduate-entry courses in Northern Ireland or Scotland as, at the time of writing there was no 4-year course in either nation.

Student loan for living costs (maintenance loan)

It is likely that paying for basic living costs will form the largest part of any debt you accumulate throughout your degree. Money for accommodation, food, transport, books, and beer will come from maintenance loans and grants, parental contributions, and, invariably, banks.

A maintenance loan is a government student loan. Along with your fee loan, it is added to your total student loan, which then increases with inflation and is paid back as you earn. The difference is that instead of being paid straight to your university, it is paid to you and is meant to cover your living expenses. You are entitled to a maintenance loan even if you are studying medicine as a second degree. The amount of maintenance loan you will be entitled to will depend on where you study and what year you are in.

In England loans are administered by the Student Loans Company: 25% of the loan is means-tested and will depend largely upon your parents' income (unless you are deemed to be independent, in which case it is assessed on your income). The maximum basic loan available in 2006/2007 for students from England studying outside of London in years 1–4 of a standard course (which is the same as that available for the first year of the 4-year fast track course) was around £4400. The minimum was around £3300. The loan is significantly more if you study in London and significantly less if you live with your parents. If you receive the maximum loan, you are also entitled to an extra week's loan allowance for every week over 30 weeks that your course lasts (roughly £75 per week outside of London). However, if you don't get the maximum loan, then you aren't entitled to any allowance whatsoever for extra weeks!

Loan amounts vary in the devolved nations. Whilst beyond the scope of this chapter, it should be pointed out that the minimum loan for students from Scotland studying in Scotland, away from their parents' home, was just £850 per year in 2006! Your loan will be reduced if you get a decent-sized grant. Grants are explained in more detail below.

Maintenance grants (or bursaries)

Maintenance grants also vary throughout the UK. These are non-repayable grants, which are generally means-tested on parental income. For example, first-degree students from England or Wales with a low parental income are entitled to a grant of £2700 per year. The situation for first-degree students from Scotland and Northern Ireland is similar, though amounts and means testing thresholds are slightly different. Check out your entitlement from your home nation and ensure you read carefully about eligibility. If your parents are to be means-tested (rather than yourself), try and get a rough idea of how much (if any) grant you may be entitled to.

First-degree students from low-income families may also be entitled to a university grant. It is well worth investigating this option, as these vary enormously from university to university. The minimum for students from England at universities in England is £300 per year for students with very low earning parents. Some offer much higher grants and higher thresholds for parental income. Contact the universities you are considering applying to for their specific arrangements.

Means-tested travel expense grants are available and the rules vary throughout the UK. For students from England in the early years of the course they are available from your local authority. However, these are also means-tested and the first £285 you incur you will have to pay yourself. Some students find it is only worth claiming when they are travelling daily. If you are in the years when the NHS pays your tuition fees, responsibility for travel expenses moves to the NHS. You are still subject to means testing, but the NHS does not apply the excess that the local authority does, so you may get full reimbursement of travel expenses (subject, of course, to means testing).

A means-tested NHS bursary is potentially available to all UK students in their fifth and subsequent years of study (including intercalating) on the 5/6-year courses, and also to students from England and Wales on the 4-year accelerated courses in years 2 to 4. The NHS bursary is fully means-tested, either on your own or your parents' income depending on your status, which means you need to be aware that you may get nothing. As mentioned above, the rules for whether you are means tested via your parents or yourself were changing at time of writing. The rules may be based on proving that you have been financially self-sufficient for a period of time, rather than on your age, so check the NHS bursary website for the latest information. Note that in the years that you're eligible for the NHS bursary your student loan will be cut in half, even if you are not entitled to the bursary because of means testing. Make sure that you are aware of this if you have a medium to high parental income so that you don't get any nasty surprises on the first day of term!

In the years that the NHS bursary is payable, extra money is available for extra weeks and for travel expenses. Even if you are means-tested out of the bursary itself you may still be eligible for means-tested travel expenses, so it's well worth applying. Apply to your home UK nation.

Commercial debt – the high-street bank

For some students, support from the high-street bank will be in addition to other forms of support, but for other students it will make up the bulk of your living costs.

At a minimum, you will probably need an interest-free bank overdraft. Most banks and building societies offer students special terms on bank accounts. These normally include an interest-free overdraft, which at the time of writing was around £2100 over the 5 years. The general deadline for repayment is within 3 years of graduation.

Keeping your bank manager happy by not exceeding the agreed overdraft limit is good practice, and also helps you avoid penalty charges and punishing interest rates. If you want to extend your overdraft, go and discuss it with the manager face to face. The bank wants your custom because you will have a good job at the end of your university career, and they are experienced at helping students out with money problems.

If you need more cash than an overdraft gives you, you may need a loan – often known as a health-care study loan or professional loan. Look around to make sure you have accessed all other sources of funding before you take out a loan, for example, hardship funds and charitable funds (see below). Many banks have specially tailored loans of up to £20,000 for medical students. The interest will be above inflation (i.e. you will pay back significantly more than you borrowed). Be aware that this loan is more expensive than the student loan offered by the government. On the flip side, as bank loans go, it is relatively cheap – medical students are considered a low risk for the bank.

The main problem with commercial debt is the repayment agreement. This is very important and it is well worth getting the longest repayment agreement available – you can always pay back quicker. Unlike governments loans, which are paid back in a manner linked to your earnings, commercial debt will be paid back over a fixed period – often starting perhaps only 6 months after graduating. Borrowing £20,000 through medical school with repayment over 7 years may mean paying back per-haps around £400 a month, including interest. That's a lot of money as a junior doctor! Ultimately, for many it will be a balance of the quality of life they want to live now versus that when they are qualified. It's a difficult decision to make and the answer will be different for everyone. Don't live on economy baked beans as a medical student if you can take out a loan, but never be blasé about debt either – it must be paid back.

As with all commercial debt, you'll be credit scored. So, if you haven't had an address in the UK for long, there have been bad borrowers in the household, or you've got a bad credit history, you might have problems. The key point is that if you think you'll need a bank loan, think about this early on so that you can do something about it.

Some students manage to have a multitude of overdrafts with different banks, moving money around to keep all of the bank accounts active (though the banks are getting wise to this now!); others have interest-free credit cards, moving balances around to get the best deals. Some pull this off with extreme success, but others get into real difficulty. Attempting this can end in tears unless you are certain you know exactly what you are doing. It may be worth just getting a bigger professional loan instead and paying the interest.

Finally, the bank account you've been with since a child and your parents have always been with is not likely to offer the best deal – forget the free teddy bear and shop around for the best deal.

Charities

There are literally hundreds of educational trust funds and charities in the UK, many of which sup-port medical students. Many are open to mature and graduate students rather than school leavers, but it may be worth trying to find some funding from these sources. General directories of charitable trusts are available in the reference section of most public libraries and some are listed in the Further Information section of this book. Spending time searching through the lists and applying for grants may be to your advantage. Many small trusts have bizarre criteria for offering awards, and you may be surprised to find that by meeting the unusual requirements you can get help towards your expenses.

Access funds, hardship funds and hardship loans

Universities receive money from the government to help students in the poorest financial situations. Applications for the money are processed locally and policies on how these funds are distributed vary widely between medical schools. It is important to be aware that this money is available as often not many people apply for it. It is especially useful if, for example, you're means tested out of a lot of support but still don't get much money. In addition, if the NHS pays for your top-up tuition fees, you can apply for a hardship grant through the NHS Grants Unit.

Work

For the majority of medical undergraduates, working during vacations in the early part of the course is a necessity. As well as casual work in bars and restaurants, some students work as healthcare assistants and medical secretaries. Work can usually be arranged through the teaching hospital or other local hospitals. The experience of working in a hospital environment in a role other than as a medical practitioner can be very valuable, but others value the opportunity to work in a different environment. As the course progresses, however, the holidays get shorter as term time extends and periods of elective study intervene, and it then becomes more difficult to find employment for these shorter periods.

You might consider taking a part-time job during term. The medical course is undoubtedly challenging and demands a lot of your time in studying, no matter how gifted you are. Because of this, some medical schools discourage students from working during term. Despite this, some students manage to do a term-time job for some of the year in earlier years. Whether you can manage this will be a personal decision, but ensure your studies come first. Also bear in mind there are many opportunities to get involved in societies, sport, and much more at university. It would be a shame to miss these opportunities due to working an excessive amount during term time, unless you really have to.

Cadetships

Some medical students sign up to one of the Armed Forces medical cadet schemes. A 'salary' is paid to cadets for 2 to 3 years. In return for this support during undergraduate training, cadets serve as an officer with, for example, the Royal Army Medical Corps for a minimum period of duty (normally 6 years after full qualification). The income cadets receive is very generous compared to other students' incomes, but the *quid pro quo* is the 6-year short service commission. You will continue to practise as a doctor, but the Ministry of Defence will require you to support military initiatives anywhere in the world. Working as a doctor in the Armed Forces can be very rewarding and challenging. It is the advice of the authors of this guide that students who embark on medical cadetships should be committed to a career in the Services after graduation, and not simply addressing the funding of their course. The Armed Forces recruit during the early years of the medical degree course and offer familiarization visits for interested students. Contact details for each service are given in the Further Information section at the end of the book.

Elective funding

Students who organise themselves well in advance can often get enough funding to pay for some (if not all) of the cost of their elective. You should have a wonderful time wherever you go, but it is helpful if you can get some funding towards the cost. If money is tight then consider the cost of living in the country that you are going to. Depending on where you want to go and what you will be studying, there are numerous grants, research awards, sponsorships, and bursaries available (the BMA holds a list of organizations that you can apply to for funds). Some will be open for all UK students to apply for, and other funds will be distributed locally. Most awards and grants are given in exchange for some sort of project report or research work. There are also some means-tested government funds available, for example for students from England on 5/6-year courses who are taking their elective as part of their fourth year of study (including intercalating) or before.

The final balance ...

Irrespective of your personal circumstances, studying medicine means undertaking a serious financial commitment. In common with many other students, you will have to face up to some debt and financial worries. By accepting this reality and planning, before you start your course, how your tuition fees, parents' contribution, bank overdraft, student loan, and bank loans will fit together over the years, you will come to terms with it better. You can find information about funding in our Further Information section. Make sure your acquaintance with debt is on your own terms. Do not avoid dealing with tough money questions and do not adopt a head-in-the-sand approach to your finances. If you anticipate difficulties during the course, take advice from the students' union welfare services, the university and your bank. Don't leave it too late to take action – there are very few miracle workers, and the people who are there to help are more likely to be helpful if they are given time.

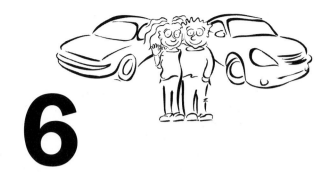

6

Life beyond graduation ...

The education of the doctor which goes on after he has his degree is, after all, the most important part of his education.

John Shaw Billings (1838–1913)

The early years

Graduating or qualifying from medical school does not, in itself, allow you to practise medicine: first you must register with the GMC. Initially, registration with the GMC is only provisional, but you can call yourself Doctor. To register fully, newly qualified doctors are required to complete 12 months of paid work and achieve defined competencies as a foundation doctor. Since August 2005 hospital trusts, in partnership with the postgraduate deanery, will offer 2-year posts which must be completed before trainees apply for specialist training. During the first year, called the F1 year, trainees will do at least 3 months in medicine and 3 months in surgery. Some rotations will be 6 months of medicine and 6 months of surgery, but most placements will be for 4 months. In the second year (the F2 year), units will be offered in other specialities such as paediatrics, general practice, accident and emergency or psychiatry. Core skills or competencies will be attained in both years of foundation training.

The ability to tailor your future career during your early working life should increase following reforms to junior doctor training. The push to modernise medical careers have introduced an integrated 2-year programme after graduation called the *foundation programme* and shorter training times to full specialization as a GP or a consultant. Key aims of the foundation programme are to ensure better supervision, clear educational and training outcomes and career mentoring and advice in the first 2 years of working. Junior doctors will also have the opportunity to 'taste' different specialities earlier in their career which should help future decisions about career.

Regardless of these changes, all foundation house officer posts must be approved by the GMC for the experience to count towards full registration. At the end of your first year of working, if you can demonstrate that you have achieved the minimum competencies, you can apply for full GMC registration. Free hospital accommodation is provided for your job because the GMC believes that the right type of experience is only gained if you are resident, so don't worry if your jobs are in parts of the country you didn't choose: there will be accommodation provided.

Applying for your first job

The process of applying for your first job was, at the time of writing, still undergoing some change but you can find detailed information in the BMA document *Guidance on applying for foundation programmes.*

In future, almost all applications to foundation programmes will occur via a UK-wide website called MTAS (the Medical Training Application Service) which was launched in October 2006. Applicants will need to register with the MTAS website before entering their final year of medical school. This will enable you to access information about the location and content of foundation programmes across the UK. Jobs are offered in regional clusters of medical schools, postgraduate deaneries, and hospitals called Foundation Schools. There are 27 Foundation Schools in the UK and you must rank all 27 schools to be sure of a job. Normally, the medical school that sends students to a hospital for clinical experience will supply the same hospital with its new house officers, but some schemes include posts that are many miles away. If you are clear that you want to work in a particular part of the country, it might be worth finding out about the specific arrangements for applying for foundation jobs in that area well ahead of time.

While some medical schools produce too few graduates to fill all the posts in their locality, all UK graduates medical students have very good prospects of getting a job as foundation programme doctors for the foreseeable future.

If you cannot get a foundation programme job in the particular town or city you would like to work in, don't worry. During the training years you can apply for jobs elsewhere in the country (and abroad). Hospitals in Australasia, for example, recruit UK doctors for short-term posts.

Life as the house dog

Working in hospitals in your first year after medical school is often the toughest part of your medical career. There is much to do and learn, and sometimes providing a service to patients and your employer comes at the cost of your continuing education. Be under no illusions that you are at the bottom of the medical hierarchy. Demands from your patients, colleagues and bosses can be overpowering. Hours of work are long (50+ per week), and working intensively at night or weekends (on call) can be exhausting. However, changes to European law that came into effect in 2005 mean that the situation is improving. In addition, current reforms aim to redress the balance and ensure that a core set of doctoring skills, as well as improved education, are gained by all foundation house officers in the future. Further information about the working arrangements for junior doctors can be found on the BMA website.

In the F1 year you will be responsible for taking histories from new patients, organising tests, following up consultants' instructions, and helping at outpatient clinics and with theatre sessions. However, there are controls and ways of reducing the strains upon you. There will probably be times when you are fed up and may want to quit medicine. Some do leave medicine, but the vast majority stays on. You will become more confident and more able to cope, and the work will eventually become more interesting (and challenging). Support and mentoring is crucial at this time as many feel the pressure of the transition from student to doctor. The BMA runs a counselling service which is available to members, 24 hours a day, every day of the year. See the Further Information section.

Beyond the house officer year

After you have completed your first year in hospital as a foundation doctor and have received registration from the GMC, you can begin to have more lengthy exposure to the career path you want. This has traditionally been in senior house officer posts through basic specialist training and, later, in specialist or GP registrar posts. If you have a strong idea about what speciality you want to practise in or you know you want to become a GP, you can begin to take the appropriate path in the second year of the foundation programme and continue through the new training grades. Don't worry if you don't know which branch of medicine you want to be in now or even, for that matter, during the first few years after graduation. Many junior doctors don't decide on their final career until well into their postgraduate training, and a core element of government reform is to ensure that career advice is more readily available. The three main areas of practice are general practice, hospital medicine and surgery. The BMA is working with government on ensuring that changes to junior doctor training and structures to specialisation do not disadvantage future generations of doctors and dovetail with existing professional outcomes.

A career in general practice

General practice is changing significantly as a result of changes to training pathways, the new contract negotiated for GPs between the BMA and government and also because of changes in government policy. Many GPs will continue to be self-employed doctors who provide general medical services to patients under a contract with a Primary Care Organisation (PCO), either as part of a general practice business partnership or on their own, and are increasingly likely to employ additional trained staff to fulfil key roles. There is also the option to work as a paid employee for a practice or PCO (which is becoming increasingly popular), or to work as a self-employed locum.

The most common route to becoming a qualified GP is to do 3 years' training as a GP registrar. At present this is divided into 2 years of hospital posts (in specialities such as general medicine, general surgery, A&E, obstetrics, geriatrics, or psychiatry) and 1 year working as a 'trainee' in a general practice surgery. However, from August 2007, with implementation of the new GP curriculum under Modernising Medical Careers, the proportion of time that will trainees spend training in a GP surgery is likely to increase.

A career in hospital medicine or surgery

In order to become a hospital consultant, junior doctors normally rotate through two or three years of SHO jobs in medical or surgical specialities. After this, and once their choice of specialty is clear, they spend between 4 and 5 years studying in registrar posts. There are specialist registrar 'rotations' which allow a doctor to prearrange 3 or 4 years of training in different hospital posts. When this training is completed satisfactorily, a Certificate of Completion of Specialist Training (CCST) is issued and the doctor can apply for consultant posts.

As with GPs, the future training paths and conditions of service for hospital doctors are also undergoing change. The BMA has agreed a new contract for consultants and there is discussion of a Certificate of Specialist Training (CST) that could be awarded for shorter periods of time served in the training grades. The BMA is opposed to the introduction a CST and continues to discuss alternative options with government.

Other career paths

General practice and hospital posts provide the greatest number of jobs for doctors in the health service, but there are many other career paths. Many doctors work in public health medicine, as medical academics, as researchers for pharmaceutical companies, for the Armed Forces and in private medicine. A great strength of practising as a doctor is the range of experience you can find in work. Flexible training is becoming more common and part-time posts are numerous. Many doctors have more than one string to their bow and it is not uncommon, for example, for a doctor to mix private work or part-time work with their main NHS job. Putting together a portfolio career as a doctor is possible. A consultant might add some medical journalism and legal work in courts as an expert

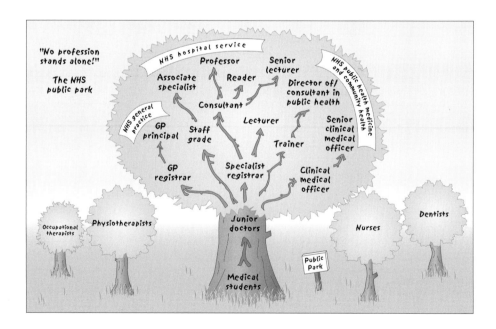

witness to their weekly duties as a hospital specialist; a director of public health might do voluntary medical work with a charity; or a GP might work part time with a local rugby club. The diagram on page 58 shows a simplified path of career options in medicine for doctors in the UK.

Continuing medical education

Don't think that studying is over once you have graduated from medical school! The GMC's view is that undergraduate medical education is just the first step toward lifelong learning. It means that doctors must continue to study to some extent throughout their working lives and are expected to keep their skills and knowledge up-to-date to remain registered as a doctor. The GMC has introduced a system of formal reassessment for all doctors on its register – *revalidation*. Many skills and much knowledge will be acquired 'on the job', but most career paths require some formal qualifications and exams will have to be passed to retain registration with the GMC. Since 2005 the Postgraduate Medical Education and Training Board has been responsible for continuing medical education, and will oversee the standards required for all specialities that will enable you get on in your career. This may include passing Royal College exams, either as a minimum requirement for membership or to supplement the minimum standards required. Both the introduction of revalidation and the establishment of the Postgraduate Medical Education Board will allow transparency in ongoing educational requirements across the entire profession.

Part 2
The A–Z of UK medical schools

How to use Part 2

Numerous factors influence which medical schools suit you most and which ones you may decide to apply to. In this chapter, we have summarized a number of important areas we think you should take into consideration before making a decision. Each medical school chapter in the following section has been deliberately divided into three sections (Education, Welfare, Sports and Social) to make it easier for you to compare different schools. A snapshot of key information for all schools can also be found at Mikey and Michelle's quick compare table on page 319.

Education

Although all students need to reach the same standard outlined by the GMC by the time they graduate, courses at different medical schools can vary considerably in the way this is achieved. More often than not the courses on offer are subject to change, and many of us at medical school are on different courses from those outlined in the original prospectus. Don't, whatever you do, get bogged down in the details of individual courses. You'll just get confused. However, it may be worthwhile considering the following areas.

Teaching

There are two broad teaching methods, either of which may be used on their own in some schools or combined to offer a mix of the two. 'Traditional' teaching relies heavily on lectures and practicals, with a large portion of the week devoted to didactic teaching where students are in lecture theatres for long periods. Problem-based learning (PBL) is the more recent approach, and usually has fewer timetabled commitments. Commonly, students work in small groups and discuss patient case studies, from which they form study agendas for the coming week. Students then work through their own study objectives, which are supplemented with laboratory sessions such as pathology and anatomy in the preclinical years. With the PBL approach, it is essential that students, and their groups, sustain a significant amount of self-motivation.

The structure of courses also varies considerably. Some medical schools maintain the traditional preclinical/clinical divide, with core science subjects, such as anatomy, biochemistry, pharmacology, and pathology, taught in the early years and speciality-based clinical subjects, such as obstetrics and gynaecology, paediatrics, and surgery, taught in the later years. Other medical schools choose a system-based approach and combine both core sciences and clinical experience in all years. Between these two extremes there are all number of shades of grey and it is worth developing an idea of which style you feel you would enjoy the most.

Anatomy teaching has also seen many changes in recent years, and in some medical schools the dissection of cadavers by students has been replaced, partly or fully, with demonstration sections (or prosections) dissected by staff before class. However, some students prefer the 'hands on' approach both in and out of dissection.

Assessment

The type of assessment varies significantly between schools. Commonly used methods include multiple-choice question papers (sometimes negatively marked), essay papers, short-answer questions, computer examinations, literature review papers, case studies, and papers which require candidates to match questions to answers, as well as many more. Some schools have final exams in the penultimate year and others have finals at the end of the last year. Increasingly, a number of schools are choosing to place a greater amount of emphasis on continuous assessment, which reduces the impact of finals at the end of the course.

When choosing which medical schools to apply for, decide whether you would prefer exams and assessments spread out during the years and the course, or whether you would prefer to take cumulative exams once everything has had a chance to fit into place. Either way, you still have to learn it all!

Intercalated degrees

This is where medical students can obtain a Bachelor of Science (BSc), Bachelor of Art (BA), or Bachelor of Medical Science (BMedSci) degree for undertaking an extra year of study (although some can be done within the 'normal' 5-year course), once they have completed at least 2 years of their medical training. These degrees can be undertaken in a variety of subjects related to medicine and provide an opportunity for students to pursue further study in an area they are interested in. Medical schools in the UK take a variety of approaches to intercalated degrees. In some (although this approach is gradually disappearing) the extra degree is open only to the academic high-flyers; some offer courses to almost any medical student; and at others it is compulsory. If you anticipate being interested in some extra in-depth research leading to a qualification, or if you think you might like to follow an academic or teaching career, think about this before you apply. Many medical schools also allow students to study for the extra degree within other faculties of the university or at other institutions.

Special study modules (SSM) and electives

Schools devote markedly different portions of the course to studying areas of special interest (SSMs) and to overseas work placements (electives). Although there is an accepted minimum provision, it is worth considering this when choosing your medical school. Some medical schools will allow 2- to 4-week SSMs in diverse medical subjects such as history of medicine, medicine and art, and modern languages, and certain schools allow students to take one or more SSMs abroad, in addition to their elective period. The vast majority of UK medical schools offer students an opportunity to spend a longer part of the course (around 2 months), known as the elective, anywhere in the world to experience medicine in a foreign healthcare setting. The exact nature of these placements varies slightly between schools. However, wherever you choose to study, these placements are seen as one of the highlights of medical school life.

Welfare

Student support

Pastoral support systems should be in place at all universities and all students should be allocated a personal tutor or 'Director of Studies'. However, standards of support vary markedly and it is well worth asking existing medical students about the provision and success of such schemes when attending the open days. Some universities will provide support through the medical faculty as well as via the main campus, and a friendly, approachable, and understanding medical faculty can make a considerable difference to a student's experience at university – especially if it is necessary for the student to manage ill health or dependants in addition to their medical studies. Most schools have in-house counselling and advice services.

At many universities freshers are allocated students from later years to be a 'mummy' or a 'daddy' – or one of each – during their first few weeks at medical school. Such schemes can be very beneficial, helping new students to settle in and providing them with support and guidance during their early years. Many students remain in touch with their 'academic families' well beyond graduation.

Accommodation

The accommodation the university provides and where it is located will have an important effect on your experience of university: remember, you will spend a large portion of your time there so you want to be happy. Important questions to ask include:

- Is accommodation provided for the first year?
- Are meals provided or is the residence self-catering?
- Is it just for medics or for a range of students?
- Is the accommodation mixed?
- Is the accommodation on campus, and if not, how far away is it?
- How expensive is the accommodation for the first and subsequent years?

Placements

Most schools will send you away from the main university hospital base for some modules. The distances involved can vary significantly. Are you the type who enjoys travelling and seeing different parts of the country or would you rather stay nearer to the medical school and spend less on travel? These are important questions to consider when applying to medical schools that have a larger number of 'peripheral' hospitals. Each chapter lists examples of the distance from campus of hospital placements and journey time to give you an indication of what to expect.

Sports and social

Most universities organise social weekends and freshers' weeks before the start of freshers' term, and this is a great way of making friends early on. The comfort of walking into the bar on the first evening of term and recognising a friendly face from such a weekend relieves some of the initial anxiety of leaving home and making new friends.

All medical schools offer medics' sports teams. Only students studying medicine will be able to represent these clubs. As almost all medical schools are now part of larger universities you will also be able to play for the university side. However, you tend to find that most medics pride themselves on playing for the medics. The camaraderie and social life are unrivalled and a constant envy of non-medics. However, this has also led to accusations of 'cliquishness'. The only limit on the number of teams you can join is the amount of time you are willing to devote to them. Most students wonder how medics can study during the day, train in the evenings, and play matches week in and week out: the answer is that you develop good time management skills. However, it is important to get the balance right. One beauty of medics' sports is that all skill levels are catered for, and as you progress in your medical career you may find you take on more responsibility for your club, from organising the mundane such as kit, to the extravagant, such as tours of Europe!

Other than sports teams, most medical schools have choirs, drama clubs, and even organise annual medic shows and comedy revues. Furthermore, most schools have medical societies that organise social events and you can also get involved with events organised by the Medical Students International Network (MedSIN), for example, Sexpression (students running sex education initiatives in their local area), or Marrow (a student-led initiative which aims to recruit volunteers to the bone marrow register), as well as others. There is something for everyone! Again, in addition to the medical school clubs, there is a wealth of university social and hobby clubs and students are always welcome to start new ones.

Top tip: Do get involved, try something new, excel at something old, but most importantly, ENJOY IT!

Aberdeen

Key facts	Undergraduate
Course length	5 years
Total number of medical undergraduates	963
Applicants in 2006	1785
Interviews given in 2006	584
Places available in 2006	162 Home 13 OS
Places available in 2007	162 Home 13 OS
Open days 2007	28 August
Entrance requirements	AAB
Mandatory subjects	2 science or maths
Male:female ratio	1:1.3
Is an exam included in the selection process?	Yes
If yes, what form does this exam take?	UKCAT
Qualification gained	MBChB

Fascinating fact: The medical school is relatively small, enabling superb care and support for students as well as the use of the outstanding clinical facilities, both locally and across the Highlands and Islands.

The grey colour and cold temperature of the 'granite city' bear no relation to the warm and friendly atmosphere and busy social life that is Aberdeen. The oldest medical school in the English-speaking world hasn't grown as much as most UK medical schools, with relatively small year sizes – generally about 175 – allowing you to get to know most of your class. The medical school is on the same site (Foresterhill) as the main teaching hospitals (20–25 minutes' walk from the main university campus, and a similar distance from the city centre), so you can go straight from lectures to wards.

Education

The scoring system used in selecting students for interview and at interview are described on the prospective students' website (see the end of this chapter). The website also includes a lot of other useful information about the application process, as well as information about studying medicine and student life in Aberdeen. Offers are made based upon combined academic, UCAS form and interview scores. Aberdeen is a member of the UKCAT consortium, meaning you do need to sit this test (see Chapter 3).

Teaching

The five years are split into four phases: fundamentals of medical science; principles of clinical medicine; specialist clinical practice; and professional practice. A core syllabus focusing on integrated systems is counterbalanced with special study modules. Students must complete each phase before passing on to the next. The course is predominantly lecture-based in the first three years, with some tutorial-based learning sessions and self-study packages. There is also a large amount of excellent small group teaching during the clinical years.

Student views and problems can be formally voiced at Staff–Student Liaison Committee (SSLC) meetings. Student representatives sit on both the year group SSLCs and the overarching MBChB SSLC (which covers the whole course). A senior student is also elected to sit on a number of other university and medical school committees.

Aberdeen received a very high rating in the last Scottish Higher Education Funding Council Teaching Quality assessment. Students experience many different learning environments such as general practice, specialist hospital wards, lecture theatres, tutorial groups and the Clinical Skills Centre. Anatomy is taught via study of prosections, models, and radiographic images in year 1. Computer-assisted learning is integrated within each phase of medical training, supplementing the compulsory ward teaching and tutorials.

Assessment

Assessment is both in-course (although most of this is formative) and exam based (written and clinical), with vivas for pass/fail candidates in summative assessments. Should you fail a degree assessment, there are three more chances to pass by way of two vivas and a further written exam. Students are supported and encouraged should this occur.

Intercalated degrees

About 30–40 students each year choose to do an intercalated degree (BSc in Medical Sciences) at the end of year 3. In order to choose this option you must have passed all exams in years 2 and 3 at the first sitting.

The BSc course starts, unusually, in April and runs until the March of the following year. The first 2 months are spent following a core syllabus, presented as lectures and small group tutorials, after which there are a number of summer exams. On returning from the summer break in September, students undertake an individual research project which is to be completed and written up for the following March. These projects are generally chosen from a list and give the opportunity for students to work in a range of different research settings.

Projects are virtually all carried out in Aberdeen, as the unusual timing of the BSc does not allow students to join intercalated courses at other UK medical schools (which normally run from September to September). A very small number of students have carried out projects abroad or at other institutions in the UK in the past, but this is not generally encouraged and little help is offered to those wishing to do so.

Some financial awards are available to help with the cost of taking on an extra year at university, generally based on either your academic grades or your project topic.

Should you chose to do an intercalated BSc, advantages include learning to work confidently as part of a team and independently, organizing your own work schedule and the possibility of having your work published. Some also feel an extra year gives you the edge by allowing you the time to mature before the hard work of year 4 begins.

Special study modules and electives

All four phases of the course include special study modules (SSMs). Prior to the final year these are chosen from lists of prescribed topics under different themes (e.g. population-based disease) and generally require the writing of a report and preparation of a presentation in a group of about 8 students. You may well not get your first choice of topic and there is little flexibility to pursue your own interests. The final phase SSM is on the theme of medical humanities. This offers students the opportunity to study subjects such as Spanish, history of medicine, anthropology, and sign language. Also during the final phase, students undertake a 7-week elective period which can be spent almost anywhere in the world. Unlike other medical schools, this includes a short research project, which contributes towards your final degree. It is not just a holiday!

Erasmus

Overseas travel opportunities are during the final-year elective and, for a limited number, the non-medical SSM.

Facilities

Library   The medical school has its own library on the Foresterhill site. Opening hours are good: 9 AM–10 PM Monday to Thursday; 9 AM–8 PM Friday; 9 AM–10 PM Saturday; 1 PM–10 PM Sunday. Texts and journals are plentiful. At the time of writing, photocopying and printing cost approximately 5p/sheet.

Computers   There are many computers available, with free internet and email. There are computer-assisted learning packages for a variety of subjects, as well as exam-style online self-assessment questions. Many lecture presentations are available on the internet. There is 24-hour access to computer laboratories on the university campus and at the medical school.

Clinical skills   The joint University of Aberdeen, Robert Gordon University and NHS Clinical Skills Centre on the Foresterhill site is equipped with models to practise almost every procedure you can think of, plus all the standard clinical equipment. It is used for teaching clinical skills and procedures to all medical students, qualified doctors, and other healthcare students and staff, with both time-tabled access and 'drop-in' sessions. Skills teaching includes examination skills, use of equipment, communication skills (interviewing simulated patients) and many practical procedures, e.g. IV access, suturing, catheterisation, defibrillation, etc. A 'Harvey' cardiology patient simulator is now used to teach all students from year 2 upwards.

Welfare

Student support

Support for medical students is lead by the clerk to the degrees in medicine, who co-ordinates the *regent* (personal tutor) scheme. Each student is paired up with a regent when they enter medical school and is required to meet with them at least twice in their first year and once in subsequent years. As with all relationships, regent–regentee relationships vary from excellent to totally dysfunctional! Students can change their regent at any stage.

All the general university support services, such as the counselling service and the chaplain, are also available to medical students. The students' association also provides welfare services. However, medical students may find the service difficult to access due to the geographical distance between the medical school and the main university campus.

Accommodation

The university has sold off a number of its halls and flats, but much of this accommodation has been bought by private companies and is still available to students. First-year students are guaranteed a place in university accommodation. Most people move into private accommodation after their first year and seem to have no problem finding somewhere within walking distance of the Foresterhill hospitals to live.

Placements

Most of year 1 will be spent at Marischal College in the centre of Aberdeen, with a small amount of time spent at the main university campus and at Foresterhill. The majority of years 2 and 3 will be spent at the medical school on the Foresterhill site, with contact with patients through placements on wards, usually two mornings a week. The aim of these attachments is to develop skills and confidence in clinical examination and history taking.

Years 4 and 5 are spent almost entirely on clinical rotations through all the specialities and general practice. During year 4, you will have to spend at least 10 weeks on attachment in Inverness and most people will spend part of their final year in Inverness, Elgin, Fort William, or Stornoway. Moreover, GP attachments in years 4 and 5 are available throughout Scotland, from Wick to West Fife. Free accommodation is provided, as is travel at the beginning and end of the attachments.

Some students will always prefer to remain in Aberdeen, but the peripheral attachments are generally popular and it is not uncommon for students to deliberately choose to spend all or almost all of their final year away from Aberdeen. There is some element of choice in when and where you do most of these attachments although, of course, not everyone's preferences can be met. One of the distinctive features of the Aberdeen course is the opportunity to have exposure to such a geographically varied range of working environments and many students feel they benefit from this.

Location of clinical placement/ name of hospital	Distance away from medical school (miles)	Difficulty getting there on public transport*
Elgin	65	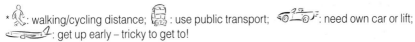
Inverness	105	
Fort William	157	
Stornoway	174 (as the crow flies!)	
GP attachments	All over Scotland	depending on distance

* : walking/cycling distance; : use public transport; : need own car or lift; : get up early – tricky to get to!

Sports and social 🏆

City life

Aberdeen is a small but busy city. With two universities, there is a large student population and accompanying vibrant nightlife. The city centre is compact and lively, with most pubs/clubs within 10 minutes' walk of each other and 20 minutes' walk from student halls. There is a good selection of bars, pubs, galleries, cinema and theatres from mainstream to alternative. Nights out need not cost you an arm and a leg, with many venues having free entry, especially before midnight.

City and surrounds

Just a short journey from the buzzing centre is the beach, with rollercoasters, an ice-rink, and a cinema. A few miles north of this traditional promenade it is possible to wander through the sand dunes of Balmedie beach, the perfect location for a summer BBQ – but you will need a car to get you there. In the other direction are the mountains and the outdoors: excellent for walking, climbing, winter sports and water sports. The northerly location means the climate can be very cold and, although there are good road, rail, and air links, Aberdeen is a considerable distance away from the rest of the UK.

University life

As the medical school is isolated from other parts of the university, medics need to make a bit of an effort to meet non-medical students, but the first year is normally spent in halls and this gives students an opportunity to meet others outside medicine. There is a small university Union in the city centre, which offers a simple and cheap starting point for nights out and club events. However, most students quickly venture out and find other favourite venues to frequent. University societies are numerous and healthy, covering a wide range of interests: sporting, dramatic, musical, outdoor, Armed Forces (army, navy and RAF), intellectual, malt whisky appreciation … the list goes on. Med-Soc holds functions every few weeks including a very popular annual ball and freshers events to introduce you to the (in)famous medic social life.

Sports life

MedSoc has its own rugby, football and hockey teams, which compete against the other Scottish medical schools. MedSoc members can join an exclusive gym in town for a massively discounted rate. University clubs offer a variety of sports from gliding, underwater hockey, archery and ultimate frisbee to the regulars such as rugby, hockey and football. Members of all levels are given a warm welcome. There are no specific medical school facilities, but the university offers an inexpensive gym, pool and tennis facilities, among others on the main campus near halls.

Great things about Aberdeen

- Friendly, small school, with teaching hospital and medical school buildings within a single site.
- Excellent clinical skills teaching and early clinical experience from second year.
- Teaching in a variety of settings, allowing students to experience not only inner-city medicine, but appreciate how medicine is delivered to patients in rural areas much further afield.
- Main exams are done by the end of year 4 – so you have got most of the knowledge and can concentrate on putting it into practice in year 5.
- Easy access to the great outdoors (beach and mountains a very short distance away; skiing 45 minutes away; sailing locally).

Bad things about Aberdeen

- No dedicated medic social centre on site.
- Geographically isolated from the rest of the university, which means the majority of your student friends are medics. This is not helped by the different timings of exams and holidays.
- You cannot organise your own SSMs until your final year.
- The intercalated BSc year runs from April to March, so it is very difficult for students to do a BSc at other universities, where BSc programmes usually begin in September.
- OK, it can be cold – but isn't everywhere in the UK sometimes?

Further information

School of Medicine Office (Admissions)
Polwarth Building
Foresterhill
Aberdeen
AB25 2ZD
Tel: 01224 553 015

Fax: 01224 554761
Email: medicine@abdn.ac.uk
Web: http://www.abdn.ac.uk/medicine/prospective.shtml

Additional application information

Average A level requirements	• AAB
Average Scottish Higher requirements	• AAAAB
Make-up of interview panel	• Two interviewers
Months in which interviews are held	• November – March
Proportion of overseas students	• 9.8%
Proportion of mature students	• 18.4%
Proportion of graduate students	• 8.9%
Faculty's view of students taking a gap year	• Acceptable
Proportion of students taking intercalated degrees	• 14.9%
Possibility of direct entrance to clinical phase	• No
Fees for overseas students	• £10,968 pa (years 1 and 2) and £20,484 pa (years 3, 4 and 5)
Fees for graduates	• £2700
Ability to transfer to other medical schools If so, under what circumstances	• Transfer is possible but uncommon and constrained by the differing structure of medical courses. Previous students have transferred for family and personal reasons.
Assistance for elective funding	• Limited funds are available locally and depend on your elective project proposal. There is a good notice board advising about external elective funding opportunities.

(Continued)

(*Continued*)

Assistance for travel to attachments	• A bus is run to and from Inverness at the start and end of the year 4 attachments. Apart from this, one return journey to any attachment will be refunded. Travel to GP attachments commutable on a daily basis from Aberdeen is refunded less £2.50 per day.
Access and hardship funds	• Access bursaries are awarded by the university across all areas of study. Limited hardship funds are awarded by the school once a year (in March) and the school recommends students for awards from other organizations.
Weekly rent	• £45–£60 if sharing private accommodation
Pint of lager	• £2.10
Cinema	• £3.50
Nightclub	• £2 though variable

Barts and The London

Key facts	Undergraduate	Graduate
Course length	5 years	4 years
Total number of medical undergraduates	c. 1500	c. 170
Applicants in 2006	2760	950
Interviews given in 2006	1100	150
Places available in 2006	277	46
Places available in 2007	277	45
Open days 2007	Three in July/August	May
Entrance requirements	AAB	2:1 in science related degree
Mandatory subjects	Chemistry and biology	
Male:female ratio	n.a.	n.a.
Is an exam included in the selection process?	Yes	Yes
If yes, what form does this exam take?	UKCAT	MSAT
Qualification gained	MBBS	MBBS

Fascinating fact: David Burckett St Laurent, a recent graduate at Barts and The London, became the youngest ever person to walk to the North Pole, raising money for charity in 2003.

The medical school that resulted from the merger of St Bartholomew's and The Royal London is centred in London's East End, one of the capital city's most exciting areas. Home to a large number of ethnic groups, this area is a fascinating place to study medicine as a result of the varied and diverse needs of its communities.

Bartholomew's is the oldest hospital in the world and is a centre of excellence for many specialist disciplines. The Royal London was the first medical school in England and is the site of our new medical school building. The new medical school building is part of a £44 million redevelopment of the School of Medicine and Dentistry's Whitechapel campus. A 1000-unit student village at the Mile End campus has also opened recently.

The school strives to be progressive, and the 2006 intake will be the eighth year to study the 1999 curriculum, which has problem-based learning at its core and a greater emphasis on the integration of clinical and preclinical elements of medical training. The first cohort of students studying under the new curriculum has qualified with remarkable results, and they are all now successful doctors in the medical arena.

The combined school of Barts and The London is part of Queen Mary College, University of London (QMUL). The merging of the Medical College of St Bartholomew's Hospital and the London Hospital Medical College united the strengths of both institutions and the skills of the staff that are involved in clinical care and internationally acclaimed research. Now, we have grown into one of the most innovative and forward-thinking schools in the UK.

Education

The medical course is designed to equip one with a fundamental knowledge and understanding of medicine, and to develop the skills and attitudes one needs in order to apply that knowledge in practice. Selectors are looking for candidates with the core qualities that a doctor must possess: good communication and listening skills; ability to relate well to their patients and demonstrate empathy and respect for them; integrity; ability to work in a team; and recognition of his/her limitations, as well as those of others. Applicants should be able to demonstrate both a real understanding of what a career in medicine involves and their suitability for a caring profession. They must have an understanding of science, but the wider their knowledge and interests, the better. Applicants to QMUL are required to sit UKCAT (see Chapter 3).

The current course is centred on the technique of problem-based learning (PBL). All students follow the same core course, and are then able to broaden their knowledge in areas of particular interest during a range of special study modules (SSMs). The traditional preclinical/clinical divide is now less distinct as the new course integrates basic medical, human and clinical sciences from the first day at medical school until graduation. Barts and The London students are placed with both GPs and hospitals during years 1 and 2, allowing early patient contact.

Teaching

In years 1 and 2 of the course teaching is systems-based, concentrating on 'Systems in Health' for year 1 and 'Systems in Disease' for year 2. There is a mixed approach, including lectures, PBL and workshop sessions, and all aspects of the body system, such as the cardiovascular system, are considered as integrated wholes. Teaching in the final three years is hospital-based, with a continued emphasis on self-directed learning. Courses in communication skills (using actors and videotaping) and ethics run throughout the five years. Dissection is no longer part of the core course, and anatomy is taught using computer-aided learning programmes, anatomical models and prosections (although you can do dissection as an SSM).

The system of teaching at Barts and The London is very responsive to student opinion, and time and effort spent fine-tuning arrangements has resulted in a course that both the staff and the students are very proud of.

Assessment

Summer exams are set for years 1–4, and 'big bang' final examinations are a thing of past with the new curriculum. Assessment is continuous, with credit being given for performance in both tutorials and examinations. Responsiveness to student feedback and opinion has resulted in huge strides being made in assessment: for example, Barts and The London is one of the few (if not the only) schools in the country where the dreaded MCQ-style questions have been phased out of the assessment programme. Even long essay questions are considered taboo. At the end of year 5 students are assessed on their 'competence to practise' as a PRHO and must pass an integrated paper and clinical exams.

Intercalated degrees

Allocation of intercalated degrees is done on a competitive basis, but all courses offered within the school will involve research-based projects. Both BSc and BMedSci courses are offered. Popular courses include experimental pathology and Bachelor of Medical Science (BMedSci), but some students have studied anthropology, psychology and even German, although this kind of choice is rare. One of the newest and most popular courses is a BSc in Sports Medicine. Previously, students were only allowed to intercalate after year 4, but the college has allowed a limited number of year 2 or 3 students to intercalate. Students can choose to stay at QMUL or go to another college for this year. If studying at QMUL, all fees for the BSc year are paid by sponsors (at the time of writing) and additional funding is also available due to the school's extensive links with the City of London.

Special study modules and electives

A wide variety of SSMs is available, including clinical, research, complementary medicine and journalism. Students are encouraged to consider organizing SSMs in subjects they find of interest if they do not find exactly what they want within the diverse selection available. Any of the SSMs, of which there are two every year, can be used as an opportunity to study abroad. It is also possible for some students to spend 3-month attachments at partner institutions in Europe.

The elective lasts 2 to 3 months, during the fifth year of the course. There are existing arrangements with institutions in other countries in Europe, and several student-led exchange programmes with institutions all around the world, which can make for a more easily organised trip. Students can go almost anywhere, as long as they can find themselves a supervisor.

Erasmus

Barts and The London has a long history of exchanging students within the Erasmus programme with the world famous Karolinska institute in Stockholm. Other regular exchanges occur with the Lund as well as several other institutions.

Facilities

Library There are three large libraries, one at each site. The two hospital libraries have wonderful architecture, history and atmosphere. QMUL is large and can occasionally be noisy during the daytime.

Availability of books is variable. Libraries are open 9 AM–9 PM on weekdays, 9 AM–4 PM on Saturdays. The QMUL library is also open on Sundays. There are two large pathology museums at the hospitals. Unfortunately, in light of the events at Alder Hey Hospital, access to these is now severely restricted.

Computers   The school is well equipped for computers on all three sites. All computing facilities and functions are available and regularly updated. Computers are increasingly used for teaching and are available during library hours and 10 AM–8 PM at weekends. There is 24-hour internet access on the QMUL campus during the week. The computer rooms at the medical schools are also open late. All rooms in student halls have now been fitted with computer access, making internet access far easier. There are also various spots in college that have wireless access, which puts the medical school ahead of most other colleges.

Clinical skills   The Clinical Skills Centre at Barts, which was one of the first in the country, is for use by both medical and nursing students. It is available to everyone in the school. First-year students learn clinical skills in an adapted ward at Mile End Hospital. All clinical-year students have access to clinical skills labs at their respective hospitals, which are also well-equipped. All students are expected to attend resuscitation courses, which are scheduled for teaching throughout the whole duration of the course. This has been a great advantage and has come in handy many times for many students.

Welfare

Student support

On the first day of college, freshers are assigned a senior student to act as their 'parent' and guide them through the first few weeks and beyond. This is called the 'mummy daddy scheme', and is considered an excellent mode of support. 'Parents' introduce their 'children' to their friends, take them out to dinner, and offer advice on all issues, from simple things such as work to more complicated matters such as their love life. This makes for a lot of integration between students from different years. All students are allocated their own academic tutor; for personal and other problems they have use of a pastoral pool of sympathetic doctors and senior lecturers. The Medical and Dental Students' Association elects a student as welfare officer, as does QMUL Students' Union. Counselling is available within 24 hours at QMUL, with a dedicated and independent advice and counselling service. Those with mental health problems can be seen in confidence by a consultant at another teaching hospital in a reciprocal arrangement with the school.

Accommodation

Students at Barts and The London can spend two to three years of their studies in college accommodation. First-year students choose whether they wish to live in Queen Mary College or University of London (intercollegiate) accommodation, and whether they wish to be catered for or to cook for themselves. Most first-year students live at the newly built Westfield Student Village which provides *en-suite*, self-catering accommodation in six different styles of building designed to create a village community feel. The other halls of residence, such as Dawson Hall, which is an old Barts residence, and Floyer House at The Royal London, are suited for clinical-year students due to their location. Dawson Hall is a very modern facility, the main attraction of which is its beautiful location near St Paul's in the centre of London. It is very hard to get into as a first-year student, so early applications are essential. It allows students to self-cater, as does Floyer House – which has recently been refurbished and is close to the Union. In central London, students from all colleges of the University of London live together in intercollegiate halls. These are a 30-minute tube ride away from college. With all residences, students should check whether or not rent is payable during holidays. As with all halls of residence in London, the cost is relatively high.

Most senior students live in the East End in shared houses. Almost everyone lives within walking distance of The Royal London and QMUL sites. Property is slightly cheaper in east London than in other parts of the capital. The Griffin Community Trust provides cheap yet luxurious housing in a very special development incorporating housing for the elderly, a community centre and flats for clinical students. Student residents spend an hour or two a week with their elderly neighbours and play bingo, watch videos or just chat. Both students and elders say how much they gain from the experience.

Placements

The medicine course is based at three sites: Barts, The London and QMUL, which are all within 3 miles of each other in the City and East End of London. They are easily accessible by tube, bicycle and bus. The medical sciences department at QMUL in Mile End is where years 1 and 2 are based currently, although this should change in the coming year with the opening of the new medical school in Whitechapel (which is widely used by all students from all years). This site has good facilities, including the Students' Union shop and computer laboratories. The final three years are spent in hospitals. Many of the district general hospitals used are in or close to the East End and are accessible by bus or tube. Several are close enough to cycle to or even walk, depending on accommodation.

Students can expect to be sent to attachments outside the main teaching hospitals. Placements are in district general and other associated hospitals (accommodation is provided free). As well as the placements below, destinations include Southend-on-Sea, Chelmsford and Harlow, although GP attachments can be arranged countrywide.

Location of clinical placement/ name of hospital	Distance away from medical school (miles)	Difficulty getting there on public transport*
The Royal London	0	🚶
Barts	2.4	🚶
Homerton	4.7	🚌
Newham	5.1	🚌
Whipps Cross	6.8	🚌

* 🚶: walking/cycling distance; 🚌 : use public transport; 🚗 : need own car or lift;
✈ : get up early – tricky to get to!

Please note that there are a number of other hospitals at which you may be placed, all of which are within 50 miles of the main campus.

Sports and social

University life

The Medical and Dental Students' Association is thriving and provides social and sporting opportunities as well as welfare services for all. The two medical student bars at Barts and The London hold regular discos and theme nights. Wednesdays (after sports matches) and Fridays are the big nights for going out. The summer ball at Barts is popular, and there are smaller balls for freshers' week, RAG week and at Christmas.

RAG week is one of the prides of the college, with medical and dental students raking in over £150,000 last year from street collections, marathon running, and a fashion show, ranking us as one of the most successful rags in the country and the biggest in London by far.

There are over 30 clubs and societies run by the Barts and The London Students' Association, which offer students the chance to develop new interests, meet people, play sport and have a good time. Among the most active societies are: the Drama Society, which stages productions every term, including the infamous Christmas show, and goes to the Edinburgh Festival; the Asian Society, which organises the famous international fashion show to celebrate diversity of culture within the school, and annually raises many thousands for charity; and the Music Society, which includes the choir, orchestra, brass groups and several bands. QMUL has more clubs and societies, if there are not enough at the medical school or if you have a particular interest not catered for.

Student social life revolves around the Association/Union buildings at both Barts and The London. The medical student president is head of the Medical and Dental Students' Association and takes a sabbatical year from his or her studies solely to represent and protect the interests of the medical and dental student community. The refurbished Association building at the London and the bar at Barts are for use by medics, dentists and their guests. In The London Association building there is a café-bar and bookshop. The official Association magazine, *M.A.D.*, comes out at least twice a term and reports on social, sporting and other events. A large Students' Union is also available at QMUL Mile End campus.

Sports life

The Barts and The London Students' Association clubs cater for nearly all sporting interests and welcomes beginners. There is an off-site sports ground and swimming pools at both Barts and The London. There are also gyms at Barts and QMUL and squash courts at QMUL, as well as tennis and badminton courts. Barts and The London have an enthusiastic rowing club based on the River Lea. Hockey, water polo, women's football and rugby have had success in recent years. The cricket club is legendary, with strong first and second teams which win titles most years.

Great things about Barts and The London 👍

- A brand new course, innovative curriculum and teaching as well as enthusiastic and approachable staff.
- All students and visitors agree that we are a very friendly community with a close-knit atmosphere and that students tend to have friends from all years.
- Reasonable rents for shared houses, considering that we are in the centre of London, and everyone lives close to each other.
- Good year-round events, and the Union bar opens with regular late licences.
- Diverse area, with a wide range of things to do and cultures to experience. The East End is very trendy, with new bars and restaurants opening all the time.

Bad things about Barts and The London 👎

- Local areas – we are surrounded by very deprived communities and, although this means good clinical experience and pathology subject matter, it can be a bit depressing. At times it is necessary to be wary, as students have been assaulted.
- Travelling – there is some travelling between sites required, and the 'rush hour' lasts for hours, although congestion charging has meant very fast bus links.
- Little interaction with non-medical and dental students in the past resulted in some rivalry between the medics and other QMUL students, although most of these issues have been fully worked out now.
- London is such a massive place that it can take you some time to feel at ease with its vastness.
- Expense – living and studying in London is more expensive than elsewhere. This is the biggest drawback to studying at Barts and The London, and in London generally.

Further information

Admissions Office
Bart's and The London School of Medicine and Dentistry
Turner Street
London E1 2AD
Tel: 020 7377 7611
Fax: 020 7377 7612
Email: medicaladmissions@qmul.ac.uk
Web: http://www.smd.qmul.ac.uk

Additional application information

Average A level requirements	• AAB
Average Scottish Higher requirements	• BB/AAA (Advanced Highers/Further Highers)
Graduate entry requirements	• 2:1 science degree
Make-up of interview panel	• Undergraduate: three (one clinical, one non-clinical and one student) • Graduate: six station OSCE plus one clinical, one non-clinical and one student
Months in which interviews are held	• November – March (undergraduate) • March – April (graduate)
Proportion of overseas students	• 8%
Proportion of mature students	• 30%
Proportion of graduate students	• 20%
Faculty's view of students taking a gap year	• Encouraged if constructive plans
Proportion of students taking intercalated degrees	• 6%
Possibility of direct entrance to clinical phase	• Yes, but only with serious extenuating circumstances
Fees for overseas students	• £13,640 (years 1 and 2), £22,330 (years 3, 4 and 5)
Fees for graduates	• £3000 pa
Ability to transfer to other medical schools If so, under what circumstances	• Students can transfer out to intercalate. Permitted only where there is a very good reason – such as the course not being available within the college, or competitive places are offered to the top 10–15 students. Students may also transfer for personal extenuating circumstances. Counselling is available for this prior to such a major decision.

Assistance for elective funding	• Several elective bursaries are available, although amounts vary. A list of potential external sponsors that have close links to Barts and The London is available. Significant sponsorship is possible but dependent on the individual's effort to obtain it.
Assistance for travel to attachments	• Travel subsidies available to all university students. Records must be kept of expenses and claimed back from your LEA with supporting documentation from the school.
Access and hardship funds	• Financial assistance for all students as well as hardship funds for medical and dental students, often left by alumni of St Bartholomew's or The London Hospital. The amounts of money are significant and the financial support easily accessible.
Weekly rent	• Average rent is between £75–£85 within walking distance of central campus and teaching hospital.
Pint of lager	• Cheap at the student association usually costing £1.10 at happy hour which is much longer than an hour!
Cinema	• Two local cinemas: Genesis, in Mile End, is about £3.50 with NUS and the much nicer UGC Multiplex in Canary Wharf, which is not much further, is £4 with NUS.
Nightclub	• Loads of nightclubs in London

Belfast

Key fact	Undergraduate
Course length	5 years
Total number of medical undergraduates	1123
Applicants in 2006	765
Interviews given in 2006	38
Places available in 2006	262
Places available in 2007	262
Open days 2007	tbc
Entrance requirements	AAA plus A at AS level
Mandatory subjects	Chemistry to A level Biology AS level
Male:female ratio	45:65
Is an exam included in the selection process?	Possible aptitude test
If yes, what form does this exam take?	
Qualification gained	MB BCh BAO

Fascinating fact: The Belfast Medical Students Association is the oldest and largest student society at Queen's.

Queen's University of Belfast (QUB) provides a relaxed and informal integrated medical course. Ninety per cent of the students come from Ireland (both Northern Ireland and the Republic), and a strong emphasis is placed on the need to balance academic studies with social interaction. The school also sits in a perfect position to access Belfast's nightlife, arguably the best in the UK. Queen's is the only medical school where it is not illegal to enjoy a good night's craic! Discussions are taking place to increase the size of the medical school, with more undergraduate places. However, as yet there have been no plans to implement a graduate accelerated course.

Education

Students with four to five A*s plus four A grades at GCSE received conditional offers in 2004; overall grades required were three As at A level plus an A grade at AS level. Chemistry and one other science at A level, and biology at A level or AS level were prerequisites. There is no compulsory interview; however, a small proportion of applicants will be called for interview. An aptitude test for medicine may also be implemented in the future, although UKCAT was not required at the time of writing. Further information is available in the prospectus or on request from the admissions office.

A six-year course (including premed year) is required for Irish Leaving Certificate students, needing four As and two Bs, and an A grade at Junior Certificate. Chemistry is compulsory.

Graduates with a minimum of three Bs or better at A level who have obtained at least an Upper Second Class honours degree would be interviewed for entry into the five-year medical course.

A traditional preclinical/clinical divide is less evident on the new course, and teaching combines a problem-based approach with more traditional lectures from year 1. Clinical skills are taught from year 1 in hospitals, in general practice and in a clinical skills centre. Each year is divided into two semesters, and the year groups are subdivided into smaller groups for teaching. In years 1 and 2 students learn the basic science of medicine with an integrated systems approach. The sociological and psychological aspects of medical practice are emphasized and special study modules are taken. In year 3 the systems are taught again, but with an emphasis on mechanisms of disease. More time is spent in hospital attachments at this stage, and year 4 students spend all their time on the wards in hospital attachments or in general practice. The final year is a consolidation process with no new subjects.

Teaching

Teaching in years 1 and 2 consists of lectures, tutorials, laboratory practicals and meeting patients, both on the wards and in general practice. There is a mixture of demonstration, dissection, and prosection for teaching, and animal tissue is used in physiology. During years 1 and 2 only half a day a week is spent on the wards. In year 3 blocks of speciality-based integrated teaching are supplemented by pathology lectures and tutorials. Teaching is very much self-directed, with the clinical aspects being taught on the wards. Years 4 and 5 are completely ward-based. Computers and clinical skills are used for training throughout the course. Ward group sizes in teaching hospitals tend to vary, but efforts are made to keep the numbers as small as possible to benefit both the patients and the students. The friendliness of the staff and their willingness to teach varies from ward to ward. Most, however, are willing to help in true Northern Ireland fashion.

Assessment

Years 1 and 2 have specific exams at the end of each semester with an overall recap exam at the end of year 2. Year 3 is examined through coursework throughout the year and end of semester/attachment clinical exams. There is a pathology written exam, covering two semesters, at the end of year 3. In year 4 exams are at the end of each 8-week block. Resit examinations start in the second week of August and last for a week or two. Most students try to give exams their best so as to maximize the holiday period. Procedure cards need to be completed as part of musculoskeletal and A&E medicine, ophthalmology, anaesthetics, fractures and obstetrics and gynaecology. Final examinations take place in two parts. The written examinations take place between January and February of the final year, and the clinical examinations are held at the end of April of the final year, although there is a possibility that this will change. During the summer between the fourth and the final year the overseas elective and clinical project is carried out, and during the final year refresher clinical placements and a clinical apprenticeship are completed.

Intercalated degrees

Between 5 and 10% of students take a BSc during their course, usually after years 2 or 3. Science degrees are available in anatomy, biochemistry, physiology, microbiology, therapeutics and pharmacology and molecular biology. In addition, the faculty are reviewing the courses offered, with a view to improving the current selection. It is possible to study degree subjects that are not available at QUB by making arrangements with another institution. Approval for this, however, has to be sought from the Dean. If there is competition for places, previous results in the respective subject will determine entry. Students from Northern Ireland may be eligible for Local Education Authority (LEA) or bursary funding for the year.

Special study modules and electives

During the summer vacation between years 3 and 4, students have the option to arrange elective placements for a period of 4 to 6 weeks at a hospital in the UK. This is optional and the student takes responsibility for organization. In the final year students are encouraged to spend their elective period overseas. Students must also carry out a 4-week clinical project, either overseas or at Queen's, followed by the production of a project report of between 6000 and 8000 words.

Erasmus

QUB is attempting to expand its Erasmus programme at present and is currently canvassing students for their opinions or interests. Opportunities already exist for students who wish to study at medical schools in Lausanne (Switzerland), Valencia (Spain), Giessen or Berlin (Germany) and Oslo (Norway). Almost all students will use the overseas elective as an opportunity to see new shores and spread their horizons.

Facilities

Library   There are two main medical libraries, the largest in the Royal Victoria Hospital (RVH) and a smaller one in the Belfast City Hospital (BCH). They both have online catalogues, with access to networked journals, Medline and other databases. They close at 9.00 PM on weekdays and 12.30 PM on Saturdays. Study space is available at BCH and at the Medical Biology Centre (MBC) outside the library opening hours. The MBC houses an anatomy study room with access to a library of microscope slides and computerized anatomical guides. Each peripheral attachment has some library provision, although this varies from hospital to hospital and medical students are more than welcome to use the libraries and facilities of the wider QUB campus. All library books are catalogued in a computerized searchable database.

Computers   The RVH and the MBC both have computer facilities available for medical students.

When the IT suites and other libraries of QUB are taken into account, computer provision is usually more then adequate, although just before an essay deadline or exam session things can tend to clog up. All computers are fully networked although certain applications for medicine can only be accessed from the MBC or RVH.

Clinical skills   The Clinical Skills Education Centre (CSEC) provides teaching on practical medicine and affords students a chance to do some 'hands-on' learning. Through a mix of simulated patients (often drama students doing some method acting or other arts students from QUB needing extra beer money!), life-like models and tuition from practising clinicians and retired consultants with a wealth of experience, students are taught various clinical skills that are assessed in the CSEC at end-of-semester examinations. Students have the opportunity to practice clinical skills at the CSEC and also on their clinical attachments.

Welfare

Student support

Each medical student is allocated to a senior doctor, known as their Faculty Tutor, whose role is to help with any problems. This scheme, previously known as the MAFIA Scheme, allows students to meet with the tutor and peers representing each year to discuss any problems or concerns they may have with any aspect of university life. Fourth- and final-year students are now required to arrange a mentor, preferably a doctor from one of their clinical attachments, to watch over their clinical progress and act as one of their references for their first foundation programme job. Staff in the faculty office are friendly and approachable, as is the current Dean. The Students' Union also has a counselling service and provides access to academic and financial advice. Rails, ramps and lifts are available in many areas for disabled access.

Accommodation

Every first-year student who comes from outside the Belfast area can apply to university halls of residence for accommodation during term time. The rooms tend to be warm and comfortable, with good food (if catered) but thin walls. Catered rooms cost between £56 sharing and £67 single per week and self-catering rooms £41–£70 per week, inclusive of heat and light. They are about half a mile from the university, but can mean a trek if an early lecture has been scheduled for the RVH. Living in halls is a great opportunity to meet many new friends, including students from outside the medical faculty. Private accommodation is available closer to faculty, although there can be no guarantees as to price or quality. Generally a room in a private house will cost between £170 and £210 per month with the average rent being £180. The Lisburn Road area of Belfast is extremely popular with medical students as it is close to the MBC, the BCH and the RVH.

Placements

In years 1 and 2 most of the teaching takes place on campus in the MBC and the BCH, with some clinical and family-attachment programmes spread throughout the greater Belfast area. The MBC and the BCH are about a 15–20-minute walk from the halls of residence. Other lectures and clinical work take place at the RVH, a 35–40-minute walk from the halls. However, a free bus runs from the BCH to the RVH every 20 minutes. From year 3 onwards students receive teaching in the RVH, and clinical attachments may be throughout the Province. The RVH recently underwent renovation, the result of which is a brand new hospital, with great teaching facilities. In addition, hospitals and GP practices outside central Belfast are used from year 3 onwards. Hospital accommodation is free and there is an allowance for peripheral GP attachments, with the furthest you might need to travel being about 80 miles from Belfast. This means spending part of the week in a peripheral hospital for a portion of the academic year – which can make a change from Belfast but can also seriously affect extra-curricular activities.

Location of clinical placement/ name of hospital	Distance away from medical school (miles)	Difficulty getting there on public transport*
Belfast City Hospital	0	
Musgrave Park Hospital	2	
The Ulster Hospital	5–6	
Craigavon	30	
Altnagelvin	72	

* 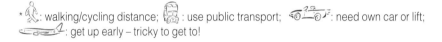: walking/cycling distance; : use public transport; : need own car or lift; : get up early – tricky to get to!

Sports and social

City life

Belfast is a lively welcoming city with much to offer visitors. The student area is only a mile away from the city centre but surprisingly self-contained – many students rarely venture out of the mainly student Malone and Stranmillis areas to Belfast's more upmarket city centre. All tastes are catered for in Belfast through a wide range of pubs, cafés and clubs, with the Students' Union hosting one of the biggest club nights in Ireland on a weekly basis. Those with a more cultural orientation will find themselves amply provided for by the range of drama, music and art available to students. The Queen's Film Theatre is an award-winning art-house cinema located within the university campus.

Although you may have your hands full coping with what Belfast has to offer, it is easy to travel further afield. Dublin is just over two hours away by train, and it is a must to visit the Giant's Causeway, the Mourne Mountains and the Fermanagh Lakes, all of which are within 1½ hours of Belfast.

University life

Student life in Belfast is largely centred around the Students' Union, a few other student venues, and the Physical Education centre. For medical students the Belfast Medical Students Association (BMSA) runs a very active and fun programme of social events, providing medicine with a social cohesion that is the envy of every other faculty, particularly the Law Society! Every year the BMSA runs a freshers' three-legged pub crawl, a mystery tour, a fancy dress party, the annual faculty ball, a staff–student dinner and regular discos which are attended by all years. The fourth year runs its own annual revue – tasteless but entertaining – and a medical charity called SWOT, which raises money by organizing blood-pressure clinics, street collections, a fashion show (with local TV celebrities) and pub quizzes. Queen's also has one of the most active MedSIN (Medical Students International Network) groups in the UK. They hosted the first ever 'CPR in Schools' national conference in 2005, and are one of the largest CPRiS groups nationwide, having trained over 300 primary schools to date. In addition, a brand new medical society was founded last year, and is fondly known as Scrubs (minus JD!). Scrubs runs workshops within the faculty that aim to teach students specialist skills, such as suturing, for the more advanced stages of their medical career. The Students' Union has three bars and runs regular discos, balls, and concerts. Like most universities, there is likely to be a society for whatever you want to do – after all we do have over 150 clubs and societies at QUB!

Sports life

There are many sports clubs at QUB, most of which compete in the Province's leagues. Near the university there are playing fields, tennis courts and a boat club. The Queen's Physical Education Centre has everything you need to keep fit. It is beside the university, is well equipped and costs 70p to get in if you are a student.

Great things about Queen's

- An updated curriculum so that students gain clinical experience from year 1 with small group teaching.
- Queen's has an international reputation for trauma care, cardiology, and ophthalmology.
- Belfast is compact as a capital city but has everything you need.
- The social life – events are organized by the BMSA on a regular basis, so inter-year relations are good.
- Relaxed and informal atmosphere.

Bad things about Queen's

- The weather – there is no danger of students blowing their allowance on suntan lotion.
- The weekends tend to be quiet. Many students go home at the weekend, particularly in the first year.
- The location of the main medical library means that students can only get to it by car at night.
- The ready availability of the 'Ulster Fry' pushes your waistband.
- The high number of students on some attachments.

Further information

Admissions Office
The Queen's University of Belfast
University Road
Belfast BT7 1NN
Tel: 028 9097 5081
Fax: 028 9097 5137
Email: admissions@qub.ac.uk
Web: http://www.qub.ac.uk

Additional information	
Average A level requirements	• AAA at A level plus A at AS level
Average Scottish Higher requirements	• AAAAA (including chemistry and biology)
Make-up of interview panel	• Four – admissions selector plus two members of academic staff and one administrator
Months in which interviews are held	• February/March
Proportion of overseas students	• 5%
Proportion of mature students	• Not known
Proportion of graduate students	• 6%
Faculty's view of students taking a gap year	• Acceptable
Proportion of students taking intercalated degrees	• 7%
Possibility of direct entrance to clinical phase	• No
Fees for overseas students	• £11,025 pa (years 1 and 2) and £20,790 pa (years 3, 4 and 5)
Fees for graduates	• £3000 (subject to annual inflationary increase)
Ability to transfer to other medical schools If so, under what circumstances	• None

Assistance for elective funding	• Yes! Plenty of different scholarships/grants.
Assistance for travel to attachments	• Can apply for reimbursement.
Access and hardship funds	• Yes, means-tested yearly.
Weekly rent	• From around £45
Pint of lager	• From £2.50
Cinema	• £4.00 at the Queen's Film Theatre
Nightclub	• £5–£15

Birmingham

Key facts	Undergraduate	Graduate
Course length	5 years	4 years
Total number of medical undergraduates	1800	120
Applicants in 2006	2700	640
Interviews given in 2006	900	80
Places available in 2006	370	40
Places available in 2007	370	40
Open days 2007	28 and 29 June	
Entrance requirements	AAB	First class life science degree
Mandatory subjects	A level chemistry and another science. Biology at least AS	A level chemistry
Male:female ratio	37:63	33:67
Is an exam included in the selection process?	No	No
If yes, what form does this exam take?		
Qualification gained	MBChB	MBChB

Fascinating fact: Birmingham Medical School has a long and distinguished history in medical research and practice. In the 19th century, Richard Harris Hill Norris first described the function of platelets in blood, Sampson Gamgee pioneered aseptic surgery and invented the surgical dressing that still bears his name, Lawson Tait was the first to successfully operate a ruptured ectopic pregnancy and Barry Haycraft performed pioneering work on blood coagulation. Nobel Prize winners Sir Peter Medawar (1960) and Sir Paul Nurse (2001) also did much of their early work in Birmingham.

Birmingham Medical School can be found on the northwest edge of the main University of Birmingham campus, just a few miles from the city centre. We are a large provincial medical school, with a huge diversity of students. We have a well-established modern course, with clinical experience introduced within the first few weeks of study. The admissions tutors strongly believe that doctors should be well-rounded individuals and not just dedicated bookworms. This is reflected in the mix of students and the lively social scene at the medical school, from sport, drama and politics to partying. From the first week as freshers, students at Birmingham can expect to work hard and play hard until their final-year dinner, held the week before graduation.

Education

The selection criteria for admission are available on the university web pages and at open days. Particular attention is paid to non-academic interests, extra-curricular activities and the personal statement and reference. The selection of students for both the graduate-entry four-year course and the standard five-year course are essentially the same. However, for the graduate-entry course, students are required to have a first class honours life science degree and a minimum grade C in A level chemistry. There are no tests in the admission procedure but the use of an objective test is 'under consideration' for the graduate-entry course.

The first two years follow a systems-based approach, with regular patient contact in general practice, beginning within a few weeks of starting the course. Full-time hospital teaching commences in year 3 in both medicine and surgery. Pathology and epidemiology are also taught during year 3. Years 4 and 5 involve rotation through specialities such as paediatrics, oncology and orthopaedics, in addition to senior medicine and surgery. Throughout the degree there is an emphasis on the social aspects of medicine, which is received well by students. Students on the graduate-entry course will study the basic sciences in their first year; in their second year they will study a course similar to the standard third year; and they will be fully integrated with the rest of the medics for their third and fourth years. Promoting and supporting diversity is something Birmingham is very proud of.

Teaching

Preclinical teaching involves lectures and follow-up tutorials incorporating problem-based learning exercises. There is no dissection at Birmingham, but we have excellent plastinated models to work with in a specially designed laboratory. Histology teaching is all done by video and accompanied by colour course booklets – there is no straining down microscopes for Birmingham medics! Hospital teaching combines bedside teaching, observation, small group teaching sessions and participation in clinics and procedures.

Assessment

Modules are examined after Christmas and in the summer term by MCQs and short- and long-answer papers, and an anatomy viva examination in the second year. Some in-course assessment is a feature of most modules. Students are expected to pass every module in order to proceed to the next year. You will also have to pass a practical exam in basic life support during your first year. Viva examinations are no longer used for borderline pass candidates and instead students can compensate losing up to 5% providing that all other modules have been adequately passed. Clinical students are examined by MCQ and OSCE.

Intercalated degrees

An increasing number of students at Birmingham are choosing to intercalate, typically after years 2, 3, or 4. This can be in the biological sciences, such as physiology, pharmacology, neuroscience or pathology, and involves a laboratory-based research project (and a chance to publish). Alternatively, you can do a 'medicine in society' intercalation, such as public health, healthcare ethics and law, behavioural sciences or history of medicine. History of medicine is particularly popular and we have an internationally renowned unit based in the medical school. 'Healthcare ethics and law' is often oversubscribed every year, due to the well-respected and hard-working department of tutors that work on ethics. The medical school encourages students at the end of year 2 to apply for an intercalation in biological sciences and at the end of year 3 to apply for an integrated health science, and priority each year will be given to the students in these year groups. Applications for biological sciences from year 4 students are discouraged. For all intercalated degrees, students must have demonstrated satisfactory academic progress in all subjects. A number of students each year opt to leave Birmingham for a year and pursue an intercalated degree at another medical school – this is allowed after permission has been sought. There is more information about intercalated degrees on the medical school website.

Special study modules and electives

Eight SSMs are completed during the course. There is a choice of many topics, with new ones starting all the time. In the clinical years, these become more clinically orientated and self-directed, and are conducted outside the medical school. Birmingham is one of the few, if not the only, medical schools to offer all three SSMs in Christian, Jewish and Islamic medical ethics. Other interesting SSMs include creative writing and drama in medicine.

Electives are taken at the end of year 4, with an opportunity to travel anywhere in the world, normally lasting 2 months.

Erasmus

Through the Erasmus and other schemes, the medical school is developing a series of exchange programmes with Lyon (France), the University of Freiburg (Germany) and Prague and Brno (Czech Republic). The medical school is currently in discussions with other universities about the possibility of expanding these exchanges. The opportunity therefore exists for some medical students from Birmingham to go to these universities as part of this exchange, to undertake elective studies or clinical placements.

Facilities

Library The library is situated within the medical school and has an extensive range of medical textbooks and journals. It has plenty of quiet study areas and computer facilities with access to Medline, the internet and library catalogues. It also has extensive photocopying facilities. During term time it is open 8.45 AM–9 PM Monday–Thursday, until 7 PM on Fridays and 10 AM–6 PM at weekends. The library contains a room with anatomy models and books aimed particularly at students in clinical years when anatomy teaching is significantly less than in preclinical years, and students feel they need to brush up on a few details.

Computers The computer cluster is well equipped, and is open 24 hours a day, 7 days a week, all year round. There is a mixture of Apple Macs and iMacs (about 100) on the east side, and about 100 PCs on the west side. You are automatically credited with free laser print credits, and you can request free top-ups on your credits once you have run out. Every computer is online and allows full access to computer-assisted learning packages that supplement the course. There are excellent, state-of-the-art computer facilities in the learning centre, located on the main university campus – printing here costs 5p per A4 sheet. Computer facilities are also available in all medical school clinical attachments.

Welfare

Student support

Students are placed into 'families', with three to four students from each year group. Each 'family' has two tutors that they can approach with problems, and the families meet throughout the year. The welfare system is being improved all the time, and students generally feel comfortable and at ease with their personal tutors. There is an effective student-run curriculum and welfare committee that is respected by staff, and students represent their year groups and feed any problems that students are facing to the academic staff.

Accommodation

Accepting a conditional offer from Birmingham guarantees you a place in university hall/flats, providing you do not already reside in the Birmingham area. All university accommodation is within 2 to 3 miles of the campus and most is within walking distance. The Vale is a complex of several halls and flats and has the greatest overall capacity. The style of accommodation ranges from large traditional halls to flats with *en-suite* bathrooms. All halls have good security and excellent committees and social events. All halls have resident student mentors who are older students in residence that provide welfare support to any student in need. The student mentor scheme is well received and allows students to have adequate information on welfare and support services within and outside of the university, and it adds to the security of living in halls. There is an excess of private rented accommodation available at reasonable prices in Selly Oak, a centre for students and just minutes away from campus. Selly Park, Harborne and even Edgbaston (which is, in parts, very posh) are also very popular – and still reasonably priced.

Placements

Situated in the suburb of Edgbaston, the university is just a couple of miles from the city centre. The medical school (which adjoins the Queen Elizabeth teaching hospital) is found at the west end of a refreshingly spacious and green campus. It has benefited from the recent refurbishment and upgrading of lecture theatres, tutorial rooms, computer facilities and student common rooms. There are four large teaching hospitals in the city of Birmingham, as well as specialist hospitals and numerous district general hospitals. Medics at Birmingham will have very few long-term attachments outside the West Midlands, and the majority of placements are within commuting distance of student accommodation. Don't be fooled by the relatively short mileage between the medical school and hospitals – the 12 miles to Heartlands can take anywhere between 15 and 45 minutes.

During years 1–4, groups of four students attend a general practice once every fortnight. This offers a valuable early introduction to patient contact and clinical skills. The family-attachment scheme is another community-based project that takes place in year 2. From year 3 onwards, students attend hospital placements full time for most of the year, with occasional teaching sessions in the medical school.

Location of clinical placement/ name of hospital	Distance away from medical school (miles)	Difficulty getting there on public transport*
Queen Elizabeth Hospital	1	🚶
Heartlands Hospital	12	🚗
City Hospital	12	🚶
Good Hope Hospital	15	🚗
Wolverhampton Hospital	20	✈

* 🚶: walking/cycling distance; 🚌: use public transport; 🚗: need own car or lift; ✈: get up early – tricky to get to!

Sports and social

City life

Birmingham is a cosmopolitan city. All the big-name stores and designer shops can be found in the city centre, most of them in the new Bullring complex – a Mecca for those who list 'shopping' as one of their hobbies. The city has a vast selection of restaurants, serving everything from Alaska cod to zabaglione, plus all the curry you could ever wish for. Birmingham boasts a vibrant nightlife, ranging from the quintessential student night to jazz clubs and trendy bars. There are plenty of theatres, and the national indoor arena, National Exhibition Centre, and Symphony Hall regularly play host to major international acts and are literally on our doorstep! The city and surrounding area are well served by public transport. There is, in fact, a train station just next to the medical school that connects to Birmingham New Street station, and from there to just about anywhere. Birmingham International Airport is also accessible directly by train. More rural locations, such as the Malverns, Stratford-upon-Avon, and the Black Country, are all easily reached.

University life

Not only is medicine the largest faculty in the university but related courses such as medical science and physiotherapy are based in the medical school. Dentistry and nursing students are also based in and around the medical school. There is considerable social integration between all these students and between different year groups. An enthusiastic medical society and final-year dinner committee ensure there is always something happening. As the medical school is located on campus, medics can easily retain involvement in university activities and social events and thus experience the best of both worlds. The University of Birmingham Guild of Students (BUGS) houses many societies that students can join and get involved in – including theatre, cricket club, karate, hang gliding abd lesbian, gay, bisexual and transgender society (LGBT), to name but a few!

The medical society organises the renowned freshers' week, regular pub crawls, wine tasting, curry quizzes, theatre trips, ski trips and a post-exam annual camping extravaganza to the Gower. An equally strong society in Birmingham is MedSIN (Medical Students International Network), which gives students the opportunity to help the local community through action projects, and also the chance to participate in national conferences and projects abroad. Calendar events held in the medical school include the musical, a very funny comedy revue, and the glamorous final-year fashion show. Many events are held in city-centre venues, which are easily accessible by public transport and cheap for a taxi home. The medical school magazine, QMM, was revived a few years ago and affords an opportunity to put pen to paper, and there is an active surgical society for those people who think they might be budding surgeons. BUGS houses the usual complement of bars, clubs and pool tables, as well as a society for every imaginable interest, from RAG committees to cocktail parties!

Sports life

The university has an excellent reputation for sport. The Athletics' Union runs an impressive range of different sporting clubs. The medics also run large clubs for hockey, rugby, football, netball, cricket, tennis and basketball. Medic rugby, hockey and netball teams have all been national medical school champions in recent years. The clubs are friendly and well-supported (especially in post-game celebrations) and cater for all ranges of ability, from absolute beginners to international players.

Great things about Birmingham

- The medical school is fair when allocating placements – if you are close to university for one rotation then you would be likely to be a little further away for the next rotation.
- First-class healthcare ethics and law teaching, beginning from year 1 and continuing throughout the course, which prepares students well for clinical and house officer years.
- The medical school is supportive of students learning about wider global health issues, has introduced a Global Health SSM and is keen to start an International Health BSc.
- Free printing in the computer cluster – no need to worry about costs!
- There is a diverse and active group of student societies within and outside of the medical school – something for everyone to participate in.

Bad things about Birmingham

- The excessive number of examinations in preclinical years can put unnecessary stress on students.
- The large intake of students can at times leave the medical school having difficulties coping with administration and timetabling, and hospital placements are at risk of becoming overcrowded.
- The wait for exam results, particularly in early years, can be rather long.

- The security guards are very diligent, so if you forget your ID card they won't let you into the medical school.
- There is little interaction with students outside of the medical school, because the medical school is physically separated from all other departments, though it is located on the main campus.

Further information

Medical School
University of Birmingham
Edgbaston
Birmingham B15 2TT
Tel: 0121 414 6888
Fax: 0121 414 7159
Email: c.j.lote@bham.ac.uk, med-admissions@bham.ac.uk
Prospectus requests: prospectus@bham.ac.uk
Web: http://www.medicine.bham.ac.uk

Additional information	
Average A level requirements	• AAB (AAA predicted grades)
Average Scottish Higher requirements	• AAAAB (AAAAA predicted grades)
Graduate entrance requirements	• Normally a first class life sciences degree
Make-up of interview panel	• Two staff and one student
Months in which interviews are held	• October – April
Proportion of overseas students	• 8%
Proportion of mature students	• 10%
Proportion of graduate students	• 10%
Faculty's view of students taking a gap year	• No problem provided constructive
Proportion of students taking intercalated degrees	• 25%
Possibility of direct entrance to clinical phase	• No
Fees for overseas students	• £12,000 pa (preclinical) £21,000 pa
Fees for graduates	• £3000

Ability to transfer to other medical schools If so, under what circumstances	• None, under any circumstances.
Assistance for elective funding	• The Arthur Thomson Charitable Trust can provide some funding to a few students.
Assistance for travel to attachments	• None is available in preclinical years. Some is available in clinical years, due to the increased amount of travelling required.
Access and hardship funds	• 'Access to Learning Fund' is available to students, and the university has a number of bursaries too. Most hardship funds are not returnable and are income assessed.
Weekly rent	• Average is £50–£60 a week excluding most bills, in private accommodation.
Pint of lager	• Cheapest can be around £1.35–£1.65 at local student friendly pubs. It is unusual to pay more than £2.80 for a pint in Birmingham!
Cinema	• £3.00–£4.50
Nightclub	• From £3 to £8

Brighton and Sussex Medical School

Key facts	Undergraduate
Course length	5 years
Total number of medical undergraduates	560
Applicants in 2006	2300
Interviews given in 2006	Information not available
Places available in 2006	136
Places available in 2007	136
Open days 2007	See www.bsms.ac.uk for details
Entrance requirements	AAB (340 UCAS points)
Mandatory subjects	Biology and chemistry
Male:female ratio	40:60
Is an exam included in the selection process?	Yes
If yes, what form does this exam take?	UKCAT in 2007
Qualification gained	BMBS

Fascinating fact: BSMS is the first UK medical school to pioneer the use of handheld computers or personal digital assistants (PDA) as an integral component of its undergraduate education programme.

The Brighton and Sussex Medical School (BSMS) accepted its first intake of 135 students in Autumn 2003. BSMS is a partnership between the Universities of Brighton and Sussex and the new Brighton and Sussex University Hospitals NHS Trust. Our students are members of both universities, and enjoy access to the academic and recreational facilities of each. The two universities have complementary strengths that will benefit the new medical school; both have biomedical research interests recognized by grade 5 research ratings. Sussex has one of England's largest Biological Sciences

Schools while Brighton has extensive and in-depth experience in the education and training of health professionals including postgraduate doctors, nurses, midwives, pharmacists, physiotherapists and medical laboratory scientists.

The two universities have adjacent campuses at Falmer, with fast rail and road links to central Brighton. Brighton is a city with a vibrant social scene to which the universities' students (comprising over 10% of the population) make a prominent contribution. The campuses also have direct pedestrian access into the planned new South Downs National Park, long recognized as an area of outstanding natural beauty. Students are based at Falmer for years 1 and 2, at the new Audrey Emerton building next to the main Royal Sussex teaching hospital for years 3 and 4, and spend their final year partly in the teaching hospital and partly in other hospitals in Sussex, Surrey and Kent.

Education

Selection for interview is based upon the strength of an individual's grades and, importantly, the personal qualities that people need and expect in a good doctor – this is normally demonstrated through the personal statement section of your UCAS application form. If a candidate is considered to be of good potential, they will be invited to attend an interview. If they impress at interview, an offer may be made to them. The standard offer for 2006 entry is AAB (at A level), although applicants that demonstrate exceptional potential at interview may be made an offer of ABB.

Within the first few weeks, students gain experience of working with patients – normally in a primary-care or community-medicine setting. Students carry out two individual family studies. In year 1 this is with a family looking after a new baby and in year 2 with a family including a dependant requiring continuing care. Students will also experience medical practice in some hospital settings, including a visit to a spinal injuries unit. In parallel, students will develop their clinical and communication skills and study the normal and abnormal functioning of the human body, using a systems-based approach. The systems modules include the core material that every doctor must know, and are centred around weekly clinical symposia that employ a problem-based learning approach. Modules also include student-selected components (SSCs) that allow students to undertake individual projects and explore selected topics in greater depth, informed by the latest research.

In years 3 and 4, a balance between clinical and academic studies is maintained. While students gain progressively more experience in clinical contexts, the requirement to integrate clinical experience with understanding of the underlying clinical and social sciences and public health issues continues. Students maintain an individual clinical skills portfolio, which becomes an important element in the assessment of progress, and a personal development portfolio, which helps students reflect on how their personal strengths are developing along with their clinical experience. Year 5 is essentially an apprenticeship year to prepare students for their first postgraduate year.

Teaching

A wide range of teaching methods are employed, with the emphasis on small-group academic and clinical teaching. Individual patient studies allow students to relate clinical findings and treatment to the principles of the underlying clinical and social sciences and so develop an understanding of the practice of medicine. It is important to integrate information from different disciplines and sources, and this is emphasized throughout the curriculum.

Tutorial groups allow the more complex topics from lectures to be discussed in greater detail. Imaging lessons are carried out in the BSMS IT suite. The study of anatomy is enhanced by cadaveric dissection (of human tissues) in the state-of-the-art dissection room that is widely considered to be one of the best in the UK.

The first two years consist of two clinical modules and six systems-based modules – this method of teaching allows the greater integration between knowledge, clinical skills, and attitudes that students will need.

The degree also gives students a real insight into the astonishing pace of development of understanding in the biomedical sciences, and prepares them for the life-long learning to which every doctor must commit themselves. Students gain personal experience in medical research as a member of a BSMS, Brighton or Sussex research team through the individual research project, completed in year 4. On graduation, students will have the necessary academic background to practice evidence-based medicine and, if desired, embark on a career combining medical practice with medical research.

Assessment

The integrated curriculum has been developed so that scientific knowledge, clinical skills, and a professional approach are combined at an early stage and are so assessed. The main formal assessments are at the end of years 3 and 5 – these test integration of clinical experience with understanding of the underlying clinical and social sciences.

The eight modules in years 1 and 2 are assessed by an end-of-module knowledge test (50% of the module grade) and a number of essays and/or presentations (which make up the remaining 50% of the grade). From year 1 students will have OSCEs (a clinical exam), where they are required to demonstrate their competence in clinical settings.

Intercalated degrees

Subject to performance, students may be offered the opportunity to take an intercalated BSc degree within their medical degree. This is usually carried out between years 3 and 4 of the BSMS course. Students who perform well in the exams at the end of year 3 are likely to be offered this opportunity.

Special study modules and electives

Student-selected components (SSCs) form part of the assessment for many of the modules. SSCs allow students to look in greater detail at an area of a module that they deem to be interesting or beneficial to their medical training. Students rank their preferred SSC option from a list of choices and are subsequently informed of the group to which they have been allocated. Group size is small and typically ranges between 8 and 12 students.

The elective is carried out during an 8-week period at the beginning of year 4; there is a minimum requirement of 6 weeks. Students are given the opportunity to work in a different medical environment to that in which they may normally work as part of their course. Students may decide to travel abroad to observe how hospitals are different in developing countries or choose to see how medical access can affect treatment in places such as Australia (e.g. shadowing The Flying Doctors). For those students who decide to stay closer to home, electives within the UK are also permitted.

Erasmus

Unfortunately there is no Erasmus scheme currently at BSMS, but it is hoped that one will be set up in the future as the school makes more links with other universities around the world.

Facilities

Library BSMS students are entitled to use both Sussex and Brighton University libraries as well as the postgraduate medical library located at the Audrey Emerton building. This gives students access to a large number of resources. The libraries also have computer rooms, quiet study areas, rooms available to hire for group work and photocopying facilities.

Computers Similarly, students have access to the computer facilities on both campuses. In addition to this, a large computer room (with over 100 computers) can be found in the medical school building at Sussex University. There are a number of 24-hour computer rooms at the University of Sussex. Another computer room can be found in the medical school building on the Brighton campus. The libraries have excellent computer facilities with a large number of computers, printers and scanners.

Clinical skills The medical school has invested heavily in 'patient-simulating' dummies, which are connected to computers – this allows the 'patient's' condition to be controlled and modified, e.g. via 'administering drugs'. On some models the heart and a variety of pulses can be felt!

Dissection consolidates knowledge taught in the anatomy lectures and is carried out in small groups in the BSMS dissection room. The room has only been operational for 2 years and is fitted with a number of dissection tables, teaching skeletons and monitors so that the dissection can be demonstrated to the class before the hands-on work commences.

Welfare

Student support

BSMS aims to give every student as much support as it possibly can. During year 1 students are assigned a personal tutor and an academic tutor who will offer support and guidance throughout medical school.

A 'parenting' or 'buddy' scheme has been organized by MedSoc at BSMS. This is a programme in which year 2 students help to show first-year students around during their first few weeks at the university.

Medical students are members of both Student Unions and are able to take advantage of both universities' student support teams if needed.

Accommodation

BSMS students are guaranteed accommodation on campus in their first year, which most students choose to take up. Students can decide whether they would rather live in the student halls of residence on the University of Brighton campus or the University of Sussex campus. All halls are self-catered and prices can range on average between £50 (basic) and £82 (flash – some even have *en-suite* facilities) a week.

Lectures are on the Sussex campus for four days and on the Brighton campus for the remaining weekday. However, it is only a 15-minute walk between the two campuses and there is currently a free bus service from the Sussex campus to the Brighton campus.

During the remaining four years of the course, students live off campus; accommodation can vary in terms of quality and price. The two universities own many houses within Brighton that they rent to students – BSMS students can apply for housing from either university.

Placements

During the first two years of the BSMS course each student is attached to two GP practices located within 20 miles of the university. Many practices are in the city of Brighton, although some can be further afield. The university provides taxis for people who have a long way to travel and reimburses students for travel outside of Brighton.

Clinical skills can be practised on the wards of the local hospitals. In years 1 and 2 students visit both the Brighton General Hospital and Royal Sussex County Hospital a number of times. In later years students will visit and may be based at other hospitals across Sussex. Two regional attachments are undertaken in year 5 in which students will experience a rotation of clinical placements in district general hospital and community settings in East Sussex and its adjoining counties. Time will be spent shadowing a foundation house officer during the regional attachments.

Location of clinical placement/ name of hospital	Distance away from medical school (miles)	Difficulty getting there on public transport*
Brighton General Hospital	4	
Royal Sussex County Hospital	5	
Royal Alexandra Children's Hospital	5	
Princess Royal Hospital	18	

* : walking/cycling distance; : use public transport; : need own car or lift; : get up early – tricky to get to!

Sports and social 🏆

City life

Brighton is renowned as a lively city, full of clubs, bars, cafés and boutiques, and attracts young people from around the country (as well as the rest of the world). Brighton is also surrounded by large areas of countryside, offering a great contrast to the vibrant city. The University of Sussex is even located in the picturesque South Downs Park.

The clubs of Brighton cater for every music taste so there really is something for everyone. It is easy to 'shop 'til you drop' as there is a large shopping centre and Brighton also boasts the famous 'Lanes' – a cosmopolitan area containing a large number of shops, cafés, bars and restaurants. Free time could be spent in the park kicking a football around, chilling out on the beach or having a laugh on the Palace Pier with all the amusements.

If you are a fan of live music then Brighton has three popular venues: The Dome, Concorde 2 and the well-known Brighton Centre; smaller venues often have local bands playing. If you enjoy sporting events, you can watch basketball (the Brighton Bears) and ice hockey at the Brighton Centre or even see Brighton and Hove Albion play football at the Withdean Stadium against other Championship teams!

If you still want to get out and explore, a 50-minute train ride will take you right into the heart of London.

University life

Brighton and Sussex Medical School is part of both the University of Brighton and the University of Sussex. BSMS students are members of both universities' Student Unions and can live on either campus, use both the universities' large libraries and join lots of clubs – and meet even more people than you would if you just went to one university!

The University of Sussex has five bars (including a cocktail bar) and even has its own nightclub on campus. Students can stand as reps for different areas of the Student Union. Furthermore, a market can be found on the Sussex campus two days a week.

BSMS MedSoc has been running for a few years and regularly organizes social events (including Christmas, Summer and 'half-way' balls and pub crawls) and fundraising events and has a number of sports teams. Other societies that are affiliated to MedSoc include the Donald Henderson Society (international medicine), the Surgical Society, the History of Medicine Society and many more. Currently the membership fee is £25 (life-long membership) and allows members discounts at all MedSoc events.

Sports life

As more students arrive at BSMS, MedSoc has begun to set up sports teams. Current MedSoc sports teams include netball, rugby and football. BSMS students may join either of the universities' sports teams (but cannot join both universities' teams for the same sport).

Some students choose to make their own 5-a-side football, hockey and netball teams and play against other teams from within the university or even the anatomy demonstrators! Due to Brighton's excellent location by the sea, there is a popular sailing club – run jointly by the two universities.

On the Brighton campus you can find the Brighton Health and Racquet Club (a private Esporta club). It offers student membership to a limited number of Brighton University students. The club's facilities include indoor and outdoor swimming pools, a sauna, jacuzzi, fitness room including weights, tennis and badminton courts, and even a dance studio.

Great things about BSMS

- Brighton is a city of great diversity; there is always something to do and there are plenty of things to get involved with.
- BSMS has only had students since 2003 and so has some of the most up-to-date and exciting technology in the medical world.
- BSMS students meet patients within the first 3 weeks at university. This allows development of communication and examination skills from a very early stage.
- Faculty members and teaching staff are friendly and easily approachable, which comes in handy for pre-exam nerves!
- Feedback from students is highly valued and is acted upon.

Bad things about BSMS

- The beach is not sandy – instead it is made up of pebbles.
- The higher-than-average price of living in the South.
- Trekking back to campus from the supermarket on a double-decker bus is always entertaining for the wrong reasons!
- Due to the timetable, it is often difficult to integrate with students on other courses!
- Brighton city centre is 5 miles away from the university campuses; however, there are excellent transport links, e.g. train and university bus services.

Further information

Medical Admissions Office
Brighton and Sussex Medical School
BSMS Teaching Building
University of Sussex
Brighton BN1 9PX
Tel: 01273 644644
Email: medadmissions@bsms.ac.uk
Web: http://www.bsms.ac.uk
　　　http://www.sussex.ac.uk

Additional application information

Average A level requirements	• AAB
Average Scottish Advanced Higher requirements	• AAB
Make-up of interview panel	• Three panel members – details available at www.bsms.ac.uk
Months in which interviews are held	• November and February
Proportion of overseas students	• 7.5%
Proportion of mature students	• 25%
Proportion of graduate students	• N/A
Faculty's view of students taking a gap year	• Acceptable
Proportion of students taking intercalated degrees	• Not yet applicable
Possibility of direct entrance to clinical phase	• No
Fees for overseas students	• £20,000 pa
Fees for graduates	• £3000 pa
Ability to transfer to other medical schools If so, under what circumstances	• Yes, as long as other medical school accepts the BSMS curriculum, i.e. what the student has learnt so far.
Assistance for elective funding	• BSMS and the Headley Trust offer assistance to some students.
Assistance for travel to attachments	• Taxis are provided for clinical attachments that are not easily accessible. Travel is reimbursed if attachment is outside of Brighton and Hove.
Access and hardship funds	• Available to BSMS students, information from Student Support Co-ordinator

(*Continued*)

Brighton and Sussex
Medical School

(Continued)

Weekly rent	• £50–£82
Pint of lager	• £1.90 upwards
Cinema	• £4.50 with NUS Mon–Thurs, Odeon • £4.30 with NUS, CineWorld at the Marina
Nightclub	• Typically between £0 and £5

Bristol

Key facts	Premedical	Undergraduate	Graduate
Course length	6 years	5 years	4 years
Total number of medical undergraduates	c. 1000		
Applicants in 2006	356	2353	517
Interviews given in 2006	29	517	48
Places available in 2006	10	216	19
Places available in 2007	10	217	19
Open days 2007	Usually June		
Entrance requirements	AAB	AAB	2:1 and BBB
Mandatory subjects	Non-science	Chemistry and one other science subject	
Male:female ratio	1:2	1:2	1:2
Is an exam included in the selection process?	No	No	No
If yes, what form does this exam take?			
Qualification gained	MBChB		

Fascinating fact: *Casualty* is filmed in Bristol; cast members and on-location filming can often be spotted around the city. Watching the show can therefore be an opportunity to spot sights as well as catch up on revision!

Bristol is a red-brick university but has a very modern and dynamic course. As well as being a close-knit medical school, there are numerous opportunities to enjoy a wide circle of friends. The city centre provides an excellent and reasonably compact environment in which to work and play. The university itself has an excellent reputation, producing high-quality research and supporting good teaching. Bristol also offers a premedical year to 10 students each year, in which the teaching is with predental students and provided by departments in the Faculty of Science.

Education

Selection is based on UCAS form and a short (10–15 min) interview. A wide range of national and international qualifications are accepted, with the normal offer being AAB at A level, which must include chemistry. If candidates offer four subjects at A level it is asked that at least one is a non-science subject. Pre-A level A grade passes are seen as advantageous but there is no minimum requirement. All candidates offered a place will have had an interview. Short-listing for interview is based on evidence of motivation and dedication to a career in medicine, and participation and achievement in extra-curricular activities. During interviews, admissions tutors look at a wide range of factors such as experience, breadth of personal interests, career aspirations, motivation, the report from your academic referee and your academic record.

Bristol introduced an integrated curriculum in 1995. The integrated course consists of three phases. Phase I, lasting two terms, acts as an introductory period and provides a basic understanding of the human body and the mechanisms of health and disease (molecular and cellular basis of medicine). Phase I also has a human basis of medicine component, where students learn medical sociology, ethics, and epidemiology. This is mainly taught in the school of medical sciences. Phase II lasts until the end of year 3 and consists of mixed clinical and theory-based systems-orientated teaching. Phase III includes teaching and clinical experience of speciality subjects (such as paediatrics, obstetrics and gynaecology). In addition, phase III includes the elective period and senior clinical attachments in medicine and surgery. Clinical contact begins in general practices in year 1, and the first hospital attachment is in year 2. During phases II and III the whole year group is regularly brought together in Bristol for lectures and tutorial teaching.

Teaching

Early-phase teaching consists mainly of lectures and practicals, supplemented by small-group tutorials and some self-directed learning. (No live animals are used in practicals, though occasionally some tissue, such as crab legs and guinea-pig ileum, is used in experiments.) Topographical anatomy is taught by young medical demonstrators using cadavers and prosections. Students have the opportunity to do a short dissection project in anatomy in year 2. Anatomy is a popular and rewarding element of the medical degree course at Bristol.

Assessment

Regular assessments are made throughout the course. Clinical attachments include projects on the preparation and delivery of a case presentation, whereas science teaching carries associated tutorial and practical work. There are usually exams at the end of each year, although continuous assessment contributes to the final-year mark. There are important exams at the end of each phase, and finals at the end of year 5.

Intercalated degrees

Undertaking a BSc is a popular option, with about one-third of students opting to intercalate. The school positively encourages students to intercalate, usually after year 2, but it is possible to do so after year 3. There is a small range of conventional science subjects to choose from, although recently programmes such as bioethics have been introduced. There is the option to intercalate in another university's degree programme, but very few students take up this option and it has to be arranged and applied for independently. The honours year gives students an opportunity to try some 'real' science in the form of a potentially publishable original research project, as opposed to the rather structured medical course.

Student-selected components and electives

Student-selected components (SSCs) are an important part of the new curriculum from year 2 onwards, allowing students to pursue subjects of special interest. Elective time is currently 8 weeks at the beginning of year 5. SSCs in years 2, 3, and 4 are marked internally and contribute to the assessment of the unit they are written for. One year 3 SSC and the year 5 elective are externally overseen by an SSC co-ordinator where students specify their own objectives.

Erasmus

There is the opportunity to take part in the Erasmus scheme in year 3, where you can study two of the four 9-week units abroad. There are firmly agreed exchanges available with Paris, Bordeaux, Strasbourg and Grenoble (France), Vienna (Austria) and Alicante (Spain). Students study orthopaedics, rheumatology, cardiovascular and respiratory medicine and surgery in their host universities from November until March. On their return, students slot back in with the rest of the year and sit exams with everyone else in Bristol at the end of the year.

Facilities

Library   The medical library is open until 9 PM on weekdays (6:30 PM during the long vacation) and 5 PM on Saturdays. The main library has longer opening hours. Popular textbooks are available from the medical library on a short-loan basis. Medline, Embase and other medical databases are on open access on library computers; email and internet connection are also available there and in the halls of residence. Students on placement are able to use their hospital library and much of the accommodation has computer facilities.

Computers   Computers are available in the medical school (including the library) and in the main library as well as a wireless network for those with laptops. There are a number of 24-hour open-access rooms dotted around the university. Computer-assisted learning packages are available in the medical library. Other terminals support internet access, email, word processing, etc. Information technology is an integral part of the new course.

Clinical skills   All the teaching centres have facilities, though the primary site is in one of the main teaching hospitals in Bristol, the Bristol Royal Infirmary. Clinical skills are taught throughout the course, appropriate to student needs at different stages, starting with adult life support and venepuncture in year 1. As students progress through the course, other clinical procedures, such as catheterisation and intubation, may be learnt in Bristol or in the medical academies (see Placements, overleaf).

Welfare

Student support

There is a personal tutor scheme in operation in Bristol, although the quality of the scheme depends largely on the tutor (or the tutee). Most students find a member of staff with whom they get on well and from whom they can seek help. The faculty tends to be supportive, provided they are informed of problems before they get out of hand. There is a staff–student liaison committee, but input does not often translate into immediate action. The university and the Students' Union both have counselling services. Access for students with disabilities may be difficult because of the layout of the university (on a steep hill). Galenicals (the medical students' society) have a specific welfare officer, and the secretary is also there to voice student opinions and views to the medical school.

Accommodation

Accommodation is guaranteed for all first-year students living outside the Bristol area so most first years live in university halls of residence. These tend to be comfortable enough and provide an excellent opportunity to bond with other freshers (both medics and non-medics) at the numerous organized events or in the hall bars. The main group of halls is located a 30–40-minute walk from the university precinct. It is possible to apply to stay in hall after the first year, but most people move into university flats/houses or into accommodation in the private sector. It is usual to pay rent over the summer and the scrum for houses starts quite early in the year. The accommodation office provides some help, but a lot depends on individual initiative.

Placements

Years 1 and 2 are spent mainly around the university campus in central Bristol. When you begin clinical speciality attachments you can be placed at one of the main Bristol hospitals or anywhere within a 50-mile radius of Bristol. Attachments start in year 3. Medical academies are established in Somerset, Bath, Weston-Super-Mare, Gloucestershire, North and South Bristol and, most recently, Swindon. The concept of an academy is a group of teachers and students (up to 80) focused on medical school activities and with equivalent resources to the home university. Students will usually spend up to 6 months at each academy; during the three years, half the time will be located in academies within Bristol. General practice attachments are also spread across the southwest. Accommodation is provided wherever it is essential for students to be away from Bristol. However, although some help is given with travel expenses, travel to and from these attachments can be an extra expense (especially if you want to come back every weekend). A car is a huge bonus, but trains or buses serve all the hospital attachments, though not all the general practice ones.

Location of clinical placement/ name of hospital	Distance away from medical school (miles)	Difficulty getting there on public transport*
Bristol Royal Infirmary	0	🚶
Frenchay/Southmead Hospitals, Bristol	6	🚌 🚶
Bath	13	🚗 🚌 🚶
Taunton/Yeovil	50	🚗 🚌
Gloucester	50	🚗 🚌

* 🚶: walking/cycling distance; 🚌: use public transport; 🚗: need own car or lift; ✈: get up early – tricky to get to!

Sports and social

City life

Bristol has a lot to offer both as a university and as a city. The university is a research-orientated institution with a excellent reputation but it also provides good teaching. The city is just brilliant fun. Mainstream attractions abound and there is plenty of 'alternative' entertainment for those who want it. It is still reasonably safe (at least in the areas frequented by students), provided appropriate precautions are taken: it is certainly no worse than most other cities in this respect.

The city centre is reasonably compact and packed with things to attract all comers. The countryside (and the attractions of the West Country and Wales) is not far away. Students tend to congregate in the areas just around the university, such as Clifton. However, there is a shift towards areas a little further away which offer cheaper rents. Clifton is the most affluent part of Bristol, offering pleasant cafés and bijou shops. Shopping, theatre, museum and music lovers will all find something to their taste. There are plenty of pubs, restaurants, clubs, cinemas (including three arthouse cinemas), parks and green spaces and all the other things you would associate with a vibrant city like Bristol.

University life

Entertainment abounds in Bristol – sometimes there seems to be too much choice! A number of big acts play at the university and at other venues throughout the city. There is a huge range of societies to join at the Union. Halls and Galenicals run a range of entertainment, organise a number of sports teams and represent students' views on a variety of committees. There are two revues for medics to take part in: the preclinical revue tends to be a rather drunken and disorganised affair, but the clinical one is a more organised and moderate event that runs for 4 nights in the Union theatre. Galenicals organizes a lot of events for medics and has its own bar which students from all year groups use.

Sports life

The university has good outdoor facilities, a tennis centre and a brand new indoor centre within the campus. Wednesday afternoons are free for sport in phases I and II and there are teams at all levels in most sports. There are a number of medics teams (including the infamous Women's Football Team) organised through Galenicals, which tend to be a bit less competitive than the university teams. They have a considerable social component as well.

Great things about Bristol

- The generally high standard of teaching and the high quality of clinical experience, especially in peripheral hospitals.
- The city of Bristol itself, with its huge range of bars, restaurants and attractions.
- The opportunity to mix with plenty of non-medics and medics from other year groups.
- A modern, clinical course in which student feedback is valued.
- An influential, active, and sociable medical student society of which 95% of medical students are members.

Bad things about Bristol

- The rather conservative nature of the university in terms of atmosphere and politics.
- The financial costs (high rents; long-distance attachments in clinical years; expensive bus fares).
- Walking up all those steep hills (Bristol is one big hill)!
- Feedback on work can take a long time and can sometimes be a bit limited.
- Huge annual scramble for accommodation at a reasonable price.

Further information

Admissions Office
University of Bristol
Senate House
Tyndall Avenue
Bristol BS8 1TH
Tel: 0117 928 9000
Fax: 0117 925 1424
Email: admissions@bristol.ac.uk
Prospectus requests: http://www.bris.ac.uk/prospectusrequest/
Web: http://www.medici.bris.ac.uk

Additional application information

Average A level requirements	• AAB
Average Scottish Higher requirements	• AAAAA
Make-up of interview panel	• Clinicians, medical scientists, GPs and non-clinical personnel
Months in which interviews are held	• November – March
Proportion of overseas students	• 5%
Proportion of mature students	• 10%
Proportion of graduate students	• 10%
Faculty's view of students taking a gap year	• Welcomed
Proportion of students taking intercalated degrees	• 30%
Possibility of direct entrance to clinical phase	• No
Fees for overseas students	• £12,400 pa (preclinical) £23,100 pa (clinical)
Fees for graduate students	• £3000
Ability to transfer to other medical schools	• At any stage, assessed on a personal level. Not many do transfer, of course, but help will be given to students having a genuine need to transfer.
Assistance for elective funding	• Many bursaries available including Medical Elective Bursary, MedChi Prize, Medical/Dental prize, and external bursary funding, e.g. from Wellcome Trust.
Assistance for travel at the start and end of each attachment	• Return travel paid for, plus accommodation provided in clinical years.
Access and hardship funds	• Available through Student Union, in line with other university arrangements.

(*Continued*)

(*Continued*)

Weekly rent	• £55–£75
Pint of lager	• £2
Cinema	• £3–£6
Nightclub	• £3

Cambridge

Key facts	Undergraduate	Graduate
Course length	6 years	4 years
Total Number of medical undergraduates	c. 1300	c. 85
Applicants in 2006	1395	210
Interviews given in 2006	Not known	Not known
Places available in 2006	280	20
Places available in 2007	280	20
Open days 2007	5 and 6 July	5 and 6 July
Entrance requirements	AAA	2:1 or above
Mandatory subjects	Chemistry and two science/mathematics subjects	
Male:female ratio	47:53	Not known
Is an exam included in the selection process?	Yes	
If yes, what form does this exam take?	BMAT	
Qualification gained	MB/BChir	MB/BChir

Fascinating fact: The teaching of medicine at Cambridge dates back to 1540, when Henry VIII endowed the University's first Professorship of Physic. Things moved quickly after that, and within only 320 years the number of medical students had reached double figures.

The standard 6-year medical course at Cambridge has two distinct phases. The preclinical course in years 1–3 is a science degree in its own right: all students intercalate (unless you are already a graduate), and there is a strong emphasis on research. The second block of three years comprises the clinical course, which has recently been extended and revamped. Students can also opt for the MB PhD course, which allows them a further 3 years during their clinical studies to complete a PhD.

In addition, Cambridge has a 4-year graduate-entry course which mixes elements from the standard preclinical and clinical courses with dedicated teaching; it is open to UK/EU graduates of any discipline. Graduate entry to the standard course is also possible, and is the only option for non-UK/EU graduate students.

All Cambridge students are members of a college, and this is the focus of social life for most pre-clinical students. Despite the intensity of the course there is ample opportunity for extra-curricular activities, not just within the colleges but also in the university and within the city itself.

Education

In addition to their UCAS paperwork, applicants to the standard 6-year course should be aware of the need to fill out the Cambridge Application Form (CAF) and sit the BioMedical Admissions Test (BMAT – see Chapter 3). Prospective students are advised to contact the university admissions office and/or their sixth-form careers department for details well ahead of time and review the prospectus on the website.

Teaching

Studying medicine at Cambridge is very much a degree of two parts, with preclinical and clinical medicine taught separately by the Faculty of Biology and the School of Clinical Medicine, respectively.

In years 1 and 2, students study anatomy, biochemistry, physiology, neurosciences, pathology, pharmacology and reproductive biology, with smaller courses in medical sociology and statistics/epidemiology, and a brief clinical-contact programme. Teaching follows the traditional format of lectures and practicals. Rather than learning anatomy from pre-prepared prosected material, students carry out the dissection themselves with six students allocated to one cadaver for the year. The main occasions when students discuss and ask questions about the lectures are the weekly 'supervisions', one for each subject.

All students (except those with a previous degree) must intercalate in year 3 and can choose from any undergraduate degree offered by the university – not just medical courses. You could apply to study, say, law or history of art or computer science; however, most students are encouraged to study one of the more scientific subjects as this is usually mandatory if you wish to do your clinical studies in Cambridge. Be aware though that patient contact is pretty minimal until you start clinical school.

Those who have fulfilled the Second MB requirements in years 1 and 2 are guaranteed a place in clinical school at Cambridge, Oxford or London – depending on your preferences, and the outcome of applications and interviews in the February prior to entry. Most of those who apply to stay on at Cambridge (roughly half the year) get to do so; the others go mainly to Oxford and London, and a few to other compatible courses, such as Edinburgh. If you apply to the Cambridge clinical course after preclinical elsewhere, it is essential to complete a BA or BSc as well as equivalents of the Second MB before starting.

A new 3-year clinical course was introduced in 2005. Teaching is still very much clinically based (wards, clinics and theatre sessions), so students get very good exposure to patients and are expected to be active in seeking out patients to clerk. After a 3-week introductory course there are three stages. Stage 1 is 10 weeks each of medicine and surgery interspersed with fortnightly GP days and regular 'review' weeks. Stage 2 is 15-months long and involves placements in specialities such as neurology, paediatrics, obstetrics and gynaecology and an elective. Stage 3 is 11-months long and contains a longer GP attachment, palliative care, A&E, critical care, senior medicine and surgery attachments. Each part of the clinical course usually starts with a block of lectures, following which students are dispersed to attachments at Addenbrooke's.

Students on the 4-year graduate-entry course are admitted to the Clinical School from the start and integrate preclinical and clinical teaching throughout the 4 years. During the first 2 years graduates attend the biological science lectures with the standard course students during term time and go to the West Suffolk Hospital (WSH) in Bury St. Edmunds (30 miles east of Cambridge) for dedicated clinical teaching whilst the standard course are taking their Christmas/Easter/summer holidays. An equivalent of Stage 1 is completed during these first 2 years. Graduates move straight to full-time clinical teaching from year 3, joining the standard course for Stage 2 with teaching both at Addenbrooke's in Cambridge and on attachment to peripheral hospitals in East Anglia. Year 4 sees a return to dedicated teaching, most of which again takes place at WSH.

Assessment

On the preclinical course exams take place in May/June at the end of years 1 and 2. These are used to assess students for both the Second MB (a GMC requirement, which is a simple pass/fail) and their BA (the Cambridge degree, for which you are awarded a class: first, 2:1, 2:2, etc.). Your classes of BA in years 1 and 2 may be taken into account by your preferred clinical school in deciding whether or not to offer you a place, but are not a 'be-all and end-all' – the final BA mark is decided by your grade in year 3.

At clinical school students sit the new Final MB, introduced in 2005. This is examined in two chunks: pathology, obstetrics and gynaecology and paediatrics finals are at the end of Stage 2, whilst medicine and surgery finals take place on completion of Stage 3. There are also assessments at the end of each clinical attachment, which have to be passed before finals.

Assessment for those on the graduate course in years 1 and 2 is similar to the standard course; however, graduates are not required to sit essay papers in years 1 and 2. Finals are identical to those undertaken by the standard course.

Intercalated degrees

Intercalation is compulsory (see Teaching above) and since it is a requirement of the BA to be resident in Cambridge you cannot intercalate elsewhere. The exception is the Cambridge–MIT (Massachusetts Institute of Technology) exchange scheme that takes three medical students each year, who are then required to stay at Cambridge for their clinical studies. Also, eight or nine clinical students each year follow the MB PhD programme, for which they apply after being accepted into clinical school but before starting the course.

Special study modules and electives

On both the standard and graduate courses there is a 7-week elective period, timetabled alongside a 2 to 3 week holiday, allowing nearly 10 weeks away in total. 95% of students go abroad. 'Special study components' (SSCs) have been introduced with the new clinical course and take place in each of the three stages, currently occupying a total of 12 weeks over the 3 years. The details of the SSCs are still being worked out; however, it is expected that students will choose from a list of options offered by the clinical school in different departments, and in the later stages of the course may have more opportunity to organize these attachments themselves. The graduate course includes two SSCs, of which one is student-selected.

Erasmus

An Erasmus exchange is not normally possible during the preclinical course due to the requirement to be resident in Cambridge, and does not form part of the clinical course. Currently the only overseas travel opportunity apart from the elective is the MIT exchange scheme described above. However, given that the Cambridge term is only 8 weeks long, there is ample opportunity to travel/work abroad during the vacations in the preclinical years.

Facilities

Library   Cambridge is not short of libraries! The medical library is based at the clinical school in Addenbrooke's, and has multiple copies of undergraduate clinical texts as well as specialist books. The University Library has some further books and each department (physiology, pathology, etc.) has its own specialized library. Each college has a library which is usually well-stocked with preclinical textbooks. Some of the college and departmental libraries have 24-hour access; the medical library is open from 8 AM to 10 PM on weekdays. Cambridge also has a public lending library.

Computers   There are computers everywhere in Cambridge and all students have an email account and access to central computing facilities. The colleges have networks available to their members, many college rooms have a network access point and most departments also have facilities which can be used by their intercalating students. The clinical school has computers reserved for the use of clinical students and a wireless area network for those with suitably equipped laptops or palmtops. There is also a set of terminals spread around Addenbrooke's hospital, allowing access to teaching resources while on the wards.

Welfare

Student support

All students are members of a college – it's where you'll live, eat and socialize, at least to begin with, and it's where your supervisions are organized. The college allocates each of its students a tutor, whose duties include welfare matters, such as finance, housing and general pastoral care, and a Director of Studies (DoS), who is responsible for students' academic progress and is there to provide educational guidance and support.

In most colleges, other contacts include a nurse, a chaplain (available for the pastoral support of students from any background) and 'porters' – generally friendly staff who act as reception and security personnel and are on hand to deal with any emergencies 24 hours a day. There are also numerous university-linked organizations involved in student support, including the university counselling service, CUSU (Cambridge University Students' Union) and various student-run bodies.

Accommodation

Undergraduates can expect to live in college for at least two out of the three preclinical years, and have college-provided accommodation, often in college-owned houses around Cambridge, for the other year. Quality and cost vary with the college, but the standard of accommodation at its worst is definitely bearable and at its best can see you in some of the finest student rooms in the country, ranging from beautiful 500-year-old conversions to new purpose-built blocks. Many colleges will also provide accommodation for the clinical years and students joining from preclinical courses elsewhere can expect to have something provided for the first clinical year at least. Students often decide to rent a shared house in the clinical years.

Placements

Lectures and practicals for preclinical years 1 and 2 are held on the science sites in the centre of Cambridge, and are within walking distance of most of the colleges. Supervisions usually take place in the colleges, but are sometimes at the supervisor's department building or another college.

All the teaching on the clinical course is based at Addenbrooke's Hospital, which is situated 2½ miles south-east of the city centre. Several students live close to Addenbrooke's and walk in; however, it can easily be reached by bus or bicycle from anywhere in Cambridge. Parking on the hospital site can be a nightmare. On the standard clinical course, students should expect to spend approximately half of their attachments in peripheral DGHs – places are allocated by the clinical school and students are rarely allowed to swap. Accommodation is provided at all placements (except in Addenbrooke's).

Location of clinical placement/ name of hospital	Distance away from medical school (miles)	Difficulty getting there on public transport*
Cambridge (Addenbrooke's)	0	
Bedford Hospital	28	
Milton Keynes General	46	
Peterborough District Hospital	41	
Great Yarmouth (James Paget)	87	

* : walking/cycling distance; : use public transport; : need own car or lift; : get up early – tricky to get to!

Sports and social

City life

With its undeniable beauty and rich history, Cambridge is an inspiring city to live and work in. Undergraduates, graduates, tourists, and the local residents provide an ever-changing and colourful population superimposed on peaceful college cloisters, colonies of bustling student houses and a busy town centre. Everything a student needs is less than 15-minutes walk away, and are certainly within a 15-minute cycle ride. Take your pick from the central market; the supermarkets and shopping centres; a wide range of chain stores; the excellent Arts Theatre; gigs at the Junction; countless pubs; several clubs; and loads of cinemas – college, art-house, and mainstream. The river gives way to open countryside, and train services to Peterborough and London's King's Cross (45 mins) give good access to the rest of the country. Cambridge also has good coach links, several city bus routes and is close to Stansted International Airport! Many students have bicycles but they are rarely essential.

Cambridge is not without the dangers of violence and crime and, like most places, these problems are often associated with last orders on a Friday or Saturday night. However, there are no very dangerous districts and students' property insurance premiums confirm Cambridge as one of the safest places in the country to live and study.

University life

The collegiate system means that in the preclinical years you get to meet students doing a wide variety of subjects, rather than just medics. Although the course does place a significant workload on you, there are a whole host of opportunities to be involved in other societies, from music and drama (ranging from the famous Cambridge Footlights to The Medics' Review comedy show, which travels to the Edinburgh Fringe every other year) to karate and gliding. There really is a society for almost every conceivable hobby and interest – be it caving or Canada, cocktails or Christmas – so the chances are you can find something you will enjoy doing.

Entertainment is provided at a variety of levels, and may be society, college, clinical school or university based. Unlike other universities, there is no central Student Union bar in Cambridge – instead, there is a bar in every college and student nights during the week at the various town and college hot spots. 'Formal hall' meals are a prominent feature of the Cambridge social scene. These are very merry three-course dinners in a college dining hall costing between £3 and £9. Students wear gowns, Latin benedictions are made and a gong sounds.

The MedSoc is the fourth-largest student society and works to make sure preclinical medics have a good time with the annual Christmas dinner, 'bops' (parties), barbecues and regular pub crawls. In addition, each college usually has its own medical society. There is much more of a 'medical school feel' to the clinical stage, with most students living nearer the hospital and away from their colleges – the clinical students' society arranges its own social events, often linking up with the doctor's mess at Addenbrooke's.

Sports life

Almost every sport is catered for and the standard in many sports is very high. At college level facilities vary, but can often include huge playing fields, gyms and/or squash courts, plus the inevitable boathouse. Thankfully, it doesn't really matter how good or bad you are and the inter-college competitions provide a great opportunity to play sport without having to commit your life to university-level training. The clinical school has a sports society (known as 'The Sharks') and there is a sport and fitness centre situated on the hospital site to which all students are given free membership. Another popular – ahem – 'sport' in Cambridge is punting.

Great things about Cambridge

- The preclinical course is regarded as one of the most comprehensive in the country – leaving you well-armed for clinical school and job applications – learning anatomy by doing the dissection yourself is invaluable.
- You can choose from a huge range of intercalated degrees, not just science subjects, and your BA gets automatically upgraded to an MA after 3 or 4 years!
- The supervision system helps to make sure that you are able to keep up with the course, and gives you substantially more individual tuition than most medical schools. It also makes sure you do the work!
- May Week (actually in June, after the preclinical exams) – a week of celebrating, winding down, and college balls!
- You get to live and study in truly beautiful surroundings with a relatively low cost of living, especially for those in college accommodation.

Bad things about Cambridge

- Highly academic and can appear a very competitive learning environment, especially just prior to exams, which for many students can be rather stressful. Good time management becomes key.
- Living in college can be frustrating, as the rules and regulations the college enforces can make some individuals feel as though they are not being treated like adults.
- The standard preclinical course is heavy on detail and can in some respects seem old-fashioned and resistant to change. Be aware that you don't get to see patients for more than a few hours a year.
- The lack of a physical 'medical school' in the preclinical years means there is no focal point for students to congregate.
- The tourists – who admittedly do generate a lot of income for the town and the colleges – manage to appear almost anywhere and at any time, including occasionally in lectures!

Further information

Cambridge Admissions Office (CAO)
Fitzwilliam House
32 Trumpington Street
Cambridge CB2 1QY
Tel: 01223 333 308
Fax: 01223 366 383
Email: admissions@cam.ac.uk
Web: http://www.cam.ac.uk/admissions/undergraduate/

University of Cambridge School of Clinical Medicine
Box 111
Addenbrooke's Hospital
Hills Road
Cambridge CB2 2SP
Tel: 01223 336 700
Fax: 01223 336 709
Email: school-enquiries@medschl.cam.ac.uk
Web: http://www.medschl.cam.ac.uk/pages/admissions/index.html

Graduate course information
Contact via one of the participating colleges:

Admissions Officer
Hughes Hall
Cambridge CB1 2EW
Tel. 01223 334 897
Fax. 01223 311 179
Email: ugadmissions@hughes.cam.ac.uk
Web: http://www.hughes.cam.ac.uk/

Admissions Officer
Lucy Cavendish College [women only]
Cambridge CB3 0BU
Tel: 01223 330 280
Fax: 01223 332 178
Email: lcc-admission@lists.cam.ac.uk
Web: http://www.lucy-cav.cam.ac.uk/
        http://www.lucy-cav.cam.ac.uk/Admissions/Postgraduate/Grad_medical_course.htm

The Undergraduate Admissions Tutor
Wolfson College
Barton Road
Cambridge CB3 9BB
Tel: 01223 335 900
Fax: 01223 335 908
Email: ug-admissions@wolfson.cam.ac.uk
Web: http://www.wolfson.cam.ac.uk/
        http://www.wsufftrust.org.uk/CGC/default.asp

Additional application information

Average A level requirements	• AAA
Average Scottish Higher requirements	• AAB
Make-up of interview panel	• Mixed clinical and nonclinical
Months in which interviews are held	• December
Proportion of overseas students	• 9%
Proportion of mature students	• 1%
Proportion of graduate students	• Information unavailable
Faculty's view of students taking a gap year	• Good
Proportion of students taking intercalated degrees	• 100%
Possibility of direct entrance to clinical phase	• No
Fees for overseas students	• £11,862 pa (preclinical) £21,954 pa (clinical) plus £3200–£3750 (college fees)
Fees for graduates	• Please contact university for details.
Ability to transfer to other medical schools If so, under what circumstances	• About 50% of students transfer for clinical studies, moving mainly to Oxford and London. • A small number of places exist for medics wishing to spend their intercalated year at MIT in the United States. Outside these schemes, transfer is not possible. • Transfer after the 3-year preclinical course, with places guaranteed at one of Cambridge, Oxford or London. Also possible to transfer to another compatible course at this point.
Assistance for elective funding	• Limited. Provided by clinical school, college and other sources.

(Continued)

(Continued)

Assistance for travel to attachments	• As for NHS Bursary in years 5 and 6.
Access and hardship funds	• Unlimited bursaries available to students who receive a full maintenance grant as assessed by LEA. Smaller bursaries available for those receiving intermediate level of maintenance grant. University-wide hardship funds also available.
Weekly rent	• £73 in college (including subsidized food at college canteens). No rent required during the vacation period. • £60–£90 in shared housing
Pint of lager	• £1.50 (colleges) to £3.50 (upmarket local venues) – take your pick!
Cinema	• Between £4.50 and £6.20.
Nightclub	• £4–£9 at local clubs. £0–£5 at college-based student nights.

Cardiff

Key facts	Premedical	Undergraduate	Graduate
Course length	1 year	5 years	4 years
Total Number of medical undergraduates	15	1500	108
Applicants in 2006	270	2800	501
Interviews given in 2006	40	896	175
Places available in 2006	15	305	70
Places available in 2007	15	305	70
Open days 2007	April and July		April and July
Entrance requirements	AAB plus AS minimum C, from 21 units	AAB plus AS minimum C, from 21 units*	2:1 degree in any subject
Mandatory subjects	One science A level	Chemistry and biology (one A grade). Minimum B at AS level	GCSE maths and English Biology/ chemistry to GCSE level
Male:female ratio	40:60	40:60	30:70
Is an exam included in the selection process?	No	Yes	Yes
If yes, what form does this exam take?		UKCAT in 2007	GAMSAT UKCAT in 2007
Qualification gained	MBBCh		

*The AS level can be a C grade unless the applicant does not take chemistry or biology to A level in which case they must take this to AS and gain a B grade. We do not accept general studies or critical thinking as an A or AS level.

Fascinating fact: The 'daddy' of evidence-based medicine and randomised controlled trials, Archie Cochrane, pioneered epidemiology as a science while working for the Welsh National School of Medicine here in Cardiff.

Following a successful merger with the University of Wales, Cardiff is now one of the biggest universities in the UK with over 25,000 students. A large number of health programmes are taught at the university: dentistry, nursing, physiotherapy, occupational therapy, radiotherapy, pharmacy and optometry as well as medicine. The close knit nature of the university makes inter-professional health education easy, and allows medics to benefit from world class research in fields other than their own.

Cardiff University is the only undergraduate medical school in Wales. Prior to 2003, Cardiff only provided the preclinical part of the medical course, with students transferring to The University of Wales College of Medicine for the remainder of their degree. Being the main medical school in Wales, Cardiff has strong links with all hospitals throughout the country, allowing medical students a massive breadth of clinical experience, from that of a bustling capital city to rural medicine in Snowdonia. As Europe's youngest capital city, Cardiff is a vibrant and exciting place to study, with a unique medical course offering a wide range of opportunities, at university and beyond.

Education

Cardiff has an integrated curriculum which blends the basic medical sciences and the clinical disciplines within a structure that combines traditional learning methods with aspects of a problem-centred approach. During the course there are three strands of learning and teaching: knowledge and understanding; skills and competencies; and attitude and conduct. Skills develop progressively throughout the 5 years and, hand in hand with these skills, is the acquisition of the knowledge base that underpins medical practice.

Cardiff also has a foundation year designed for students who have demonstrated high academic potential but who do not meet the specific subject requirements for entry to the 5-year medical programme, i.e. those who have non-science subjects or a combination including no more than one of biology, chemistry and physics. Students on the 1-year modular programme study 12 modules alongside students of other science disciplines. Normally modules include biological and chemical sciences or other subjects such as mathematics. Modules are also available in other subjects (e.g. psychology and languages). The combination of subjects is selected according to the student's prior qualifications. About 16 students are admitted to this every year, who then automatically progress on to the 5-year course.

September 2004 saw the first intake into the new 4-year graduate-entry programme. The first two years of the course follow a problem-based learning style of course, based at Swansea University. At the end of these two years the students will have to meet the same learning outcomes as the year 3 students in Cardiff, after which they complete the same final two years as those on the 5-year course in Cardiff.

Teaching

A combination of lectures, tutorials, small group sessions and self-directed learning makes up the bulk of the learning. Anatomy is learnt by hands-on human dissection and taught using demonstrated dissection and prosections. Various computer-assisted learning programmess are used, mainly as a revision medium and for tutorial support. Firm sizes vary depending on the hospital: five to six in the main teaching hospitals, and usually two in the district general hospitals (although one-on-one teaching is increasingly possible during the senior years).

Assessment

Major examinations take place at the end of years 1, 3 and 5, with in-course and on-going assessment used more in years 2 and 4. Resits are available in all years. The three sets of exams make up the Primary MB, Intermediate MB and Final MB. Whilst the majority of exams are formal written papers, OSCEs and other clinical exams form an increasing part of assessment as students progress through the course. It is generally accepted that the toughest year for students is year 3, followed by either year 5 or 1.

Intercalated degrees

Intercalated degrees are available to a third of the year, and can be done after years 2, 3 or 4. The choice of subjects includes basic medical sciences (anatomy, physiology, biochemistry, genetics), or more clinically orientated degrees (such as sports science and psychology). Intercalated degrees can be pursued at any university in Wales, and occasionally at other institutions throughout the UK.

Student selected components and electives

Special study components make up 24–30% of the timetable throughout the 5 years. In year 2, many students take a 6-week language SSC, in anything from Welsh to Spanish. In years 1 and 2, students are attached in pairs to an expectant family. The students follow the family over a period of 9 months, charting the development of both the child and the family, and presenting a detailed report at the end. Likewise, in year 3, students are attached to a patient recently diagnosed with cancer somewhere in south Wales. They accompany the patient through their experience of cancer for nine months, learning not just the clinical effects of the disease, but also the social and emotional toll of cancer. A reflective and academic oncology project is submitted, which forms a major part of the Intermediate MB assessment.

An 8-week period of elective study, either in the UK or abroad, is undertaken at the start of the final year as part of the normal block rotation. This is normally a clinical experience, undertaken anywhere in the world (that's safe!) and students now produce a reflective learning diary rather than the original research formerly necessary.

Erasmus

The medical school participates in the EU's Erasmus programme. Opportunities exist in all major European countries, from Sweden in the north to Italy in the south, and from Spain in the west to Romania in the east. About 30 students are selected each year following tough competition.

Facilities

For years 1 and 2, students are based at the School of Biosciences (BIOSI) in the city centre at the main university campus. For year 3 onwards students are entirely based at the medical school at the University Hospital of Wales (UHW) for lectures and classes, with clinical placements throughout the country.

Library   A specialist library exists at BIOSI for year 1/2 medics and other bioscience students. Specialist librarians and a large number of group study rooms are all within the building. A room with 50 PCs is reserved for BIOSI students only during the day, and there are three 24-hour PC rooms, each with 200+ computers. Journal and book availability is pretty good. A large clinical library is available at UHW for 12 hours a day, with every possible speciality covered. It is the major medical library for the whole of Wales with massive postgraduate as well as undergraduate coverage. There are also libraries in all the major hospitals throughout Wales, which students can use if they're away form Cardiff on placement. Book and journal coverage is excellent. A large 24-hour 40-PC room is located in UHW.

Computers   There are good computer facilities on site, and in most outlying hospitals. Some tuition is given initially, with more specialized (other than statistical) teaching being given when needed. All assessed work must be word processed and normally has to be submitted electronically.

Clinical skills   Practical skills are taught from year 2, when students undertake a compulsory basic life support course. A new clinical skills lab is used to teach a variety of skills, from venepuncture and suturing to breaking bad news.

Welfare

Student support

The School of Medicine at Cardiff University is very student-friendly and actively encourages and acts upon the views of its students. Weekly meetings between student reps and the deanery staff occur where students' grievances are voiced in an informal setting. Students are also represented on all the curriculum-planning committees. Being part of Cardiff University allows students access to its general counselling and welfare services, as well as pastoral care within the faculty. Provision for disabled and dyslexic students is generally considered excellent.

Accommodation

Accommodation is provided by Cardiff University in year 1. There is space for all first-years in halls. The standards are high, with over 60% of accommodation being less than five years old, and two-thirds is *en-suite*. There is ample good-quality private housing for rent, with prices ranging from £45 to £65 a week. Cardiff Council runs a house renting registration scheme, which aims to monitor and license rented accommodation in the city. Most halls are with a 10-minute walk of BIOSI, and for subsequent years, students often live near to the city centre for year 2, moving up to near UHW from year 3 until the completion of the course.

Placements

The medical school is based on two sites, approximately 1.5 miles apart: the Cardiff School of Biosciences (a part of Cardiff University Cathay's Park campus) and the Heath Park Campus (jointly occupied with the University Hospital of Wales). Community-based teaching in practices in and around Cardiff forms a substantial part of the course. Hospitals throughout Wales are used for teaching, ensuring an excellent student:patient ratio. It also provides an opportunity for students to see all of the different parts of the nation, and gain more of an idea where to apply for jobs a few years down the line. In year 1, students spend 7 to 10 days on clinical placement, which is designed to introduce that particular speciality to the student and show the relevance of the science learnt to date to clinical practice. In year 2, all students spend a period of 3 weeks shadowing a nurse or student nurse somewhere in Wales. The aim is to enable the doctors of the future to have a better understanding of the profession they perhaps work most closely with.

Bangor is the most distant of the DGHs used, being 260 miles away from Cardiff. Attachments in general practice include some time spent at a rural practice somewhere in Wales. Travel subsidies are available from the college, and accommodation is provided in all DGHs that are not within a 1-hour commute from Cardiff. All placements for years 1–3 are with commuting distance of Cardiff. Whilst the medical school provides coaches to all placements in years 1 and 2, most students from year 3 onwards find it necessary to have their own car, given the enormous geographical distribution in placements for students.

Location of clinical placement/ name of hospital	Distance away from medical school (miles)	Difficulty getting there on public transport*
University Hospital of Wales, Cardiff	0	🚶
Royal Glamorgan Hospital, Llantrisant	12	🚗
Princess of Wales Hospital, Bridgend	20	🚗
Singleton Hospital & Morriston Hospital, Swansea	40	✈️ 🚗
Ysbyty Gwynedd, Bangor	260	✈️ 🚗

* 🚶: walking/cycling distance; 🚌 : use public transport; 🚗: need own car or lift; ✈️ : get up early – tricky to get to!

Sports and social 🏆

City life

Cardiff is a very student-friendly city. The presence of four universities (Cardiff, UWIC, Royal Welsh College of Music and Drama and Glamorgan on the city outskirts) makes for a student population of over 60,000. In a city bustling with so many students, there is a lot of provision for their needs. Most clubs, pubs and theatres host student nights and offer special rates for NUS card holders. The city also has plenty of parks and open spaces, with the enormous central Bute Park full to bursting during the summer with students trying to revise for finals whilst getting a tan! As the capital of Wales, Cardiff has all the attractions that you would expect of a large city, while being small enough to make you feel at home. The local countryside is very beautiful, ranging from the mountains of the Brecon Beacons to the beaches of the Gower, and, for outdoor activities and sports, Cardiff is second to none. The city is developing with amazing pace under the direction of the new Welsh Assembly Government. The swish Cardiff Bay area is the place to eat and to live when you want to splash out or finally become a young professional doctor. The bay boasts the brand new Wales Millennium Centre, now one of Europe's premiere opera, music and theatre venues. The Millennium Stadium regularly hosts all the leading bands of the UK and beyond, as well as major national and international sports fixtures. Oh, and Dr Who is based and filmed in Cardiff – what more could you want?!

University life

Medical students are members of their own students' club, which provides sporting facilities and teams, its own fleet of minibuses, and its own bar, where drinks are often the cheapest in Cardiff. The students' club organizes one staff/student dinner a year, six balls and many other social events, ranging from top-name bands, comedians, long-distance pub crawls and tours around the UK – all attended by a mix of medics, dentists, nurses, radiographers and physiotherapy students. A wide range of clubs and societies is available, including climbing, orchestra, canoeing and martial arts. There are also religious groups such as the Islamic Society and the Christian Medical Fellowship. Each year the students organize a charity revue called Anaphylaxis and runs Medrag to raise money for local charities. In 1992 the Students' Union started its own charity, BACCUP. Each year a limited number of healthcare students from Cardiff University have the opportunity to travel out to Belarus to work in an orphanage for children with special needs. Students also have access to all of the facilities offered by Cardiff University and its Students' Union.

Music plays a large role in university life, with all standards being catered for. There are jazz bands, choirs, rock bands and classical music groups for those only beginning music, right up to groups performing on national radio. The proximity of the Royal Welsh College of Music, the BBC and the Welsh National Opera makes Cardiff an artistic place to be for any student with an interest in performing music, as well as listening. There is also a dedicated medic's choir and orchestra. Many of the UK's premier bands have originated from south Wales, often starting their careers at the city's must-visit Bar Fly bar.

Student life can be very hectic, juggling work commitments with the variety of sports and clubs offered by the students' club. The majority of teams, clubs and societies are fully funded by the club, including the provision of minibuses for the use of its members. MedClub provides a friendly, social and cheap venue for the post-match celebrations and a very cheap source of alcohol for those not partaking in the sporting scene! It is also the venue for some of the craziest scenes you're likely to find during freshers' week. There is also the impressive Cardiff Students' Union, with its two bars, 1800-capacity nightclub, live music venue and snooker/pool hall. As a capital city, Cardiff also offers excellent sport, leisure and recreational facilities. The Millennium Stadium currently hosts the FA Cup and the Worthington Cup Finals and Six Nations rugby, as well as a number of live music gigs. Cardiff also has a great range of shops, pubs, clubs and a redeveloped seafront at Cardiff Bay. Living in Cardiff also allows easy access to beautiful and varied scenery, including the Brecon Beacons National Park.

Sports life

The student club has a large number of teams, some of which gain great success far beyond that expected of a small university. Our rugby team has won the Med Schools Cup nine times in its 10-year history and also won the BUSA shield in 2004. Most teams compete in the various BUSA inter-university competitions, inter-medical school competitions and some local leagues. The students' club also has pool tables. Besides the facilities on offer by the dedicated Students' Union for medics and other healthcare students, students have the benefit of using the sports and Union facilities of Cardiff University. There are two gyms, one on the site of the main halls, the other in the main campus in the city centre. Both are open for 14 hours a day and allow students to work up a sweat at about £1 a go.

Great things about Cardiff

- Students are members of the Students' Union at Cardiff University, allowing access to both Med Club and the bars and nightclub at Cardiff University. This also allows medical students to socialize with non-medics as well as medics.
- A lot of interactions (socially and academically) between students of all years, and with dental, nursing and physiotherapy students.
- All the advantages of living in an expanding and vibrant capital city without the usual costs.
- Using all Welsh hospitals keeps firm sizes low and student/patient ratios high.
- An excellent course with a great balance between problem-based learning, lectures and clinical experience.

Bad things about Cardiff

- The large year group size means it can be difficult to get to know all fellow students individually.
- The wait for coursework to be returned is often long.
- Distances between hospitals and the accessibility of some rural hospitals make travelling very awkward and time-consuming, unless you have a car.
- Clinical placements in years 4 and 5 can make it hard to see your non-medic friends (and medic friends not with you on placement) regularly.
- The weather – boy does it get windy!

Further information

Undergraduate Admissions Officer
University of Wales College of Medicine
Heath Park
Cardiff CF4 4XN
Tel: 029 2074 2027
Fax: 029 2074 3690
Email: uwcmadmissions@cf.ac.uk
        medical-school@cardiff.ac.uk
Web: http://www.uwcm.ac.uk

Additional application information

Average A level requirements	• AAB
Average Scottish Higher requirements	• AAAAB to include chemistry
Make-up of interview panel	• Undergraduate: three – to include at least one clinician and one current 4- or 5-year student • Graduate: two – one academic and one clinician
Months in which interviews are held	• November – March (undergraduate) • February (graduate)
Proportion of overseas students	• 7%
Proportion of mature students	• Not known
Proportion of graduate students	• 7%
Faculty's view of students taking a gap year	• Acceptable if student is spending time in a positive way
Proportion of students taking intercalated degrees	• 15%
Possibility of direct entrance to clinical phase	• No
Fees for overseas students	• See website for details
Fees for graduates	• See website for details
Ability to transfer to other medical schools If so, under what circumstances	• Applications to transfer will each be considered in their own right. Financial and family health reasons are usually accepted. However, transfers require a mutual acceptance from the receiving medical school.
Assistance for elective funding	• Several bursaries available to compete for.
Assistance for travel to attachments	• Free transport provided to placements in year 3, clinical placement costs reimbursed in years 4 and 5. A car-sharing scheme is in the pipeline!

Access and hardship funds	• Financial contingency funds available to those in serious financial difficulty.
Weekly rent	• £50–£60
Pint of lager	• £1.50
Cinema	• £5
Nightclub	• £5

Derby

Key facts	Graduate
Course length	4 years
Total number of medical undergraduates	181
Applicants in 2006	1033
Interviews given in 2006	237
Places available in 2006	91
Places available in 2007	91
Open days 2007	May (for those students with an offer of a place) General open days to be confirmed
Entrance requirements	2:2 degree in any discipline
Mandatory subjects	N/A
Male:female ratio	59:41
Is an exam included in the selection process?	Yes
If yes, what form does this exam take?	GAMSAT
Qualification gained	BMBS

Fascinating fact: Derby is as far south as Bonnie Prince Charlie and his army reached.

Editor's note: If you are considering applying to Derby it is worthwhile reading the Nottingham chapter too, as, due to the proximity of the cities, there will be a large amount of relevant information in it.

The graduate entry medicine (GEM) course at Derby is situated in a purpose-designed medical school (opened in 2003) in the grounds of the Derby City General Hospital. Students study for 18 months in Derby and then join the same 30-month clinical practice course as the Nottingham undergraduates. Successful students graduate with BMBS degrees from the University of Nottingham. Entrants are graduates of any discipline who are selected by interviews offered to those achieving high enough GAMSAT scores (cut-off varies each year). Derby and St George's operate a joint admissions process so candidates who apply to both places may be interviewed at either. Applications may be made to both the 5-year Nottingham course and 4-year Derby course without prejudice to either. It may be helpful to read the Nottingham chapter in addition to this.

Education

The preclinical course lasts for 18 months and is based around problem-based learning (PBL). A PBL group usually consists of seven students and a facilitator, who may or may not be a clinician. PBL is good fun but demands a certain amount of private study to be effective. There is a new case each week over three sessions with lectures specific to each case supporting the week's work. PBL cases are divided into successive blocks: foundation, musculoskeletal, respiratory, cardiovascular, alimentary, renal, neuroscience, endocrine and cancer. Anatomy is taught in lectures and workshops where you handle prosected material. Anatomy teaching is one of the most enjoyable parts of the course.

The highly prided personal and professional development (PPD) programme is composed of clinical skills workshops, lectures and GP placements. Clinical skills workshops teach basic procedures, such as listening to heart sounds and taking blood pressure, as well as communication skills. There are sessions linked to each block covering the examination skills for that system, and at the end of each block there is a 'patient with …' session where patients with relevant conditions come in and discuss their experiences.

There are nine visits to your designated GP surgery, to observe and practise basic examination and history-taking skills, during the preclinical months. These visits form the basis for some case write-ups as part of your PPD portfolio in both years of the PBL course. The clinical practice course is as described for Nottingham.

Teaching

Teaching is largely by clinicians practising in the Derbyshire area. There are a few in-house academics for core material, while some travel from Nottingham to lecture. Feedback is sought on lecturer performance and lecture content and changes are made where necessary from year to year. The quality of overall lectures is considered overall to be high by existing students.

Assessment

After the first 18 months of the course, anatomy, physiology and psychosocial aspects are assessed with a set of final written exams (short essay and multiple choice). Students may also have an objective structured clinical examination (OSCE) at this time, but it is usual to complete assessments of clinical skills as an ongoing part of the course and an OSCE is only run if necessary. A PPD portfolio must be submitted for review at the end of years 1 and 2. Failing the portfolio is virtually the only barrier to progression at the end of year 1. A formative exam is set at the end of each PBL block, the results of which are indicative only and do not contribute to the final degree mark. The clinical years, the final 30 months, are assessed as described for Nottingham (see the Nottingham chapter for more information).

Intercalated degrees

These are not available since all entrants are graduates. Unlike the 5-year Nottingham students, GEM students do not obtain a BMedSci degree.

Facilities

Access to the building is available 24 hours a day, 7 days a week. The library, lecture theatre and anatomy suite have set hours of access. Walk-in access is available to anatomical learning aids throughout the day. Each group of seven students has exclusive access, via key code, to their own PBL base room; each is equipped with two computers (with CD-RW), tables, white boards, lockers and a set of core textbooks. Students also have access to a café area with sofas. There is a pool table in the building for student use.

Library The library is very well stocked with the latest editions of many texts. All of the core texts are multiple-stocked in both the short and week-long loan sections. The library will often purchase books suggested by users. There are few paper journals held but online access is available for many more. Photocopying facilities and 10 computers, linked to a printer, are available. The library is open until 9:45 PM on weeknights and is also open at the weekends. Library staff run skills sessions on, for example, using online databases. GEM students also have full access to the Greenfield Medical Library, at the QMC in Nottingham, and may use the library of the Derby City General Hospital. There is a public library in the city centre.

Computers There are over 100 computers available in the computer rooms, with a laser printer, colour inkjet printer and quiet work desks. All computers in the building are linked to the University of Nottingham network with fast broadband Internet access. PowerPoint lecture presentations are available from the GEM website, along with a vast amount of learning resources. The PBL scenarios, and all associated learning materials, are also on the website. Email is widely used for communication within the school, along with the bulletin board on the GEM website. Access is available to the computers at all times, and most have 250MB ZIP drives and USB ports.

Clinical skills centre Extra practice with medical equipment can be booked between 9 AM and 5 PM.

Welfare

Student support

Because the course is quite small, staff and students have a friendly and close relationship on first-name terms. Each student is assigned a personal mentor – a member of staff available to help with both personal and academic issues – and students meet with them after each block to formally review progress and set goals. Meetings are relaxed and staff are very approachable. Each year 1 PBL group has a parent group in year 2. A counsellor is available at the medical school site and all of the university and Students' Union services described for Nottingham are also available to GEM students.

Accommodation

Accommodation at Brookside Hall is available in year 1. Brookside Hall was built in 2001 and is composed of self-catering houses with six or seven students, each with a private bathroom. Each room has phone and dial-up points with broadband coming. About half the new intake opt for university accommodation each year and the rest usually share private accommodation. Many students purchase houses or flats during the course, but there is also a wide range of rented accommodation available to suit most tastes.

Placements

The placements are the same as described for the Nottingham students, as what follows also appears in the Nottingham chapter.

The teaching hospitals are all located within 1 rush-hour drive of Nottingham. Transport is provided for clinical visits in years 1 and 2. The smaller hospitals are generally friendlier (as they have more time to talk to you), but sometimes more work is expected from you. Students usually arrange to share lifts, as some hospitals can be very difficult to travel to via public transport. Accommodation is provided free of charge in Lincoln, otherwise you are expected to travel daily. At Nottingham students can state preferences for where their attachments are. It is unlikely that any student will have all their attachments in Nottingham itself, so a degree of travelling is inevitable.

Location of clinical placement/ name of hospital	Distance away from Nottingham medical school (miles)	Difficulty getting there on public transport*
Nottingham City Hospital	5	
Derby Royal Infirmary	20	
Derby City General Hospital	25	
Kings Mill Hospital, Mansfield	30	
Lincoln Hospital	45	

* : walking/cycling distance; : use public transport; : need own car or lift; : get up early – tricky to get to!

Sports and social

City life

Derby is a compact city with historical areas and newer areas. There are several regeneration projects ongoing and the city is generally pleasant and welcoming. Derby has well-connected train and bus stations, with a return bus ticket to Nottingham costing between £2 and £6.50 depending on time of travel. Buses back from Nottingham operate through the small hours on Saturday and Sunday mornings, with a journey of about 20–30 minutes. Most major high-street names can be found and there are strangely almost as many banks as shops! A multitude of pubs and bars, many with late licences, cater for those who like a quiet drink almost as well as those who like to dance and karaoke into the night. The medical school is about 40 minutes' walk away from the centre of Derby. A retail park, with a Sainsbury's, Boots and B&Q, is found near the school, and Tesco is within driving distance (although I once walked it in the blistering summer's heat – never again!). Buses into the city centre from near the medical school or halls are frequent and cost £1.90 return at most. Parking near the medical school in the hospital staff car park costs around £110 for a permit that lasts a year. The surrounding area of Derbyshire is very beautiful and rambling is popular.

University life

All students are automatically members of the University of Nottingham Students' Union but travelling can become tiresome without a car. Affiliate membership of the University of Derby Students' Union can be bought for a small fee and provides access to their societies and sports facilities. GEMSoc is the in-house society for arranging social and sporting events. The anatomy society GEM Cutters provides an opportunity to perform dissection. GEM students are proactive in arranging entertainment, often for charitable purposes, and recent years have seen a charity slave auction, a cheese and wine evening and a gruesomely funny end-of-year revue, to mention but three.

Sports life

Football, hockey, netball, squash and tennis are all played. Hockey and football tours were held in 2005, taking in Budapest and Dublin amongst other places. The course seems to attract active people and there are many walkers, cavers and climbers. A small karate class is held weekly and there are salsa dancing and yoga classes. Anything that isn't already happening is easy to set up as there are usually at least a few people interested. There is often the opportunity to challenge the Nottingham undergraduates and to train with them.

Great things about Derby

- Attractive new purpose-designed building.
- Excellent teaching and facilities, with dedicated staff.
- Wide mix of students with different degrees and life experiences.
- Close community atmosphere.
- Much of the teaching is by clinicians who are very enthusiastic about the course.

Bad things about Derby

- You can feel fairly isolated from the main university and Students' Union.
- A few people find the city lacking in excitement.
- The course is relatively small and some may find it insular.
- Living and working with medics can lead to medicine overload!
- As with many other universities, there are too many students to compete with in the clinical years following the UK expansion of medical student numbers.

Further information

Nottingham

Admissions Officer
Faculty Office
Queen's Medical Centre
University of Nottingham
Nottingham NG7 2RD
Tel: 0115 970 9379
Fax: 0115 970 9922
Email: medschool@nottingham.ac.uk
Web: http://www.nottingham.ac.uk

Derby

Admissions Officer
GEM Course Office
The Medical School
Derby City General Hospital
Uttoxeter Road
Derby DE22 3DT
Tel: 01332 724622
Email:gem@nottingham.ac.uk
Web: http://www.nottingham.ac.uk/mhs/gem

Additional application information	
Average A level requirements	• N/A
Average Scottish Higher requirements	• N/A
Make-up of interview panel	• Clinicians, academics and lay people
Months in which interviews are held for 2007 entry	• March – April
Proportion of overseas students	• Only open to EU students, no international students
Proportion of mature students	• All graduate students – age range 21+
Proportion of graduate students	• 100%

(Continued)

(Continued)

Faculty's view of students taking a gap year	• Acceptable provided constructively used
Proportion of students taking intercalated degrees	• 0%
Possibility of direct entrance to clinical phase	• No
Fees for overseas students	• N/A
Fees for graduates	• £3000 pa
Ability to transfer to other medical schools If so, under what circumstances	• No
Assistance for elective funding	• Not directly, but students are invited to apply for elective prizes.
Assistance for travel to attachments	• No, students must apply to their LEA and the medical school will validate the claim.
Access and hardship funds	• Yes, but must be paid back in the future. All cases dealt with anonymously.
Weekly rent	• £60 (self-catering halls) • £50–£70 (private)
Pint of lager	• £1.40 Union bar • £2.20 city centre pub
Cinema	• £4 with NUS card
Nightclub	• Free–£4 Monday to Friday

Dundee

Key facts	Preclinical	Undergraduate
Course length	6 years	5 years
Total number of medical undergraduates	5	770
Applicants in 2006	158	1533
Interviews given in 2006	8	469
Places available in 2006	Up to 10	154
Places available in 2007	Up to 10	154
Open days 2007	To be confirmed	
Entrance requirements	AAA	AAA
Mandatory subjects	Non-sciences	Chemistry
Male:female ratio	1:4 (actual)	44:56
Is an exam included in the selection process?	Yes	Yes
If yes, what form does this exam take?	UKCAT	UKCAT
Qualification gained	Entry to 5-year MBChB course	MBChB

Fascinating fact: Dundee is home to Professor Sir David Lane, ranked in the top 10 biochemists in the world, and discoverer of the ubiquitous p53 cancer gene.

Dundee is a modern, friendly, progressive and forward-thinking medical school with an international reputation. The new curriculum was introduced in 1993. Dundee medics have a reputation for being friendly, fun-loving and down-to-earth. Intake is approximately 40% Scottish, 35% Northern Irish, 5% Republic of Ireland, 10% English and 10% overseas. Dundee is extremely supportive of graduate/mature students and encourages applications from a wide variety of backgrounds. Over 16% of every year are graduate/mature students, and each year also has about seven entrants from the premed course. The curriculum offers good staff–student participation and has achievable learning goals with a realistic workload. Students obtain real clinical experience with direct patient contact from the start of year 1. Clinical teaching is phased in from year 2, and by year 4 the content is 100% clinical. The twelve Dundee learning outcomes, now adopted by all Scottish medical schools, direct learning and assessment throughout the course.

Problem-orientated, student-centred and community-based, the medical course at Dundee closely follows recommendations from *Tomorrow's Doctors* made by the GMC. The Dundee course was rated 'Excellent' in 1997 by the Scottish Higher Education Funding Council Quality Assessors.

Dundee is an exceptional place to study medicine, not just in terms of the high quality of the teaching programme, but also the facilities available. Ninewells Hospital and Medical School, the largest purpose-built teaching hospital in Europe, is the centre of many areas of pioneering research in cancer, keyhole surgery, heart disease, drug development and medical education.

Education

The first cohort from the new-style course graduated in 2000 and the integrated course is well established. Teaching is structured around body systems. Phase I is an introduction to the basic principles of anatomy, biomedical science, safe medical practice and psychosocial and disease mechanisms, and runs during the first semester. Phase II runs from Christmas in year 1 to the end of year 3 and concentrates on learning about abnormal structure and function. Phase III (years 4 and 5) deals with diagnosing and treating abnormal structure and function. Student-selected components comprise approximately one-third of the undergraduate course.

Teaching

The integrated, systematic course at Dundee is under constant review to improve and develop its design.

The main component of the first three years (phases I and II) is an integrated body systems course dealing with normal and abnormal structure, function and behaviour. Contributions come from anatomy, biochemistry, physiology, pharmacology and behavioural sciences, and there is a systematic study of clinical medicine, including health promotion and disease prevention. Early contact with real and simulated patients is promoted in the learning environments of community, hospital ward and clinical skills centre.

Phase III consists of a range of clinical experiences, skills and knowledge which are built around 12 learning outcomes gained in phases I and II. All students are provided with a study guide, including timetables, a summary of clinical skills, tutorial questions, problem-solving cases, a recommended reading list and a list of online resources.

Teaching is delivered through lectures and in small groups. In order to illustrate the clinical relevance of the teaching, patients are brought along to the lecture theatre to demonstrate examinations, signs and symptoms and treatments. Dissection classes accompany the anatomy lectures to aid the integration of theory and practice. Time is also spent seeing patients on the wards and in an outpatient clinic setting, learning clinical skills in the clinical skills centre, and in general practice/primary care. To promote multidisciplinary aspects of the healthcare team, teaching takes place jointly between the medical, nursing and midwifery students at appropriate times in the course.

During years 4 and 5 (phase III), students further advance their understanding of medicine through clinical attachments and learning through 100 core clinical problems, which bring together your experiences in the attachments. The core component of the programme emphasizes the competencies necessary for a newly qualified doctor to work in the hospital or community.

Year 4 comprises 10 rotations, each lasting 4 weeks, and students are able to choose their own rotations for some of these attachments. There is less formal teaching during year 4, but tutorials on the core clinical problems are provided by rotation supervisors. Year 4 students also receive a Themed Therapeutics study guide and can attend optional tutorials throughout the year.

Year 5 officially begins with an elective on which a report must be submitted. The remainder of year 5 comprises 7 rotations of 4-weeks duration. Students pick their rotations from a list, but there is also the option to self-propose rotations. The shadowing rotations allow students to become *au fait* with the jobs they will be doing when they graduate, and are usually spent in the hospital where the student has obtained a job for the foundation house officer year.

Dundee has a very active peer tutoring programme, in which year 4 and 5 students hold tutorials for year 2 and 3 students to clarify difficult points and to go through case scenarios/exam-style questions. The junior students find this very valuable and the senior students enjoy teaching. The medical school provides support for the programme through the curriculum secretary, who posts sign-up lists, photocopies materials for the tutors and organizes the tutorial groups, tutorial times and venues.

Assessment

A range of assessment methods is used including written tests, patient management problems, clinical examinations and portfolios. The initial phases of the course are currently being restructured so detailed information on assessments in the first three years is not yet available.

The medical finals at Dundee are currently split into two parts. Part 1 is taken at the end of year 4 and comprises two CRQ papers and an OSCE (practical component). Part 2 comprises a portfolio examination at the conclusion of year 5.

Intercalated degrees

Most students wishing to complete an intercalated degree do so between years 3 and 4. However, it is also possible to take it between years 4 and 5, in a range of medical subjects. Students can opt to take an intercalated degree at one of the London medical schools.

Special study modules and electives

Student selected components (SSCs) comprise approximately one-third of the undergraduate course and can be chosen from a wide selection of modules, or by your own design. Some SSCs may be undertaken abroad, e.g. the 7-week elective in phase III or medical French followed by a clinical SSC in France. Others are mini-research projects that may be published in scientific journals. Prizes are awarded to students for work of particular merit in SSCs.

Staff are very supportive of individually designed SSCs arranged in their clinics, laboratories and wards.

Year 5 kicks off with a 7-week elective from July to September, which includes a 2- or 3-week vacation. It is up to you to organize your own programme.

Erasmus

The medical school does not participate in the Erasmus scheme. However, SSCs provide an opportunity to travel abroad and the medical school offers an SSC in France.

Facilities

Library   Year 1 books are housed in a large multi-faculty library on the main campus. Year 2–5 books are housed at the Ninewells medical library. Normal opening hours for the Ninewells library are Monday, Wednesday, Friday 9 AM–5 PM; Tuesday and Thursday 9 AM–10 PM; Saturday 12 noon–5 PM; closed Sunday. The main campus library is open 9 AM–10 PM during term time; Saturday 12 noon–5 PM; Sunday 12 noon–7 PM. There is good availability of reference books, but be prepared to reserve some books in advance. Library opening hours increase as the academic year progresses.

Computers   There is extensive computer access at both Ninewells (open 8 AM–11 PM all week) and the main campus. The computers in Ninewells are modern, with flat screens, and provide fast internet access with designated areas for wireless connection, which can also be found in the main campus library. Facilities include computer-assisted learning (CAL) tutorials, microbiology laboratory summaries, MCQs, MRI/CT/X-ray imaging and revision sessions.

Clinical skills   The purpose-built clinical skills centre opened in 1997. It provides multi-professional teaching to small groups in areas such as: communication and history taking; professional attitudes and ethics; physical examination and laboratory skills; diagnostics and therapeutics; practical skills; and resuscitation. The clinical and administrative staff are very supportive, and run a book-in service for clinical skills revision sessions. Facilities include: access to anatomical models and mannequins; diagnostic, therapeutic and resuscitation equipment; videos; simulated and real patients; and telemedicine links.

Welfare

Student support

The staff at Dundee are friendly and approachable. They make an effort to ensure that all students receive the clinical training, core knowledge and time for small group work required by the new curriculum.

Each student is assigned a personal tutor. There is a special-needs coordinator based at Student Welfare on the main campus. The Dean operates a student-friendly, open-door policy and lecturers and clinicians are equally approachable.

All medical freshers are sent a student-produced *Student Survival Guide*, which covers academics, social, sport and local transport. The Dundee University Medical Society (DUMS) run a Senior–Junior scheme. All new students who want to participate are paired with a senior student who gives them academic advice and, perhaps most importantly, introduces them to the social scene.

The faculty at Dundee are very keen to receive student feedback and always strive to improve aspects of the course in response. The Medical Students Council (MSC) regularly attend faculty meetings to voice student opinions and also run a careers fair, women in medicine evening, annual symposium, electives evening and PRHO meetings for students.

A good indicator of staff–student relations is the number of staff who regularly attend year club and Medical School balls.

The medical school has good wheelchair access.

Accommodation

A programme of new building work is currently underway (for completion in 2006) for over 1000 new bedrooms, all with *en-suite* shower/toilet and IT network.

Dundee University currently has eight self-catering residences. Each residence comprises of a number of self-contained apartments accommodating between 2 and 12 residents with shared kitchen facilities. Residences built within the last 10 years offer *en-suite* shower and toilet within each single bedroom (Belmont, Seabraes and West Park Villas), while the older residences have shared shower and toilet facilities and a limited number of twin occupancy rooms. All the residences are furnished and a limited cleaning service is provided for shared kitchens and common areas. The accommodation is let for the full academic year, i.e. 37 weeks from the beginning of the session and includes freshers' week. The university (via the website) provides information about rent levels and full breakdown of services provided. Private accommodation costs £45-£80 per week depending on your requirements.

Placements

There are occasional hospital and GP placements in year 1, but years 2–5 are hospital based. Many students walk (30 minutes), cycle or drive to the hospital but numerous buses run (approx. fare £1.10) and there is now a free university bus running from campus to Ninewells and back throughout the day. Car parking is available at £1.50 per day (£23 per month by direct debit for unlimited entry to staff car parks).

In years 2 and 3, ward teaching is at Ninewells Hospital. Up to 5 months of year 4 can be spent away from Dundee on out-blocks if desired. Rotations in district general hospitals and general practice are set up around Scotland (including the Highlands and Islands) and the north of England, with free accommodation provided. Travel expenses can be reimbursed by applying to the NHS directly for student funding. The university only reimburses for travel during rural GP placements. A computer-matching system allocates students to their peripheral attachments on a best-fit basis so most students can stay in Dundee if they wish, although for many the experience of peripheral hospitals is a highlight.

Location of clinical placement/ name of hospital	Distance away from medical school (miles)	Difficulty getting there on public transport*
Ninewells	3	
Perth	22.5	
Queen Margaret, Dunfermline	45.3	
Airdrie	78.2	
Whitehaven	206.7	

* : walking/cycling distance; : use public transport; : need own car or lift;
 : get up early – tricky to get to!

Sports and social

City life

Dundee is Scotland's fourth largest city and has a beautiful location on the Firth of Tay. Local sights include: the riverside itself; the neighbouring seaside town of Broughty Ferry with its sandy beaches, castle, shops and pubs; Tentsmuir Forest Park and beaches; Carnoustie; St Andrews (15 miles away); numerous golf courses; and fantastic sunsets. Glasgow, Edinburgh and Aberdeen are all within reach for a weekend jaunt, being a 1–1½-hour drive/train journey away.

Dundee is currently undergoing a facelift to transform it into a modern, up-to-date city. A new shopping centre, the Overgate, opened in 2000, vastly improving Dundee's shopping facilities, while the past 18 months have seen the opening of many new trendy shops, cafés, bars and clubs in Dundee's West End.

Despite these ongoing changes, Dundee remains very student-friendly, and the area around the university is very much a student community. Taxis are affordable, and bars cater for students through abundant drinks promotions. Property prices in Dundee are also still reasonable, although they have increased considerably in recent years.

University life

Dundee University Medical Society (DUMS) sponsors freshers' week events, and puts on many social bashes and trips throughout the year. DUMS tends to form a large part of a medic's social life, especially in the earlier years. Each year also has its own year club, which organizes events, e.g. end-of-year balls, fancy-dress parties, nights out, pub visits, golf and slave auctions – to raise money for charity. Ceilidhs (Scottish dancing) are very popular and are a great ice-breaker – lessons are given for the uninitiated. Each year club organises a halfway dinner (a weekend away at a hotel with a ball, etc.) guess when – halfway through the course – and their own graduation ball (there is also a university graduation ball).

The Student's Union building has undergone major refurbishment in the past 2 years. The new Air Bar opened in September 2004 and the existing bars and clubs have also been dramatically overhauled. They were always good but are now even better – very modern and trendy. The Student's Union regularly hosts packed-out club nights through the week, and is very popular with medics and non-medics alike. Local pubs abound (some hosting live music) and the beer is cheap. The Dundee Repertory Theatre is active nationally, and hosts plays, musicals and jazz festivals. The popular Dundee Contemporary Arts Centre (DCA) provides two screens for art-house films, a large art gallery, café and wine bar, all right beside the university. Unfortunately, Dundee only has one multiplex cinema, which is located on the outskirts of the city and can be difficult to get to without a car. The Duncan of Jordanstone Art School is part of the main campus, adding diversity to the student population, and their summer degree show is always a sell-out. The university also has the usual wide variety of societies and sporting organizations.

Sports life

Dundee has some of the most modern and extensive sports facilities in Scotland – indoors and outdoors. On campus there is a sports centre with two multi-purpose halls, gymnasium and fitness suite, a 25-metre pool with sauna and 4 floodlit all-weather tennis courts. Off campus there is a 33-acre sports ground for all major team sports, a water activities centre for sailing on the estuary and the countryside nearby provides outdoor activities all year round – canoeing, skiing, rambling and climbing, horse riding or pony trekking.

The university has a very active and varied sports scene, with over 40 sports clubs in existence providing a good level of competition at both Scottish and National university level. The medical school has its own teams in football, rugby and netball. Competitions are organized against other Scottish medical schools. Medics often play for both the medical school and the university, with the medical school teams being a little less competitive in spirit than the university teams.

Great things about Dundee

- Good teaching on an established new-style course with early patient exposure.
- Good social life based around DUMS and a friendly bunch of staff and students means that you can always find something to do.
- Dundee is a cheap, safe and fun place to live.
- The clinical skills centre is excellent.
- Dundee is surrounded by beautiful countryside, with access to skiing, hill walking, water sports and places such as St Andrews are close by for day trips.

Bad things about Dundee

- It can take some time to get used to the local accent.
- Dundee is not a great centre for shopping.
- There is no major airport in Dundee.

- It does get cold and windy over the winter.
- It can be difficult to park at Ninewells.

Further information

Information Centre
Admissions and Student Recruitment
2 Airlie Place
The University of Dundee
Nethergate
Dundee DD1 4HN
Tel: 01382 384697 (admissions)
    01382 384160 (prospectus requests)
    01382 388111 (international)
Fax: 01382 388150
Email: srs@dundee.ac.uk
Web: http://www.dundee.ac.uk

Additional application information	
Average A level requirements	• AAA
Average Scottish Higher requirements	• AAAAB (pre-medicine course) • AAABB (medicine course)
Make-up of interview panel	• Faculty members
Months in which interviews are held	• January – March
Proportion of overseas students	• 7.5%
Proportion of mature students	• 2.5%
Proportion of graduate students	• 13%
Faculty's view of students taking a gap year	• Will be considered
Proportion of students taking intercalated degrees	• 12%
Possibility of direct entrance to clinical phase	• No

Fees for overseas students	• £8000 (premedical year) • £12,800 pa (preclinical years) • £19,800 pa (clinical years)
Fees for graduates	• £2700 pa (paid by all UK/EU students)
Ability to transfer to other medical schools If so, under what circumstances	• Students are free to transfer to other medical schools if another school has a place for them.
Assistance for elective funding	• Dependent on faculty funds
Assistance for travel to attachments	• No – responsibility of LEA/ELB/SAAS, but accommodation is provided.
Access and hardship funds	• There is a university hardship fund available.
Weekly rent	• £60–£90 (furnished)
Pint of lager	• £2.00
Cinema	• £3.50 with student ID
Nightclub	• £3.50 with student ID

Dundee

East Anglia

Key facts	Undergraduate
Course length	5 years
Total number of medical undergraduates	651
Applicants in 2006	1500
Interviews given in 2006	700
Places available in 2006	168
Places available in 2007	168
Open days 2007	In July and October
Entrance requirements	AAB at A2, plus B at 4th AS level
Mandatory subjects	Biology or human biology
Male:female ratio	Information not available
Is an exam included in the selection process?	Yes
If yes, what form does this exam take?	UKCAT
Qualification gained	MB/BS

Fascinating fact: James Paget, who was born in 1814 in Great Yarmouth, is eponymously associated with various conditions, including Paget's disease of the bone and nipple! A three-star hospital named after him hosts UEA medical students.

The University of East Anglia is one of the new medical schools, set in a scenic campus environment in Norwich. The syllabus is exciting and innovative, with the university offering early access to patients (in week 1), as well as unique ways of learning to become a competent doctor. The university motto is 'do different', and the students and staff are a credit to this saying. Apart from a very strong support structure, the university hospital (only a 10 minute walk away) offers an ideal opportunity to socialize and to learn from junior doctors in the Norfolk region. Placement is not limited to hospitals either, UEA links you with general practice and community care so you can get a feel of other areas of medicine. The latest GMC report confirmed that the course will get its seal of approval at the end of the year, and the first cohort of students will be entering practice in 2007. It is an exciting time to be at UEA, a university which truly prides itself in being different.

Education 🔖

A range of qualifications are accepted including A levels, degree courses, nursing diplomas and access programmes, but candidates must have a strong background in biology – a grade B or above in A2 biology or human biology. Applications are scored according to evidence of being a team member as well as working in a self-directed environment, motivation, responsibility and personal effectiveness. Admissions tutors are looking for motivated well-rounded individuals who will flourish at UEA, who can be effective both independently and as part of a team.

The curriculum is innovative, and in some respects controversial, in that the structure places patients at the centre of learning. Clinical exposure starts from the beginning of the course with integrated teaching at university, general practice and hospitals. Communication skills and an understanding of people are paramount to the way this course addresses issues surrounding patient-centred medicine.

Teaching

The course is systems-based and is divided into 14 units (e.g. locomotion, paediatrics), each lasting around 13 weeks. A majority of time is spent in university-based teaching, with 1 day a week in primary care and the remaining 4 days in university, as well as 4 weeks of each unit in secondary care.

The university teaching block is the time to acquire knowledge and understanding of the unit being studied so that this can be implemented during clinical time in primary and secondary care. A typical week consists first of PBL group sessions, with each member having responsibility for preparing their topic to present and explain to the group, as well as maintaining their own broader reading of the week's theme. Lectures (the whole year group) and seminars (groups of around 30) take place throughout the week and provide formal teaching. Students decide which seminars to attend – it is not possible to attend all of them. This is deliberate and allows the group system to be more effective with students feeding back to their peers and learning to rely upon each other as well as reducing total contact time for each student. Anatomy seminars are an exception and are compulsory. Cadavers are used to illustrate relevant anatomy.

Each student also meets their Inter Professional Learning group on a weekly basis. This is a group composed of medical, nursing and midwifery students and other allied health professionals. These sessions take a similar format to PBL sessions and are aimed at improving understanding of the different roles of healthcare professionals.

One day a week students see patients who are relevant either to that week's theme or the unit in general, as well as observing GPs and other professionals, practising clinical skills and taking part in group teaching.

There is a continuous block of 4 or 5 weeks spent at the Norfolk and Norwich University Hospital (NNUH) in Norwich or the James Paget Hospital (JPH) in Great Yarmouth. Time is spent observing clinics and surgery, seeing patients, and learning and practising clinical skills.

In preparation for the transition from student to doctor, UEA students will shadow a junior house officer in the months before they graduate. Where possible, the school intends this to be with one of their NHS partners in the region.

Assessment

Students are required to take part in formal assessment procedures in a number of formats during the MB/BS programme.

- Mini-OSCEs: they consist of six 5–10-minute stations and assess communication, clinical skills and medical knowledge for a unit.
- Integrative Period Portfolio Report: a reflective appraisal of the year. Students write about personal experiences, illustrating that the GMC's expectations of what makes a good doctor are being met.
- Integrative Period OSCE: this is a larger OSCE consisting of 18–24 stations of 5–10-minutes duration. It assesses all aspects of the course completed thus far.
- Integrative Period Advance Notice Paper: this comprises two parts – extended matching questions (EMQs) and advance notice questions (ANQs). The ANQ is based upon 6 PBL-like scenarios. These scenarios are provided 2 weeks before the assessment. The student prepares notes that are brought into the exam. The actual ANQ is based upon three of the scenarios.

All assessed work during the units is awarded Pass/Fail. The integrative period assessments are awarded Distinction/Pass/Fail. Two or more distinctions are required to obtain an overall distinction for the year.

Intercalated degrees

There are currently no students undertaking intercalated degrees at UEA. These will start in September 2006.

Special study modules and electives

All students are required to take student selected studies (SSS), which are divided into presentation and research. In years 1 and 2, titles of presentations are prearranged but students formulate their own titles from year 3 onwards. Ten-minute presentations take place at the end of each unit in front of peers and tutors with 5 minutes for questions afterwards. Presentations are formally assessed.

The research element in years 1 and 2 involves learning how to critically appraise scientific papers and is formally assessed at the ends of units 1–5 in years 1 and 2 via a written appraisal of a given paper. While to most students it is not the most interesting assignment, its usefulness comes into light during year 4, when students have to design and conduct their own research project.

In years 3 and 4, students study a subject outside medicine (SOM), which range from astrology to languages, creative writing to geology. Assessments vary in nature.

The current year 4 students are looking forward to their 8-week elective at the end of the 2005–06 academic year.

Facilities

The medical school building was built in 2002 and holds spacious seminar rooms equipped with state-of-the-art equipment. There is a small common area in the lobby with hot drinks, water and snack machines. Space can be limited at times.

The medical school utilizes university facilities so lectures and seminars are split between various buildings.

Library   UEA boasts a large, well stocked library. A new £2m library extension is nearly completed and some improvements have already been noticed. Medical textbooks have a lot more shelf space and supplies have doubled! We also have access to the hospital libraries.

Computers   The course relies on a virtual learning environment called Blackboard so computer access is essential for all students. The medical school building offers 24-hour access but it gets busy during lunchtimes and minutes before student deadlines! There are also terminals and round-the-clock access at UEA's library. At the NNUH there are networked computers exclusively for students on placement. Network access is available (and free) in all campus residences.

Clinical skills   The medical school works very closely with the NNUH, who have set aside a designated 'ward' specifically for student teaching. It includes a well-equipped clinical skills lab with a variety of equipment, from prosthetic arms for blood taking to dummy models for rectal examination. The JPH, which shares the responsibility for hospital teaching during attachments, also has an excellent clinical skills lab.

There is a structured clinical skills programme extending across the 5-year course, with gradual additions to the student 'armory'. Skills begin basic, with hand-washing and observation skills, and progress with relevant units, for example: venepuncture during haematology, catheterisation during urology, and so on.

Communication skills are core to the medical education ethos provided at the UEA and are taught extensively in year 1, with supplementary training periodically thereafter both to refresh and build upon the students' proficiency. The sessions are predominantly conducted in small student groups and incorporate trained actors who role-play the parts of patients.

Welfare 🏠

The majority of students are mature although the percentage of school leavers has increased slightly. The great diversity of students is one of the great strengths of UEA.

Several medical school students are parents and they are happy with structures in place regarding childcare. A brand new campus nursery opened in September 2005 offering more than 100 places. It is relatively inexpensive and the university provides additional financial support for students ineligible for government help. There is also a newly opened nursery at the NNUH. The medical school ensures that students with small children do not travel too far on placement.

Student Support

Medical school staff are friendly and approachable and make a point of getting to know students individually. Each student has a personal advisor from the academic or clinical staff with whom they can discuss personal or academic issues.

A mentor scheme run by medical students ensures that everyone has a supportive peer in the year above them as a first point of contact for help and advice. This improves integration between years.

The medical school also uses UEA's support services. The Dean of Students is responsible for university welfare and extensive services are also provided by the Union of Students. Problems on campus are addressed by resident tutors, senior students living in halls, and the Chaplaincy is also located on campus.

Accommodation

The accommodation on the UEA campus combines nature with architecture. The famous Ziggurat residences (Norfolk and Suffolk Terrace) are listed buildings. Campus accommodation is guaranteed to first-year students and all residences are self-catering. Some are *en-suite* while others have shared bathroom facilities. There are also twin and shared rooms available.

A UEA medical student needs a longer accommodation contract compared to others (42 weeks versus the normal 38). The university tries to keep health professional students together so you won't be on your own for the extra teaching weeks.

The Village, Nelson Court and Constable Terrace residences (*en-suite* flats with a shared kitchen) giving a greater feeling of independence from the rest of university with all the advantages of proximity to the university or Norwich. New residences have recently been built with a mixture of *en-suite* and shared bathroom facilities and are self-catering.

The university has guest facilities, with parents able to stay at the Nelson Court Guest Suite.

In addition there is an extensive range of privately let housing in Norwich. The main student area is 'The Golden Triangle', which is 30 minutes' walk from UEA and has bus routes into campus.

Placements

Each PBL group is allocated a GP surgery at the beginning of the year, which they visit once a week to cover the week's practical learning objectives. These occur in surgeries across Norfolk, Suffolk and Cambridgeshire.

Students attend secondary-care attachments within each unit, which take place either at the NNUH or the JPH. The corresponding hospital department is responsible for organizing various activities and teaching sessions (ranging from sitting in clinics to major surgery). There is a degree of flexibility in the timetable, allowing students to accommodate their particular areas of interest.

The medical school provides transport to all placements that are not within walking or cycling distance.

Location of clinical placement/ name of hospital	Distance away from medical school (miles)	Difficulty getting there on public transport*
Norfolk and Norwich University Hospital	1	🚶
James Paget Hospital	32	🚌
General practice attachments	Across Norfolk and Suffolk	🚌

* 🚶: walking/cycling distance; 🚌 : use public transport; 🚗: need own car or lift;
✈: get up early – tricky to get to!

Sports and social

City life

Norwich is not just the 'capital' of Norfolk but a vibrant regional city attracting visitors from across the world. Steeped in history, there are two magnificent cathedrals, a Norman castle and numerous medieval buildings. Admiral Lord Nelson went to school in Norwich and once famously remarked: 'I am myself a Norfolk man ... and glory in being so.'

Shopping is another attraction. Norwich has a large open-air market and two shopping centres – Castle Mall and the new Chapelfield Centre. One local journalist described it as a scheme that would 'not look out of place in a European capital city'. A medieval church and a mosque nestle up against Chapel Fields. Visitors can experience the strange juxtaposition of getting to the shops via a churchyard full of elegant Regency tombstones.

Norwich's club land is the centre of East Anglia nightlife, although students used to big city life often complain that it's still 'a bit quiet'. Norwich's pub/club scene offers a whole range of student nights and low prices. There are 22 'microbreweries' in Norfolk and real ale is extremely popular in many drinking holes.

Norwich's surroundings are some of the most attractive and unique anywhere in the world, from the waterways of the Norfolk Broads to the vast expanses of the North Norfolk coastline. Rail links to London, Cambridge and the Midlands are good, and many students find it an attractive residence post-graduation.

University life

The social life of medics and other healthcare students is organized by MedSOC (Medical Society).

So far this has been lively and varied, from karaoke nights to informal anatomy classes. Themed nights (including a Footballers' Wives night) are particularly memorable, not forgetting the Christmas balls and spectacular Halfway Ball for third years.

Another core society is MedSIN. Formerly the Medical Students International Network, this national society is open to all Union members. For budding surgeons there is the student-run Surgical Society and those with a speciality interest can join the obstetrics and gynaecology student interest group. There are also over 100 societies, so whatever your interests you're bound to meet like-minded people.

UEA is a self-contained campus with post office, grocery store, book shops and travel agents. In the centre of this thriving metropolis stands the Union bar – providing solace after a gruelling day of lectures and seminars with its cheap alcohol, large-screen TVs and pool tables. The party continues after closing time upstairs in the Large Common Room (LCR), UEA's recently refurbished campus club, guaranteed to provide a memorable night with music, comedy or film. There are numerous eateries and it is famous nationally for the quality of its gig programme – Coldplay, The Darkness, Katie Melua, and Jools Holland have all played at UEA.

The Sainsbury Centre for Visual Arts was architect Norman Foster's first public building and houses the Sainsbury family's extensive arts collection. Students can enter free.

Sports life

From aerobics to athletics, korfball to karate, there is something for everyone. UEA runs an inter-school competition called Ziggurat Challenge in which the medical school finishes consistently in the top three.

Medical sports teams are developing as school numbers increase. Clubs include netball, men's and women's football and rugby teams. Whilst the emphasis is on fun and socializing, all teams train regularly, play in local leagues as well as national medical competitions and have tours planned at home and abroad for the coming seasons. Students also play the hospital and teaching staff annually at football and cricket.

UEA boasts 40 acres of dedicated sports field in addition to Astroturf, brand new tennis courts and local access to water sports. The incredibly popular UEA Sports Park, a Sport England Centre, possesses an Olympic-sized swimming pool, indoor arena, gym, climbing wall and national standard athletics track. All students have free access to the Sports Park and discounted activity rates. Off-peak use of the gym and swimming pool is £1.25.

Great things about UEA 👍

- Clinical teaching and patient contact from week 1.
- Excellent facilities at teaching hospitals coupled with superb teaching.
- A school small enough for staff and students to know each other.
- A campus set in gorgeous countryside.
- A gig programme that no other university can beat.

Bad things about UEA

- Overcrowding! But expansion of the school will be completed by 2007.
- GP surgeries can be miles from the university.
- Campus car parking is a nightmare.
- The school loves feedback forms.
- Concrete – you either love it or hate it.

Further information

The Undergraduate Admissions Office
Faculty of Health
Edith Cavell Building
University of East Anglia
Norwich
Norfolk NR4 7TJ
Tel: 01603 591072
Fax: 01603 597019
Email: med.admiss@uea.ac.uk
Web: http://www.med.uea.ac.uk

Additional application information	
Average A level requirements	• AAB + B at 4th AS
Average Scottish Higher requirements	• AAAABB (standard) AAB (advanced)
Make-up of interview panel	• OSCE style, panel of seven including mix of academic staff and active NHS practitioners/ clinicians
Months in which interviews are held	• January – March
Proportion of overseas students	• 13%
Proportion of mature students	• Information not available
Proportion of graduate students	• Information not available
Faculty's view of students taking a gap year	• Acceptable, but interested in candidate's plans for gap year
Proportion of students taking intercalated degrees	• None at present

(Continued)

East Anglia

(*Continued*)

Possibility of direct entrance to clinical phase	• No / Not applicable
Fees for overseas students	• £17,100 pa
Fees for graduates	• £3000 pa
Ability to transfer to other medical schools If so, under what circumstances	• Due to the unique nature of the course, it may be difficult to transfer to other schools.
Assistance for elective funding	• None as yet.
Assistance for travel to attachments	• All transport is provided.
Access and hardship funds	• Plenty of access through the main university.
Weekly rent	• £48–£78, bills included for campus residences
Pint of lager	• £1.70–£2.10 on campus • £1.60–£2.20 city centre pub
Cinema	• Campus: £2.75 (or £12.50 for the year) • City: £3.60–£5
Nightclub	• £2–£6

Edinburgh

Key facts	Premedical	Undergraduate
Course length	6 years	5 years
Total number of medical undergraduates	1332	
Applicants in 2006	308	2713
Interviews given in 2006		64
Places available in 2006	Premedical offers made	218
Places available in 2007	to applicants without	218
	the right subject combination, but who would otherwise be made an offer to the MBChB undergraduate programme	
Open days 2007	3 - see website	
Entrance requirements	AAAB	AAAB
Mandatory subjects	GCSE: maths, English, language or dual award combined science	A-level chemistry and one maths/ physics/biology
		Biology at least at AS level
		Applications welcomed from non-medical graduates
Male:female ratio	Not provided	37:63
Is an exam included in the selection process?	Yes	Yes
If yes, what form does this exam take?	UKCAT	UKCAT
Qualification gained	MBChB	MBChB

Fascinating fact: Former students of the University of Edinburgh Medical School have made historic contributions to scientific thought and the practice of medicine. For example, the use of antiseptic was pioneered by Joseph Lister, and James Simpson was the first to use the anaesthetic chloroform to relieve pain in labour.

Although it is one of the oldest medical schools, Edinburgh has shed the traditional preclinical/ clinical course in favour of a new integrated curriculum that started in October 1998. With a strong research tradition (reflected by 40% of students taking an intercalated BSc), Edinburgh seems to attract high academic achievers and a lot of students from England and Northern Ireland. The recent opening of The New Royal Infirmary means that Edinburgh's medical students have the privilege of being taught in this state-of the-art facility.

Education

The new curriculum is taught in teaching hospitals, in district general hospitals and on attachment in GP practices. It is taught in an integrated fashion, with themes of clinical skills and communication skills running across all 5 years. Studying starts with the normal function of the body, building through to disease processes and clinical systems. Although there is some clinical involvement in the early years (particularly in general practice settings), the bulk of clinical placements are in years 3 to 5.

Teaching

The general trend is towards lectures and tutorials in the first couple of years, with formalized en-masse teaching being replaced by ward-based teaching later on in the course. Although there is some problem- or case-based work, most of the teaching is by formal lectures and small group sessions. These are balanced between tutorials and group work, with facilitators, with the aim of gaining not only knowledge but also team-working skills. Anatomy is taught with prosected material and computer-assisted learning programmes, rather than by traditional dissection of cadavers by students themselves.

Assessment

Exams have traditionally been at the end of each term and count for at least 60% of the course mark. There is an increasing amount of continuous and modular assessment in the new curriculum.

Intercalated degrees

At Edinburgh there is a well-established Honours year programme and a large number of students intercalate every year, so those choosing to intercalate take the extra year with many year group colleagues. Acceptance onto an intercalated honours course is on a competitive basis (academic performance over the first two years is taken into account), and the vast majority of intercalating students usually do so after year 2. There is a wide range of degrees to choose from, including those with components in Leiden (see Erasmus below) as well as the option to study at a different UK university if your ideal course is not offered at Edinburgh.

Special study modules and electives

Electives take place in year 5 and last for 2 months. The medical school is very flexible about what you do and where you go – just as long as it is medically related. There are also several periods for special study modules, starting in small groups in years 1 and 2, and leading to an independent research project for 14 weeks in year 4. The elective is a great opportunity to do your own ground-breaking research (in a subject of your choosing) at a university renowned for it!

Erasmus

There is the opportunity to study part of some intercalated BSc subjects in Leiden (Netherlands). Outside the Erasmus scheme, you are able to do your elective virtually anywhere in the world that you want, so long as the medical school approves it.

Facilities

Library   The medical collections are found alongside those for most other subjects in the main library, which is situated centrally and is easily accessible from most student accommodation. There are also smaller collections of medical texts found in libraries at the main teaching hospitals. The availability of recommended textbooks on short loan is fair, and the main library is open 8.30 AM–10 PM Monday to Thursday, 8.30 AM–7 PM on Friday, 9 AM–5 PM on Saturday, and 12 noon–7 PM on Sunday. However, holiday opening times vary and students on peripheral rotations in years 4–5 sometimes need to be well organised to get to the library within opening hours.

Computer facilities   There is a dedicated computer laboratory in the medical school with 100 PCs (and more in the library, throughout the university, and at the teaching hospitals); programmes needed for study are available, including word-processing, email, internet and specially designed computer-assisted learning. It does not currently have 24-hour access, but this should be remedied soon.

Clinical skills   There are clinical skills centres at both the main hospitals, which are used for learning clinical skills. These facilities are available to all medical students for personal practice outside timetabled hours, and are also used for formal teaching throughout the medical degree course.

Welfare 🏠

Student support

The medical school can seem a bit harsh and traditional when you first arrive. As well as a dedicated Dean of Student Affairs responsible for the welfare of all students, each student has a Director of Studies responsible for monitoring his/her progress and providing pastoral care, which effectively acts as a safety net to identify and deal with problems. A hands-off approach tends to be taken by the medical school, which on one level gives you freedom and independence, but can leave you feeling like a small drop in a big ocean. However, if you have genuine difficulties then the school really is extremely helpful and genuinely flexible. The school has good relations with the local Medical Students Council and a comprehensive *Student Handbook* is published jointly every year.

Accommodation

University accommodation in halls or flats is guaranteed in year 1. However, demand from all students for halls (which are of a good standard) is greater than the places available, and after year 1 most students get a group together and rent a flat from a private landlord or the university. Some students also choose to take out a mortgage to buy their own flats, renting rooms to other students. An advantage of Edinburgh is that most of the student accommodation is very central for the university and the city, and almost invariably within 15–20 minutes' walking distance. However, the cold winters do put up your heating bills. Halls cost between £111 and £132 per week, and include most meals, cleaning, heating and internet. A room in a private flat costs between £250 and £380 per month, and will usually not include bills.

Placements

For years 1 and 2 medics are a real part of the university, with the medical school being centrally placed in George Square. It is very handy for all the library facilities, computers, Unions and halls. However, now that the New Royal Infirmary is open, services are gradually being moved there (about 4 miles from the city centre) and it remains unclear how much of the school will remain on the university site and how much will move out. The feel of things, particularly in the early years, is bound to change. In the last three years of the course, most time is spent in the hospitals and occasionally away from Edinburgh, so medics can begin to lose touch with their student roots and see less of their colleagues.

In year 1 students go into general practices for two well-received community-based practicals. Time in year 2 is spent in local GP practices learning clinical skills. In year 3 you have clinical rotations and may have the rare clinic outside the city. In years 4 and 5 students may have their 6-week clinical blocks in peripheral hospitals and GP practices up to 80 miles from Edinburgh. There are normally at least two students on each placement, and accommodation is provided free of charge. As there are fewer students you get much more involved in the team, and the teaching is generally as good as (if not better than) in the central teaching hospitals. However, although most can be reached easily by train or bus, transport to one or two sites can be inconvenient if you don't have a car, and many students group together to get lifts.

The two main teaching hospitals are the New Royal Infirmary and the Western General Hospital, which are both about a 25-minute bus ride away (about 80p) from the city centre. Both have an atmosphere of pioneering, cutting-edge medicine and surgery. The facilities for students are adequate. There is a tremendous range of patients to learn from and ward groups are normally small (six or seven students in year 3 – but sometimes bigger – and two students per ward in years 4 and 5). If you put the effort in you'll get a lot out of it.

Location of clinical placement/ name of hospital	Distance away from medical school (miles)	Difficulty getting there on public transport*
New Royal Infirmary	3.5	🚶 🚌
Western General	2.5	🚶 🚌
GP placements in 1/2 year	between 0 and 10!	🚶 🚌
Peripheral placements in years 4 and 5.	between 20 to 120	🚌 🚗 ✈️

* 🚶: walking/cycling distance; 🚌 : use public transport; 🚗: need own car or lift; ✈️: get up early – tricky to get to!

Sports and social 🏆

City life

Edinburgh, the city of festivals, is a great place to spend 5 years of your life. The university is centrally located, with the medical school at the heart of the university. Although it is the capital of Scotland, Edinburgh has more than its fair share of English and overseas residents, so there is a very cosmopolitan atmosphere. For the first 2 years you really blend into mainstream student life, but the clinical years are time-consuming – spent in different rotations and hospitals – meaning that medical students tend to gradually drift away from the main student body. However, there is a strong community spirit within each year group, and no shortage of medic societies, sports clubs and socializing opportunities.

Edinburgh has the advantage of being a compact and generally safe city where everything is within walking distance. It is a lively cosmopolitan capital city with a good pub and club scene, theatres, cinemas, shopping and a lot of tourist attractions. Although it is a huge tourist trap (especially during the Military Tattoo and the International Festival and Fringe in the summer), the paths of tourists and students don't really cross. Between the three universities there is a large student population, which is very well catered for. Edinburgh has one of the highest concentrations of pubs in a city centre, and most are licensed to 1 AM (clubs open to 3 AM). Green space is found at the Meadows and Holyrood Park. Both are excellent areas for friendly football, rugby, hockey, American football, korfball matches, etc. Edinburgh is well connected for getting to most other parts of the UK, and the great outdoors is not too far away if you want to get away from it all for some fresh air. Many great locations for outdoor activities such as mountaineering, mountain biking and various water sports are not too far from the city.

University life

The medical students' council, Royal Medical Society (which has rooms open to members for 24

Edinburgh

hours) and each year's final year committee organize social events, talks and balls. There is also a medics choir and orchestra, an active Christian Medics group, and the medical school magazine *2nd Opinion*. In short, if you want it, it is probably there (and if it isn't you can set it up!). Apart from traditional medic activities (various balls, plays, revue, academic families), most students find their own entertainment in the wider city and university rather than relying exclusively upon medical societies. The Union is one of the largest in the country, offering a good range of societies and good venues.

Sports life

The medics rugby team is well organized and successful, with a formidable reputation both on and off the field. A mixed hockey team and a netball team have recently been formed, and what they (sometimes) lack in skill they make up for in character. There are various year football and badminton teams. Medics tend to play a more active part in the wider university sports scene rather than just staying within the medical school. Most sports people who represent the medical school will also play for the main university and/or local clubs. As well as a variety of sports clubs, the university now has a fully refurbished gym with lots of shiny new equipment, a sports injury clinic, and a schedule of well-run exercise classes popular with students and members of the public.

Great things about Edinburgh

- Edinburgh is a vibrant and lively university and city with excellent shopping, pubs, and clubs. The Festivals and Hogmanay are an extremely important part of the city's spirit, and the new Scottish Parliament has added to the city's charms.
- Edinburgh is renowned for its ghosts and is thought to be one of the most haunted cities in the world. There are many scary and exciting tours, many of which enter into the vaults under the city!
- Edinburgh hosts a lot of innovative and world-respected research projects in clinical medicine and surgery. You will be taught by some very big names!
- You can drink in pubs and restaurants 24 hours a day if you know how (and want to).
- The medical students have a very good collective spirit, especially in the first three years, without being too cliquey.

Bad things about Edinburgh

- Large numbers of tourists, festival luvvies and the New Year Hogmanay invasion.
- Peripheral attachments in the latter years mean that the year group doesn't meet up very often.
- The support network works well in a crisis, but you can feel a bit anonymous to the school at other times.
- Without a car, travelling to a few peripheral hospitals can be awkward.
- It can get quite cold and windy in winter, when the nights draw in.

Further information

Admissions Office
College of Medicine & Veterinary Medicine

Room GU315
Chancellor's Building
49 Little France Crescent
Edinburgh EH16 4SB
Tel: 0131 242 6407
Fax: 0131 242 6791
Email: medug@ed.ac.uk
Web: http://www.mvm.ed.ac.uk/studying
http://www.ed.ac.uk/

Additional application information

Average A level requirements	• AAA and B in fourth AS level subject
Average Scottish Higher requirements	• AAAAB
Make-up of interview panel	• Interviews not normally held for school-leaving or overseas applicants
Months in which interviews are held	• Check website
Proportion of overseas students	• 9%
Proportion of mature students	• 10%
Proportion of graduate students	• 10%
Faculty's view of students taking a gap year	• Applications from undergraduates who wish to defer entry for a year are welcome. Deferred applications will not be accepted from graduate, mature or overseas applicants.
Proportion of students taking intercalated degrees	• 40%
Possibility of direct entrance to clinical phase	• Yes, for students from St Andrews, Oxford and Cambridge
Fees for overseas students	• £12,450 pa (premedical year); £15,300 pa (years 1 and 2); £25,850 pa (years 3, 4 and 5)
Fees for graduates	• £2700

(Continued)

(Continued)

Ability to transfer to other medical schools If so, under what circumstances	• Unusual, however special circumstances will be considered by the college.
Assistance for elective funding	• Funding and advice are available through various organizations such as the Royal Medical Society.
Assistance for travel to attachments	• Free buses run between city hospitals.
Access and hardship funds	• Available – enquire through tutor system.
Weekly rent	• £40–£80
Pint of lager	• £1.50 to £3.00
Cinema	• Loads, most offering student discounts
Nightclub	• Huge variety, every taste catered for

Glasgow

Key facts	Undergraduate
Course length	5 years
Total number of medical undergraduates	1307
Applicants in 2006	2065
Interviews given in 2006	1165
Places available in 2006	223 Home/EU, 18 Overseas
Places available in 2007	223 Home/EU, 18 Overseas
Open days 2007	Open day 5 September, applicant visit day 20 March
Entrance requirements	Minimum of AAB at A Level
	UKCAT score
	Personal statement and reference
	Interview
Mandatory subjects	Chemistry and one of maths, physics or biology. General studies not acceptable as a third subject at A2. GCSE pass in English required. If biology is not studied at A2 level, it should be taken at GCSE or AS level.
Male:female ratio	35:65
Is an exam included in the selection process?	Yes
If yes, what form does this exam take?	UKCAT
Qualification gained	MBChB

Fascinating fact: Dr Ian McDonald, pioneer of the ultrasound, and the neurosurgeon Professor Graham Teasdale, responsible for the Glasgow Coma Scale, are both famous medics linked to Glasgow.

Glasgow medical school has historical origins in the 17th century and is well renowned for its teaching and research excellence, particularly in the fields of cardiovascular disease and cancer. The new Wolfson Medical School Building, situated on the main university campus, opened in 2002 with state-of-the-art facilities. These include a well-stocked study landscape, suites for problem-based learning and vocational studies, lecture rooms, and a clinical studies area with a ward.

Education

The new problem-based learning course, now in its 10th year, has achieved a fine balance between vocational and scientific aspects of medicine. It well equips the modern medical student with the skills necessary to pursue a career in medicine today. Applicants need to sit UKCAT (see Chapter 3).

Teaching

The mainstays of the course are problem-based learning sessions. These involve groups of around 8 students, guided by a facilitator, tackling two medical scenarios each week. There are also some supporting labs (fixed-resource sessions) and lectures (plenaries). In later years lecture weeks are added to revise core science and give focus to clinical learning.

Patient contact and practical skills are now taught from week 1 as Glasgow's progressive course seeks to blur the traditional preclinical/clinical divide. Hospital-based teaching still forms the majority of years 4 and 5.

Assessment

Continuous assessment occurs every 5-week block (in years 1 and 2) through coursework essays. There are also two formal written exams on the full curriculum at the end of year 1. An additional exam, testing the student's ability to work through a problem, is taken year 1. This is the medical independent learning exam (MILE), in which a scenario is handed out and the student has 24 hours to work through it and produce a set of pertinent questions that he/she must answer along with a summary of the subject tackled.

An objective structured clinical exam (OSCE) is also part of the assessment from year 2 onwards. Years 4 and 5 are treated as a continuum consisting of ten 5-week blocks: three in medicine, three in surgery, and one each in general practice, child health, obstetrics and gynaecology, and psychiatry. An OSLER (objective structured long examination record), case studies and a supervisor assessment are used to judge suitability to pass each clinical block. If the student does not pass a clinical block they must arrange a meeting with the head of the year and will also have to repeat the block before they can progress to the next year. These final 2 years also include four special study modules, outlined below.

Intercalated degrees

There are both 1- and 2-year intercalated degree options. One-year courses are available in clinical or science subjects and lead to a special degree type open only to medical students: the BSc (Med Sci) Hons in Clinical Medicine. The student chooses one of nine modules: cardiovascular studies; cancer studies; neuroscience; mechanisms of disease; developmental medicine; public health;

sports medicine; immunology; and psychological medicine. These modules involve the teaching of underlying science and completion of a research project which accounts for 60% of the degree mark. In addition, the degree has a core curriculum which all students undertake, comprising statistical methods relevant to medical research, journal clubs presented by students and teaching on experimental procedures and techniques including advanced IT. The degree is designed to better equip the student to undertake and critically appraise medical research. The two-year BSc (Hons) option is only available in science subjects. Intercalated degree courses are undertaken between years 3 and 4 of the MBChB.

Special Study Modules and Electives

Special study modules (SSMs) cover a wide range of subjects and constitute approximately 20% of the overall course time (one 5-week block in year 2, and two blocks in each year thereafter). Students choose from a list of options and may decide their own from year 3 onwards. Almost any topic can be proposed, including non-medical subjects such as French or philosophy. SSMs can also be taken abroad in years 3–5. There are two 4-week electives during the summers of years 3 and 4, which can also be spent abroad. An SSM can (timetable permitting) be amalgamated with an elective to provide a greater depth of study in a topic of interest.

Erasmus

There are no overseas travel opportunities due to the vast opportunities provided by the SSM and elective systems.

Facilities

Library The main university library, with an excellent range of reference books and journals, is open until 11 PM on weekdays and during the day at weekends. The new medical school's study landscape is well-equipped with three floors of extensive library and computing facilities along with smaller seminar rooms, which can be booked for group study. There is 24-hour access during term time, with each student being issued a swipe card upon matriculation.

Additional study facilities are available on campus (24-hour access in Unions) and in all hospitals, some of which are open 24 hours.

Computers There is good provision of computers in the main university library, with over 300 PCs available. The last year has seen the introduction of WiFi with 'hot spots' across campus for those with enabled laptops. The medical school study landscape provides over 100 flat-screen multimedia PCs that allow students to access a range of electronic learning facilities. The central teaching hospitals have approximately 20 PCs each for dedicated student use and the peripheral hospitals are generally adequate, with most now linked to the campus network.

Clinical skills Students are taught clinical skills from year 1, including first aid and basic/advanced resuscitation training. The new medical school building includes a fully equipped ward and side rooms contain audiovisual facilities to enable students to study their own performance in a simulated clinical environment before being confronted with a real hospital situation. Other new facilities include a cardiology patient simulator (known as Harvey) which can mimic symptoms of 26 cardiac diseases.

Welfare

Student support

Glasgow is renowned for its friendly and relaxed atmosphere, and the medical school is no exception. Each student is allocated an Adviser of Studies to offer advice and support. The students' representative council (SRC) provides excellent guidance on such topics as finance and housing. The SRC also arrange academic guidance if you encounter problems at university and run a free minibus service between campus and student halls. Glasgow has a free counselling service and operates a telephone nightline from 7 PM to 7 AM every night. The university health service offers a general consultative service, with more specialist branches such as travel clinics and occupational health.

Accommodation

Glasgow has a large number of local students, but guarantees accommodation to first-year students moving to the city. The quality is generally good with many of the halls divided into small hostels or flats consisting of a few single rooms with the occupants sharing a kitchen/diner area. The majority of places are in self-catered halls of residence as there is only one catered hall left. A year's fee ranges between £2200 and £3700 and must be paid in three instalments by direct debit. The university has little control over private sector flats but there is an accommodation office to help you. Rents can be highly variable, with a good guide being £40 (plus bills) per week for a 52-week lease on a university flat, and £55–75 (plus bills) per week for private flats.

Placements

Glasgow has a large, attractive campus in the West End of the city, two miles from the centre. Six large teaching hospitals within the Glasgow area and 13 District General Hospitals (DGHs) provide the mainstay of the teaching. Hospitals used include the Glasgow Royal Infirmary, the Western Infirmary, Gartnavel, Southern General and Stobhill Hospitals. Some of the DGHs are some distance away, but free accommodation is provided and the facilities, whilst free of silk sheets and champagne, are clean and warm. Groups of students number between five and eight with a drop to one or two per ward by the final year allowing for more involvement, better teaching, and less fighting for interesting cases.

For placements outside the university, peripheral attachments can take you to Paisley (8 miles) or as far as Dumfries in the Scottish borders (80 miles away). However, there are many hospitals and general practices in the Greater Glasgow area and GP practices are invariably local.

Location of clinical placement/ name of hospital	Distance away from medical school (miles)	Difficulty getting there on public transport*
Royal Alexandra (Paisley)	8	
Monklands and Wishaw	20	
Ayr	40	
Inverclyde	30	
Dumfries	80	

* : walking/cycling distance; : use public transport; : need own car or lift; : get up early – tricky to get to!

Sports and social 🏆

City life

As Scotland's biggest city Glasgow is truly international, with a large city centre containing all that you might require. A cursory tour of the city's highlights, including the university building, will soon reveal why Glasgow was the 1999 City of Art and Design and 1990 European City of Culture. Lots of students are accommodated in West End flats close to the university, great pubs, shops and a lively club scene.

You are never short of something to see or do, from the well-established Kelvingrove Gallery (reo-pened in July 2006), which houses one of the best art collections in the UK, to the new Museum of Modern Art and there would be another 24 public art galleries/museums still to visit. Glasgow also boasts some of the best shopping in Scotland and a leading club/pub scene.

The city hosts many international sporting events, frequently involving athletics and, in 2003, held the Champions League Final. If you want a change of scene, getting out of Glasgow is easy enough, with access to some of the best hill-walking, climbing and skiing in the UK, a mere 1 to 2 hours away. Other Scottish cities are also close at hand, with Edinburgh and the new Parliament only 45 minutes away. Buses and trains leave every 15 minutes.

University life

The Medico-Chirurgical Society (Med-Chir) is an educational and social society set up and run by medical students. It meets every Thursday, with refreshments and talks from a range of speakers on a variety of entertaining topics. It also arranges events, including trips abroad, the annual ball, the annual revue and a musical culture night. Each year has its own year club to organise club nights, ceilidhs and balls, and to raise money for a massive graduation ball. Our medical students' maga-zine, *Surgo,* will also keep you updated on all the activities and gossip within the faculty. Unusually,

Glasgow has two unions: Glasgow University Union (GUU) and Queen Margaret Union (QMU), both with bars, clubs, catering facilities and a regular programme of bands, balls and special events. The GUU has a debating chamber and Glasgow University has won the World Debating Championships more times than any other university.

Sports life

The sports centre at the heart of the campus has recently undergone a massive refurbishment pro-gramme. The facilities include a 25m pool, sauna, weights room, squash courts and sports hall. For only £30 per year you can have unlimited access to the sports facilities, as well as a wide range of daily classes in aerobics, muscle conditioning and circuits. There is also a large off-campus sports facility housing tennis courts, floodlit hockey and football pitches and another new gym. There are more than 25 sports clubs on offer, from the traditional rugby and swimming, through to sailing, pot-holing, cheerleading and ultimate frisbee. Med-Chir also has medics' football and rugby teams.

Great things about Glasgow

- The West End provides the perfect combination of shops, bars and restaurants, all contained within walking distance.
- Superb facilities: two great unions, accommodation, sport complex, main library and a well-equipped new medical school building.
- One survey found Glasgow University to have the best social life for students in Scotland.
- Teaching by internationally acclaimed experts.
- Acclaimed as a music/club venue: King Tut's, The Arches, Barrowlands …

Bad things about Glasgow

- It's not Barcelona – bring the rainbow scarf your granny made.
- Some of the district hospitals are far away.
- Some people dislike problem-based learning.
- Glasgow city has a student population of 150,000 so you might have to queue to get into your favourite club.
- Beware a Scottish breakfast – it is helping to make the west of Scotland the heart disease capital of Europe.

Further information

Admissions Enquiries
Wolfson Medical School
University of Glasgow
University Avenue
Glasgow G12 8QQ
Tel: 0141 330 6216
Fax: 0141 330 2776
Email: admissions@clinmed.gla.ac.uk
Web: http://www.gla.ac.uk/faculties/medicine/medicalschool.html

Additional application information

Average A level requirements	• Minimum of AAB
Average Scottish Higher requirements	• Minimum of AAAAB
Make-up of interview panel	• Two members of the Admissions Committee
Months in which interviews are held	• November – March
Proportion of overseas students	• 18 places available
Proportion of mature students	• No set quota
Proportion of graduate students	• No set quota, but current intake approximately 35–40 per annum
Faculty's view of students taking a gap year	• Acceptable if used constructively
Proportion of students taking intercalated degrees	• Current limit of 70 per annum
Possibility of direct entrance to clinical phase	• Dependent on student numbers
Fees for overseas students	• £19,600 pa (2006)
Fees for graduates	• £2700 pa (2006)
Ability to transfer to other medical schools If so, under what circumstances	• Transfers are unusual, but Glasgow would certainly consider an individual's needs and circumstances.
Assistance for elective funding	• Faculty and specialist society support available and advertised.
Assistance for travel to attachments	• None from faculty. Dependent upon SAAS or LEA support with its concomitant regulations and restrictions.
Access and hardship funds	• The university has a hardship fund for home students only (i.e. not EU or international).
Weekly rent	• £65 approx.

(*Continued*)

(*Continued*)

Pint of lager	• £1.70–£2.20
Cinema	• £3.50–£4.50
Nightclub	• £3–£8, with big dance events at The Arches as much as £20

Guy's, King's and St Thomas'

Key facts	Premedical	Undergraduate	Graduate
Course length	6 years	5 years	4 years
Total number of medical undergraduates	36	c. 2000	80
Applicants in 2006	423	4020	1165
Interviews given in 2006	c. 140	1150	201
Places available in 2006	40	332	24 (+4 MaxFax)
Places available in 2007	40	332	224 (+4 MaxFax)
Open days 2007	July/August	July/August	July/August
Entrance requirements	AAB + AS (B)	AAB + AS (B)	2:1
Mandatory subjects	None	Chemistry and biology	None
Male:female ratio	67:33	35:65	63:37
Is an exam included in the selection process?	Yes	Yes	Yes
If yes, what form does this exam take?	UKCAT	UKCAT	UKCAT
Qualification gained	MBBS		

Fascinating fact: Guy's Hospital, with its 30-storey 'tower' boasting spectacular views of Tower Bridge, the Tower of London and St. Paul's Cathedral, holds the record of being the tallest hospital in the world. The Gordon Museum of Pathology, located at the Guy's Campus, has a unique range of specimens dating back to the 18th century.

Medicine has been taught at the site of Guy's campus since 1726, making this medical college one of the oldest in the country. King's College London School of Medicine at Guy's, King's and St. Thomas' hospitals, popularly known as GKT, was formed in August 1998 by the merger of the United Medical and Dental School (UMDS) of Guy's and St Thomas' Hospitals and King's College School of Medicine. The result is a medical school enriched with a long history and tradition, which also embraces modern technology and innovative methods of teaching. This combination makes the college an ideal place for those who want the best of both worlds.

An intake of nearly 400 students makes the medical school one of the biggest in the UK, and makes King's College, as a whole, the largest centre for healthcare teaching in Europe. Both King's and GKT emphasize personal academic development with, for example, its strongly supported intercalated BSc programme, and encourages students to participate fully in extra-curricular activities. King's College also holds four Medical Research Council grants – more than any other university in the UK.

Education

Applicants to King's College need to sit UKCAT (see Chapter 3). The course is split into two main sections. Years 1 and 2 place an emphasis on the basic medical sciences in the form of PBL. Each week a new scenario is introduced by a clinician, and students are then taught the basic medical science behind it, followed by a final summing-up session where everything is brought together and put into clinical context. There is also early patient contact, with communication teaching taking place in a GP setting from year 1. The course is organized into systems, i.e. cardiovascular, musculoskeletal, etc. All the core basic science teaching takes place at the Guy's Hospital campus.

Clinical disciplines are taught in the latter three years on the wards of St Thomas' Hospital, King's College Hospital, Guy's Hospital, University Hospital Lewisham and also in the community. The long-established systems-based clinical course has been designed to complement the course structure from the earlier years. The core clinical subjects are delivered and examined during years 3 and 4. The final year consists of an 8-week elective, followed by attachments in the community and attachments shadowing medical and surgical foundation programme doctors in district general hospitals.

GKT has a strong commitment to widening access to medical degree courses. A small number of places are available on an access programme, which is designed to help bright and talented young people from low aspiration backgrounds become doctors. The programme will eventually allow for up to 50 extra undergraduate places in medicine and will be for talented pupils from South London who would not normally achieve the necessary grades to apply to study medicine. The course is based on a standard MBBS course but takes 6 years rather than 5, because of the addition of special modules in the first 3 years.

A new graduate-entry programme has been introduced and is designed to encourage access to medicine for graduates in the arts or other healthcare professionals. The course is shortened to 4 years and after a unique first year, the students join the regular 3-year clinical programme. At the time of print, from 1200 applications only 27 were successful in gaining places!

Teaching

There are a mixture of lectures, tutorials, and practicals, together with computer-assisted learning. Anatomical dissection is still a valued part of preclinical teaching.

Teaching during the clinical course has changed. Under the new curriculum students are divided into two phases, clinical science and clinical apprenticeship. During the clinical apprenticeship phase students are able to devote their time entirely to hospital work, clerking patients and receiving bedside teaching. During the clinical sciences phase students can spend time learning the core subjects and undertake special study modules (SSM).

Assessment

Essay and short-answer questions are now rare during years 3–5. Written examinations during the clinical years are now mostly computer-scored multiple-choice question. OSCEs (objective structured clinical examinations) are the main practical examinations during the clinical years, starting with a short communication skills OSCE in year 2. Year 3 students have mini-OSCEs at the end of each rotation and, if they pass these, they can avoid sitting the rather long and traumatic end of year OSCEs.

Intercalated degrees

There are well-supported intercalated degree programmes at the college. There is a wide range of options to choose from, including many outside medicine such as medical law and ethics and philosophy. If a subject is not offered at King's, students are permitted to enrol in BSc programmes at other universities. As the BSc is not compulsory, and students are allowed to undertake a degree programme after years 2, 3 or 4, students have the unique freedom and flexibility to tailor their BSc to suit.

Special study modules and electives

About 20% of each year is devoted to SSMs. There is a considerable range of subjects available and this is increasing every year. As the school is part of a multi-faculty institution, many non-medical SSMs are available, e.g. modern languages and the popular history of medicine. Students may also design their own SSM if the subject they wish to study is not on offer.

The 8-week elective period is an opportunity to travel to far-flung destinations (or just down the road) to study in fields of medicine of your choosing. Assessment of how time is spent on the elective, to discourage the temptation to just lie to a beach, takes the form of a poster presentation. Various awards and sponsorships are available to help students fund their electives.

Erasmus

Despite the end of GKT participation in Erasmus schemes, the school has special links with numerous medical schools around the world, including the Johns Hopkins University in the USA, and the University of Hong Kong. As GKT is twinned with these institutions, there are special allocations for GKT students who want to do their electives there. Accommodation will also usually be arranged for you, and extra bursaries may be available to help with travel costs to these colleges. Students also have the opportunity to arrange their peripheral placements in one of the twinned institutions during year 4.

Facilities

Library Libraries at Guy's are open between 9 AM and 9 PM on weekdays, 9 AM and 5 PM on Saturday, and 1 PM and 5 PM on Sunday; there is also a large 24-hour study room. At King's College Hospital the library is open until 9 PM on weekdays and 1 PM on Saturday. Students also have access to the King's College London library at the old Public Records Office on Chancery Lane, which is open until 9 PM from Monday to Thursday, 6 PM on Friday and 5.30 PM on Saturday and Sunday. All libraries have a good range of books and journals.

Computers All campuses have a large number of computer stations, with access to email, the internet and computer-assisted learning programmes designed in-house. There are 24-hour computing facilities at Guy's, Kings and St Thomas' campuses. The virtual campus is a specialized area of the King's College London website for the GKT schools of medicine, dentistry and biomedical sciences and enables students to download lecture notes, register for course components or obtain details, but unfortunately not the answers, for their exams.

Clinical skills A clinical skills centre opened at Guy's in 1999. It is the largest of its kind in Europe, and is available every weekday from 9 AM to 5 PM. Students can book individual rooms in small groups or with their tutor. There are also various laboratories at the three main hospitals. These are great, with latex models of every imaginable part of the human anatomy on which students can practise their clinical skills, such as taking blood pressure or suturing. In the past, King's students on accident and emergency attachments practised suturing pigs' trotters before being let loose on the population of south London!

Welfare 🏠

Student support

Students are assigned to a personal tutor to support them throughout the course. Welfare and counselling services are available on the Guy's campus, where there is a welfare officer available every day. All sites are friendly environments with lots of support from the faculty and staff, as well as the Students' Union which provides student representation on a wide range of matters. The BMA representative also complements the Students' Union in looking after the medical students' welfare. There are also other forums that look after the academic welfare of the students, including the Student Medical Elective Committee (SMEC) and the Student Staff Liaison Committee (SSLC).

Multi-faith pastoral care is provided on all campuses, as well as many student-run religious groups covering the main religious faiths.

Accommodation

College accommodation is available in many different parts of London. Some is on or near campuses; on-site accommodation is available on the Guy's campus whereas other accommodation is much further away. The quality and cost of private accommodation can vary a lot in the central Guy's/St Thomas' area, but cheaper, good-quality accommodation is more readily available in the Denmark Hill area and at Hampstead. Students can opt for intercollegiate University of London accommodation, although this tends to be some distance from any of the campuses.

Placements

Students in years 1 and 2 are taught at the newly developed Guy's Hospital campus at London Bridge. The campus is shared with other departments in biomedical sciences and dentistry. Most of the Guy's campus has been refurbished to accommodate the large number of students, and many facilities are new. A large new building houses most of the disciplines, with state-of-the-art library and computing facilities. Most clinical teaching takes place at St Thomas' Hospital, King's College Hospital, Guy's Hospital and University Hospital Lewisham. Students can also access King's College's other campuses, including the Strand campus and Waterloo campus. Psychiatry teaching is at the infamous Maudsley Hospital, and at the Institute of Psychiatry, which has been awarded the status of five-star top research institute in the United Kingdom.

As well as placements at the central teaching hospitals in years 4 and 5, there are placements in district general hospitals in southeast England. This relieves some of the pressures at the central London teaching hospitals and provides access to high-quality teaching; clinical workloads tend to be lower, and consultants are able to devote more time to students. Peripheral placements also expose students to the more common conditions that are not seen at the tertiary referral centres at the large teaching hospitals.

Location of clinical placement/ name of hospital	Distance away from medical school (miles)	Difficulty getting there on public transport*
Woolwich	5	
Bromley	8	
Canterbury	30	
Brighton	50	
Salisbury	90	

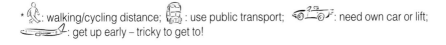

* : walking/cycling distance; : use public transport; : need own car or lift; : get up early – tricky to get to!

Sports and social 🏆

City life

Most of campuses are close to the centre of London, with all of London's attractions within easy reach by public transport.

University life

The old medical schools always had thriving social scenes, with numerous balls, weekly events, annual revues and RAG week. The social scene at GKT typifies this and GKT medical students still hold the world record for having the largest number of people naked on live TV! GKT also boasts that it has the best university Diwali Show. There is a vast selection of clubs and societies to join, including orchestras, bands, singing, dancing, drama and musical theatre groups. Everyone can usually find something that interests him or her, or comrades with which to start up a new society. The Students' Union runs its own bars, shops, cafes, nightclubs, and gym. Student bars are present on all campuses and there is the main medics night spot in the basement of Guy's Hospital. If that's not enough, all students have access to the University of London Union (ULU) with its own range of facilities.

GKT gives students access to a large multidisciplinary institution while retaining the friendliness of a medical school. With its almost enclosed courtyard, promenade, and park at London Bridge, the Guy's campus is regarded as the closest thing to a campus university in central London.

Sports life

GKT proudly boasts having the oldest rugby team in the world, associated with long and strong traditions which you will quickly find out once you join the college. The scene in general is healthy, and particularly strong sports include football, hockey, netball, tennis, badminton, rowing and squash. GKT has sports grounds at Honor Oak Park in south London, Dulwich, and Cobham in Surrey, which provides facilities for rugby, football and hockey. However, the sale of Cobham grounds to Chelsea FC by the college has severely limited the number of games played there. King's College also has sports grounds in Surbiton. There are gyms at the Guy's and St Thomas' campuses, and also at the Stamford Street halls of residence. For swimmers, there is a pool at Guy's.

Great things about GKT 👍

- GKT hospitals are all world-renowned.
- Excellent range of learning and social facilities at the medical school campuses, with more on the way.
- The new school is part of a multi-faculty institution. Students will have the opportunity to mix with a variety of students from other courses, and have access to a wide range of facilities.
- Good sports clubs with lots of history and traditions.
- Welfare and student support mechanisms are well-established with proven efficacy.

Bad things about GKT

- Cost of living in London and travelling to far flung clinical placements.
- Student accommodation can be a long way from your campus.
- Large number of medics in each year group can lead to it being a bit cramped and impersonal.
- The medical school can be a bit bureaucratic.
- Some feel there is a lack of teaching on pharmacology.

Further information

Student Admissions Officer
The Hodgkin Building
Guy's Hospital Campus
King's College London
St Thomas' Street
London Bridge
London SE1 9RT
Tel: 020 7848 6501
Fax: 020 7848 6510
Email: guysadmissions@kcl.ac.uk
Web: http://www.kcl.ac.uk

Additional application information

Average A level requirements	• AAB/B
Average Scottish Higher requirements	• Premedical: AA/BBB (Advanced Highers/Highers) • Undergraduate: AA/BBB (Advanced Highers/Highers)
Graduate entry requirements	• 2:1 degree
Make-up of interview panel	• Chair and interviewer (sometimes an observer as well)
Months in which interviews are held	• December – May (Premedical) • November – May (Undergraduate) • February – April (Graduate)
Proportion of overseas students	• Information not available
Proportion of mature students	• Information not available
Proportion of graduate students	• Information not available
Faculty's view of students taking a gap year	• Encouraged
Proportion of students taking intercalated degrees	• Please contact university for more information
Possibility of direct entrance to clinical phase	• Yes (start of year 3)

(Continued)

(Continued)

Fees for overseas students	• Premedical: £13,936 (years 1, 2 and 3) £25,844 (years 4, 5 and 6). Undergraduate: £13,936 (years 1 and 2) £25,844 (years 3, 4 and 5). Graduate: £13,936 (year 1) £25,844 (years 2, 3 and 4).
Fees for graduates	• £3000
Ability to transfer to other medical schools If so, under what circumstances	• Yes, for intercalated BSc or for clinical years.
Assistance for elective funding	• Good – both college awards and advice for external sources.
Assistance for travel to attachments	• No – and some attachments are far away.
Access and hardship funds	• Excellent student support and hardship facilities.
Weekly rent	• £80 (London prices!)
Pint of lager	• £2.00 (ditto)
Cinema	• £5 upwards
Nightclub	• Free–£15

Hull and York

Key facts	Undergraduate
Course length	5 years
Total number of medical undergraduates	556
Applicants in 2006	1300
Interviews in 2006	c. 500
Places available in 2006	141
Places available in 2007	141
Open days 2007	Hull: 24 March, 7 July York: 2 July
Entrance requirements	AAB at A2 (to include an A grade in biology and A/B in chemistry, excluding general studies) and a B grade in a 4th subject at AS. All applicants must have taken the UKCAT
Mandatory subjects	Chemistry A2, biology (or human biology) A2
Male:female ratio	40:60
Is an exam included in the selection process?	Yes for all applicants applying for 2007 entry
If yes, what form does this exam take?	UKCAT
Qualification gained	MBBS

Fascinating fact: Hull is the home of the world's smallest window, which can be found in the George pub in the Land of Green Ginger.

September 2003 saw the long-awaited opening of the Hull York Medical School (HYMS) and its first 136 students take up their places on a new and exciting programme of medical education. The first intake students are now in their fourth year. HYMS is a collaboration between the long-established universities of Hull and York. Both have a wealth of experience in health and bioscience education and the medical school is very much a natural progression in their development.

HYMS is a place of innovation. It accommodates the growing need for doctors in the UK whilst striving to set the pace in delivering a curriculum and education that will equip them for the realities of 21st century practice, by ensuring they truly are the doctors of tomorrow.

Education

Applicants will need to sit UKCAT (see Chapter 3). Students are divided equally between two campuses at Hull and York universities during phase I. Despite the physical separation for years 1 and 2, staff and students work hard to ensure complete continuity in teaching, resources, timetables and social activities at the respective locations. Both sites have new custom-built facilities (such as video links) and the constant movement of faculty staff between the two locations guarantees that students have good access to most members. The running of parallel timetables and employment of moderators insures HYMS students receive the same education and opportunities regardless of where they are placed. In years 3, 4, and 5 Hull and York groups combine and together follow a programme of community and hospital-based study in centres throughout East and North Yorkshire and Northern Lincolnshire.

The course content is organized around the study of body systems and the 5-year course is divided into three phases. In phase I (years 1 and 2), basic sciences are studied in the context of clinical medicine. In phase II (years 3 and 4) the course becomes multi-centred with teaching in hospitals, general practices and community placements across North and East Yorkshire and Northern Lincolnshire. Clinical teachers deliver the programme and students benefit from low student/teacher ratios and plenty of opportunity for learning in hospital and primary care settings.

Phase III, year 5, gives students extensive clinical experience in medicine, surgery, and general practice. Phase III also provides the opportunity for an elective period of 8 weeks, where students are able to travel abroad if they wish to experience medicine in a different part of the world.

Teaching

The curriculum at HYMS is designed to make education interesting and exciting. In phase I, virtual patient case studies are used each week as a framework in which to conceptualize and explore the science. Concomitantly, clinical placements provide the opportunity to transpose the theory into medical realities.

A broad range of teaching methods are employed at HYMS to meet the variety of learning objectives set by the curriculum. These include PBL and self-directed learning, which are the mainstay of education, but also there are lectures, and a staff-supported resource laboratory, which contains visual aids such as anatomical models, X-rays and computer packages. A new anatomy museum provides use of prosections. Typically, a lecture is delivered by a speaker at either Hull or York and beamed into the other end by an impressive video conferencing link. Technological teething problems have now all but subsided and, likewise, stage fright, as students across campuses regularly engage in discussion via the video system. There are also biopracticals which consist of some teaching where students learn about different aspects of physiology through performing experiments, for example, finding out about values of lung function by spirometry. Workshops are an innovative way of expanding gained knowledge in clinical contexts, for example, the use of ethics in clinical practice.

Patient contact is made from day one. Clinical placements start from the beginning of year 1 with weekly half-day attachments within a small group. In year 2, a full day per week is spent with patients and in phases II and III clinical experience becomes much more intense with the majority of the final year spent on placements. The early placements provide an excellent opportunity to improve communication skills and give a welcome taster of the latter course years. The importance of engaging with patients and considering the panorama of psychological, social and biological factors of illness is given strong emphasis at HYMS, and is reflected in the fully integrated course where complementary disciplines are learned together.

Assessment

Assessment addresses the learning outcomes of each stage of the course using a combination of factual tests: multiple-choice questions (MCQs), modified essay questions (MEQs), and matching-type questions and also practical patient-based assessments (OSCEs). Exams are conducted at the end of the summer term. Students also keep a computer-held portfolio of learning and reflective writing as a record of progress. Formative assessments allow students to gauge their progress, without contributing to the final degree mark, and occur at the beginning of the summer and spring terms. These help students to recognize their strengths and weaknesses and to guide their work objectives accordingly.

Intercalated degrees

Selected students may devote an optional year, usually between years 2 and 3 (although it is also possible between years 4 and 5), to study for an Honours degree in the biomedical or health sciences or another appropriate subject (which may be an arts/humanities/social science subject). These can be taught- or research-based. They take the form of 120 credits: 40 are research-based and the remaining 80 are taught-based. Out of the 80 taught-based credits, 20 credits are at level 2 and 60 credits at level 3, requiring more critical analysis. Entry for the degree is competitive and is based on good performance in the previous exam. Six students over the two sites were allowed to intercalate in the inaugural year of the course, although undoubtedly the numbers will increase.

Special study modules and electives

Special study modules (SSMs or SSCs) provide an exciting opportunity to pursue new interests or develop existing ones. Comprising about a fifth of the course they are highly valued by HYMS students and can cover a broad range of disciplines. These could be basic or social sciences, medical specialities, or non-medical subjects such as languages or the arts. Students in years 1 and 2 take three SSCs a year, one in each term. In the clinical years they continue, and students are expected to complete four in each year of phase II.

The elective is an opportunity to spend 8 weeks experiencing any medical speciality(s) in any part of the world in year 5.

Erasmus

There is no opportunity to participate in an Erasmus programme at Hull/York although students can travel abroad for their elective.

Facilities

Both Hull and York have custom-built or modified buildings and bear testimony to a substantial budget well spent. Within the buildings are the PBL rooms, which constitute the students' favourite resource. All who see them agree: we are spoilt. Students are divided into groups of about eight for PBL sessions and are allocated a PBL room which contains an up-to-date, high-tech networked computer for each group member, a large and incredibly useful array of interactive learning packages, wall-to-wall white boards and most importantly the learning support of peers in your group. Friendships and learning relationships develop quickly and strongly within these groups. PBL members have access to their own room 24 hours a day. This is where students do the majority of their study, securing it as a respected learning environment, a source of note sharing, and, rumour has it, a pizza-delivery place for those working into the night!

Library   The library resources are abundant and joint access to both the Hull and York libraries, regardless of your home campus, translates to access to over two million books. This is before the surrounding hospital and local affiliated libraries are considered. Although, of course, you do have to travel to the libraries to actually get hold of the books you want. There is a substantial collection of medical and health-related papers and periodicals at both universities. Students also have access to a large number of electronic journals, multimedia CDs, videos and the Cochrane database. At York, the medical library is part of the university's JB Morrell library. Term-time opening hours are 9 AM–10 PM and weekends are 11 AM–6.00 PM. Hull's Brymore Jones library is open Monday–Thursday 9 AM–10 PM, Friday and Saturday 9 AM–9 PM and Sunday 1 PM–9 PM.

Computers   In addition to the HYMS buildings, medical students have full 24-hour access to other computing resources across both Hull and York campuses. University and HYMS email accounts are provided. IT training and language courses are open to students at both campuses.

York runs an excellent information literacy course, ILIAD. The Languages for All programme enables students to learn a foreign language whilst studying for their degree. Hull gives all students the opportunity to develop or gain language skills and hosts the Language Institute, one of the largest and best-equipped learning centres in Britain.

Clinical skills   Students take part in weekly clinical skill sessions to learn communication skills whilst taking medical and social histories from actor patients. They perform clinical examinations on healthy volunteers. Skills learnt from these sessions can be transferred to real-life patients in clinical placement sessions.

Welfare

Student support

Student welfare and a caring supportive environment are very important at HYMS. We are acutely aware that the most valuable commodity we have is each other and a formidable support network comes from fellow students and the academic support gained by close contact with staff.

In addition to departmental and academic support, both Hull and York offer a range of specialist services. At the beginning of term you are introduced to the support facilities rather than having to seek them out when you need them most. These include chaplains, counselling staff, health professionals and disability services. York has the added bonus of strong support via the college network and all HYMS welfare services are supplemented by the welfare work of the Students' Union.

A buddies scheme is now in operation at HYMS, under which first-year medical students are allocated a second-year medical student buddy. This informal relationship allows the first-year student to gain the benefit of the experience of other students and to integrate the two years.

Accommodation

Accommodation is guaranteed for all medical students at both campuses. Most students are offered rooms in halls of residence on campus; however, a small number of off-campus places are within easy reach of the medical school. Students can indicate which hall they would prefer to be in on their application form.

Placements

Clinical placements start from the beginning of year 1 with weekly half-day attachments within a small group. Attachments increase in frequency and duration throughout the course. In years 3, 4, and 5 Hull and York groups combine and follow a programme of community and hospital-based study in regional centres throughout East and North Yorkshire and Northern Lincolnshire. Free accommodation is provided during phase II regional placements by the Trust that place you where you are not normally based. Accommodation is not provided for students during years 1 and 2 as partner hospitals are all in close proximity to the medical school.

Location of clinical placement/ name of hospital	Distance away from medical school (miles)	Difficulty getting there on public transport*
York NHS Services Trust	varies	
Hull Royal Infirmary	3 (approx. from campus)	
Castle Hill Hospital Hull	4 (approx. from campus)	
Primary and secondary care placements near three partner hospitals	near to medical schools	

*: walking/cycling distance; : use public transport; : need own car or lift; : get up early – tricky to get to!

Sports and social

City life

Hull, once a hideout for beatniks and intellectuals, is now a living catwalk for the cool and the trendy. Indeed, Hull is the focus of an ongoing multimillion urban regeneration project. Unfortunately, it suffers from preconceptions that are far off the mark. Students love to live and study here. Graduates gush with praise and fondness and the new HYMS intake are already displaying ferocious loyalty and affection for the place. The nightlife at Hull is nothing short of legendary, with numerous venues in the city centre and its very own on-campus nightclub recently voted the best university venue in the UK. Hull is unbelievable value for money. Lower accommodation costs will be difficult to come by at another university and if you are coming from London, expect another three pints for your fiver.

Hull University holds a global reputation not only for academia, but also for friendliness. Its graduates are consistently among the top 10 UK universities for graduate employment and the university places strong emphasis on students excelling both in and out of the classroom.

York is a beautiful city. Steeped in history and encircled by ancient walls, it boasts some remarkable architecture including its impressive landmark Minster, the largest gothic cathedral in Northern Europe, and winding medieval streets called the 'Shambles'. A strong tourist industry ensures it bustles with life throughout the year and hosts a remarkable array of shops, restaurants, pubs, bistros and sights. York has a distinctly cosmopolitan feel, catering for every interest. The Theatre Royal, Grand Opera House, art gallery and a wide variety of live music venues enrich the staple student regime of clubs and kebabs. The university has a collegiate system which ensures friendships can run far beyond the medical school. Socializing tends to take place in the college bars or the city centre, but York's proximity to Leeds and Manchester ensures there are bigger nights out not too far away.

Hull and York are both couched in some of the most spectacular countryside in England. Surrounded by the Pennines, Dales, North Yorkshire Moors, and the seaside towns of Whitby, Robin Hood's Bay and Scarborough, there are many opportunities to explore and appreciate the area. York also has the advantage of being placed halfway between Edinburgh and London, each of which are about 2 hours away by train. The regular and cheap ferries running from Hull to Amsterdam require little promotion.

University life

With the array of extra-curricular opportunities existing between Hull and York and HYMS, social calendars require some organizing. The enthusiastic Medsoc, a body of eight students from both campuses who arrange events ranging from visiting speakers to charity pub-crawls, does this. Enthusiasm and talent are not in short supply and all students are working hard to bring to life plans for unisex sports teams, a medics band, a Christmas revue and a HYMS newspaper. As a new school, clubs and projects are evolving to reflect students' interests and talents and we eagerly await the new intake to supplement and enrich the current stream of activity.

Links with the BMA and other medical schools are growing and HYMS is eager to establish itself in the wider community of medical students and health professionals. HYMS has been shown a warm welcome by York Medical Society and the local trust. Outside lectures, close contact is maintained between both students and staff by the web-based discussion boards and regular social activities.

Common rooms outside HYMS provide a place for a coffee, chat or break should one be needed, and they are great for socializing.

Sports life

The sporting facilities at Hull are excellent with gyms, jacuzzis, an AstroTurf and squash courts. The Athletic Union currently has around 50 different sporting clubs. A magnificent new sports stadium and *The Deep*, an innovative ocean discovery centre, are just two of the exciting new developments marking out the future face of the city. In York, there is an abundance of facilities accommodating the golfer, cyclist, swimmer, climber, gym fanatic and hardened gambler – we have one of the finest racecourses in the country.

Great things about Hull and York

- You are spoilt with the huge amount of resources available to students.
- Clinical placements from the very beginning of the course give invaluable early experience.
- Hull's Asylum nightclub was voted the best Students' Union venue in the UK.
- Professor Paul O'Higgins and Dr Menos Lagopoulos are our eminent tutors in anatomy. They are an unmissable double act.
- HYMS is a close community where a culture of cooperation, not competition, reigns.

Bad things about Hull and York

- Self-directed and problem-based learning requires adaptation from A level-style syllabus and teaching.
- Although students state a preference for the campus they would like to be placed at, allocation is largely by ballot. Certain individual personal circumstances are taken into account.
- The refusal of students and staff to accept that the video link is not TV: and no, your mum cannot see you wave. Will the novelty ever wear off?
- The consequences of freshers' week or, to be more specific, three freshers' weeks. Hull starts term a little earlier than York does and HYMS fits into the former's timetable. What this translates to is a freshers' week at HYMS, one at Hull University and a later one at York University.
- In the clinical years there is considerable travelling between the hospital and GP placements, so transport is an important issue and most students end up buying a car.

Further information

Admissions and Schools Liaison
University of York
Heslington
York YO10 5DD

Tel: 01904 321 690
Fax: 01904 321 696
Email: admissions@york.ac.uk
Web: http://www.hyms.ac.uk

Student Recruitment and Admissions Service
University of Hull
Kingston upon Hull
Hull HU6 7RX
Tel: 01482 466 497
Email: admissions@hull.ac.uk
Web: http://www.hyms.ac.uk

Additional application information

Average A level requirements	• AABB
Average Scottish Higher requirements	• AAAAB (taken in a single attempt)
Make-up of interview panel	• Two people: one clinician and one non-clinician
Months in which interviews are held	• December and February
Proportion of overseas students	• 7.5%
Proportion of mature students	• 30%
Proportion of graduate students	• 32%
Faculty's view of students taking a gap year	• Encouraged
Proportion of students taking intercalated degrees	• 2%
Possibility of direct entrance to clinical phase	• No
Fees for overseas students	• £20,000 pa (fixed for five years)
Fees for graduates	• £3000 pa
Ability to transfer to other medical schools If so, under what circumstances	• Transfer to other medical schools is not available (due to the integrated nature of the course).
Assistance for elective funding	• None

Assistance for travel to attachments	• All travel expenses are met. Petrol is reimbursed at 23p a mile.
Access and hardship funds	• Hardship funds are available through the universities independently of the medical school.
Weekly rent	• Hull £50–65 per week. York £60–£70
Pint of lager	• Carling £1.40 and Stella £1.60 Student Union • £2–£2.50 city centre pub
Cinema	• UCG and the Odeon cinema cost approximately £3.50
Nightclub	• £2–£5 – the Asylum in the University has been voted best university nightclub in the UK. There are many others as well

Imperial College London

Key facts	Undergraduate
Course length	6 years
Total number of medical undergraduates	c. 2000
Applicants in 2006	c. 2200
Interviews given in 2006	700
Places available in 2006	326
Places available in 2007	326
Open days 2007	14 February, 25 April and 4 July
Entrance requirements	AABB
	Graduates need 2:1 degree and three Cs at A level
Mandatory subjects	Biology, chemistry
Male:female ratio	44:56
Is an exam included in the selection process?	Yes
If yes, what form does this exam take?	BMAT
Qualification gained	MBBS+BSc

Fascinating fact: The triangular teabag was invented at Imperial College!

Imperial College School of Medicine (sometimes known as ICSM rather than Imperial) is a fairly young institution, established in 1997 from the medical schools of St Mary's, Charing Cross and Westminster. However, despite the name change, the ideals and traditions of the old institutions have been upheld and built upon by the new school, creating its very own identity. For years, Imperial has been renowned for shaping a special kind of student (and eventually doctor): friendly, enthusiastic, and fun. The Faculty of Medicine at Imperial College is one of Europe's largest institutions – in terms of staff and student population and research income. The Sir Alexander Fleming building at the Imperial College site in South Kensington is very central and only a stone's throw away from Hyde Park, with first-year halls of residence close to this site. Imperial is now one of the largest medical schools in the country, proudly producing its own breed of doctors since 1994, and the non-course elements such as sport and music are flourishing in their new environment. Which other medical students graduate in the Royal Albert Hall?

Education

Imperial provides the new generation of medical students with a modern and integrated course which they can learn and thrive in, based on the curriculum outlined in the GMC document *Tomorrow's Doctors*. Imperial offers a 6-year course that is exemplary with both high performance in university league tables (top medical school in *The Guardian* in 2005!) as well as in research, where it is a world-class leader. Subject-based teaching has given way to modern and wide varieties of teaching with systems-based teaching, where the emphasis is on understanding and not just reciting knowledge and with a focus also placed on communication skills, ethics and law. Integrated teaching begins from the first day, with early exposure to general practice combined with both laboratory and clinical skills sessions. Studying at Imperial means unprecedented access to teaching from the UK's best – you can study cardiology at the best cardiac centre in the country, HIV at Chelsea's specialist unit, renal medicine at the country's biggest transplant centre, to name just a few. The well-tailored and enjoyable course has now matured and improved, year upon year, with the helpful and insightful comments of the pioneering students.

Teaching

A mixture of exams and continuous assessment is used to monitor students' progress. Didactic teaching is the mainstay of teaching at Imperial, with problem-based learning small group sessions also in place to reinforce learning. Students are encouraged to use computers and clinical skills laboratories, which are located on all campuses. Lectures and hospital attachments occur during all parts of the course, but as you progress more time is spent on the wards. Anatomy is taught from year 1 by dissection of cadavers as well as use of pre-dissected cadavers which you are guided through by an anatomist (usually a surgeon in training). These are fun weekly sessions which have been lost at many medical schools, but Imperial is proud to maintain this traditional aspect as students constantly comment on how useful dissection teaching is.

Assessments

End-of-year exams form the basis of assessment in years 1–3, with more regular assessments after most attachments as you progress into the clinical years. Formative exams in year 1 are useful to gain an idea of what is expected at medical school, as it is very different to what most have experienced before. Exams can include multiple-choice questions, extended-matching questions, short-answer questions and essays. Clinical exams take the role of the modern OSCE (observed structured clinical examinations). Retakes are offered after all end-of-year exams if things don't go to plan and are usually held in the September before the following academic year. Vivas (oral examinations) have been mainly phased out at Imperial, but remain in place for borderline candidates after the retakes. Assessments on the BSc take place throughout the year with in-course essays and also end-of-year exams. For those undertaking a research project, this is also assessed.

Intercalated degrees

Imperial is one of very few universities that offers a compulsory intercalated BSc degree and this can only be an advantage to set students in good stead for the future. The honours degree in year 4 offers students a chance to study in greater detail a subject that they have encountered during their years at medical school and enjoyed, or even take on a brand new discipline. An example of a new subject is management, which is undertaken at Imperial's renowned Tanaka Business School. The system available at Imperial is extremely flexible and as well as offering a great number of degrees from neuroscience to genetics, from paediatrics to psychology, and from biochemistry to obstetrics and gynaecology, there is also the possibility of studying the BSc at a different university, if you fancy a completely different environment for a year. The flexibility extends within each degree itself as students can choose to work on research projects finding themselves at the cusp of scientific knowledge with the prospect of publication, or opt to expand their horizons by studying taught modules that can include humanities and the social sciences.

Special study modules and electives

There is an 8-week elective in the final year where you are encouraged to learn and explore how medicine is practised abroad. Students have gained priceless insight and experience from their electives, be it in Cape Town or the Congo, Auckland or Alaska. Imperial offers many grants and funding assistance each year to students undertaking valuable study abroad, which helps ease the cost. An SSM in the final year covers a 3-week block in a topic of your choice. There is a wide range of specialities to choose from, ranging from alternative medicine to sports medicine to radiology.

Erasmus

Although Imperial as a university participates in the Socrates and Erasmus schemes, the school of medicine does not. However, students get the opportunity to spend time abroad not only on their elective, but some students may undertake their research projects abroad. Even students who stay in London for their projects may still get the chance to present their research findings at international symposia, which in the past have included Las Vegas and Amsterdam. Imperial also operates an exchange programme with the Tokyo Medical and Dental School.

Facilities

Library   There are libraries at all sites (including peripheral ones), most of which are open from 9 AM to 9 PM on weekdays, with times varying at weekends. In the summer term, the Central Library on the South Kensington campus operates a 24-hour opening policy, handy for those in exam season should they wish to spend their insomniac hours revising some physiology. The libraries do hold reference copies of all recommended texts, but loan copies can disappear quite quickly. All libraries also hold videos of clinical lectures, so that if you miss one or don't understand one, you can always review it at your leisure. Imperial also has the technology to 'beam out' centrally-given lectures to the peripheral hospitals so that you never miss important lectures if you are on an outside placement.

Computers   Emphasis on IT in the Imperial course extends to including many state-of-the-art learning programmes on all topics ranging from embryology to nephrology, as well as access to hundreds of electronic journals. All computers are modern and up-to-date with CD writers and DVD playing facilities, and IT training is also provided formally in year 1. There are computer facilities for Imperial medical students at all peripheral attachments as well. Printers and photocopiers are available at all sites using a 'pre-pay' card system that is convenient and easy to use.

Clinical skills   There are clinical skill labs at all central hospitals and peripheral hospitals. Students are encouraged to use them as part of their training in both timetabled and student-arranged sessions. They are very well equipped and good fun to use – many are supervised so that you can obtain help if you need it. You can practise everything from taking blood to doing a rectal examination on latex dummies. These help you build confidence before doing procedures on real patients, and always come in handy when it comes to preparation for exams.

Welcome 🏠

Student support

Students in the first years, who are based at South Kensington, can feel remote from the medical environment. During freshers' fortnight, each fresher is allocated a 'mum' or 'dad' student from the years above. Your 'parents' are there to help you adjust to university and medical school life. They also help you to ease into the social life and can offer advice and tips about the course; they may even cook you dinner and show you why medic life is so renowned!

Each student is also allocated a personal tutor, who should be available for personal, academic or financial advice. They are keen to be contacted, so never hesitate to approach them should a difficulty arise. There is also a head of pastoral care who can be contacted in the event of your tutor not being available. Imperial offers fantastic counselling and welfare services to all students. For those who would prefer to talk to a student instead or in addition to their tutor, the Student's Union has a welfare officer who is available at any time a friendly ear is needed.

Accommodation

The accommodation at Imperial cannot be matched. Not only are most of the halls located within 5 minutes of where your lectures will be, but it will be the only time in your life (for a long time anyway) that you will be able to afford to live in an SW7 postcode area (that means very nice indeed). All first-year students have a guaranteed place in halls and the pricing reflects whether the room is shared, single or *en-suite*. Aside from the advantage of being able to fall out of bed into your lecture theatres, all of Imperial's halls are located in plush surroundings.

Private sector accommodation is expensive if you want to live near to Imperial College in South Kensington. However, as you will spend the majority of your time from year 2 onwards based in Hammersmith, most students live in and around Hammersmith and Fulham where rent is less expensive but still quite high.

Placements

The school uses a wide range of centres across central and west London for teaching. The main teaching hospitals – Charing Cross (Hammersmith), Chelsea and Westminster (Fulham) and St Mary's (Paddington) – are supplemented by peripheral district general hospitals and teaching hospitals in Middlesex and Surrey. The impressive Sir Alexander Fleming building at the main Imperial College site is where students spend most of years 1 and 2. This is where lectures take place and where you will also find the Students' Union office and a café.

Students experience a wide range of clinical attachments, starting with GP practice placements in year 1. Initially, many attachments will be near to Imperial, but as you proceed into your specialist clinical studies they may be further afield (outside central London).

One of the many advantages of living in London is the tube, which gives easy access to virtually every location in the capital. There are good public transport links between all sites, and a London Transport discount scheme reduces the travel costs. Where there is difficulty getting home from peripheral sites (for example, if you are on call), free accommodation is provided.

Location of clinical placement/ name of hospital	Distance away from medical school (miles)	Difficulty getting there on public transport*
Charing Cross	4	🚶🚌
Chelsea	1.5	🚶
St. Mary's	1.5	🚶
West Middlesex	6	🚌 🚗
Northwick Park	9	🚗

* 🚶: walking/cycling distance; 🚌 : use public transport; 🚗: need own car or lift; ✈: get up early – tricky to get to!

Sports and social

City life

Nothing written in a short paragraph could do justice to the plethora of activities, events, venues, clubs and locations that London offers. Literally anything you ever want to do is on your doorstep, from the big exclusive clubs (many of which we hire for our balls) to galleries and theatres. Suffice to say that if you went to a different restaurant, cinema, bar, museum, or club each day for the 6 years you are here, you still wouldn't have seen it all!

University life

Medical school life is famously hectic and this is no less true at Imperial. Many of our events are steeped in tradition but we still have plenty of additions to increase the multitude of opportunities available. We have a Students' Union which operates its own clubs and societies to help Imperial medics maintain a separate identity from the rest of Imperial College students. However, medical students are still able to take advantage of Imperial College Union and its teams and clubs (of which there are over 300!). Clubs range from individual countries' societies to ultimate frisbee. Whatever your creed, colour, faith, political persuasion or niche interest, Imperial can guarantee that there will be a club/society to suit you!

We also have our very own newly refurbished student bar, The Reynolds, at the Charing Cross campus, which hosts regular events including film nights, Paramount Comedy Channel nights, regular Wednesday Sports nights as well as Imperial's renowned 'bops'. These produce a good turn out of students from all the years, often in amusing fancy dress. Highlights of the year include the whole of freshers' fortnight (especially the Roadshow, the Doctors and Nurses pub crawl and the outstanding freshers' ball), the inter-year rugby match, RAG week, including the Circle line pub crawl, 'Bumps', countless plays and concerts and, of course, our legendary black-tie balls. There are plenty of medical student events spread through each term, organized by either the medical school union or individual clubs and societies, to ensure that everyone plays just as hard, if not harder, than they work!

Sports life

Imperial College medical school teams have grounds at Teddington (previously home to England RFC), Chiswick and Richmond, whilst Harlington is the largest of our sports grounds (also serving as the training ground of Chelsea FC). Students can also use one of three Imperial College-owned sports centres at various campuses, as well as the brand new flagship Imperial Sports Centre, which provides the South Kensington campus with some of the best sporting facilities in London.

The Imperial medics rugby team (old boys include JPR Williams) has already made a name for itself at a European level, and the school frequently holds many United Hospitals trophies. A substantial financial rugby scholarship is also awarded annually to the fresher who has made the greatest impression at the club. Rowing at Imperial College is world-class, having produced Olympic gold medallists, and the training facilities reflect this with a boathouse in Putney and a University of London boathouse in Gunnersbury. Women's sports are well-established, with hockey and netball being among the most popular. Other sports include football, water polo, cricket, golf, mountaineering, windsurfing and mixed lacrosse, to name but a few. The variety of sporting choice is paralleled only by the mixture of abilities: from the social players to the semi-professionals and internationals, all are welcome and encouraged.

Great things about Imperial

- The opportunities available here will ensure you leave with the greatest of experiences.
- State-of-the-art audiovisual systems, meaning that if you are at one site and the lecture is at another it can be beamed to your site.

- You can choose between the close-knit medical community at the medical school, the larger Imperial College environment, or metropolitan city life.
- The award-winning Sir Alexander Fleming building at the South Kensington Imperial College site, as well as Chelsea and Westminster Hospital (known as the 'Hilton Hospital') means salubrious surroundings.
- The pick of the crop of teaching hospitals in the heart of London – St. Mary's has won national recognition for its clinical excellence.
- Students live in the vibrant, safe, cosmopolitan area of west London – and halls in year 1 in South Kensington make celebrity spotting a frequent occurrence.

Bad things about Imperial

- The course is academic; however, expect the demands to be great and the rewards high.
- Travel between sites adds to the expense of studying and can be stressful.
- Split teaching at different sites can divide the year group up.
- Imperial College is sometimes pictured as boring and academic. But remember that's not the medics!
- Expensive, polluted, overpopulated, time-consuming, dirty old London.

Further information

School of Medicine
Imperial College
London SW7 2AZ
Tel: 020 7594 8056
Fax: 020 7594 8004
Email: admitmed@imperial.ac.uk
Web: http://www.imperial.ac.uk

Additional application information	
Average A level requirements	• AABB
Average Scottish Higher requirements	• AAABB + AAB in Advanced Highers
Make-up of interview panel	• Chair, two members of the selection panel and a senior medical student
Months in which interviews are held	• January – April
Proportion of overseas students	• 6%
Proportion of mature students	• 7%
Proportion of graduate students	• 7%

Faculty's view of students taking a gap year	• Welcomed – applicants must state in UCAS personal statement how they propose to spend their time. Deferred applications not normally accepted from graduate, mature or overseas applicants.
Proportion of students taking intercalated degrees	• 100% (suitably qualified students may apply for exemption from BSc year and if granted exemption will follow a five-year course and will be awarded the MBBS degree only)
Possibility of direct entrance to clinical phase	• No (apart from an agreement with Oxford and Cambridge to fill a quota of transfer places)
Fees for overseas students	• £21,350 (years 1, 2 and 3) • £31,900 (years 4, 5 and 6)
Fees for graduates	• £3000 for Home/EU, as above for overseas. • The above fees are for 2006 entry. The fees for 2007 have not yet been announced.
Ability to transfer to other medical schools If so, under what circumstances	• If the student has the agreement of the Head of Undergraduate Medicine in exceptional circumstances.
Assistance for elective funding	• Based on contribution to medical school and/or hardship reasons.
Assistance for travel to attachments	• None available.
Access and hardship funds	• Several funds are available to all students.
Weekly rent	• £50 (triple room in halls) –£120 (private with en-suite bathroom)
Pint of lager	• £2.80
Cinema	• £7.00
Nightclub	• Free–£20

Leeds

Key facts	Undergraduate
Course length	5 years
Total number of medical undergraduates	1250
Applicants in 2006	3058
Interviews given in 2006	782
Places available in 2006	238
Places available in 2007	238
Open days 2007	June and September
Entrance requirements	AAB
Mandatory subjects	Chemistry
Male:female ratio	36:64 (for first year)
Is an exam included in the selection process?	Yes
If yes, what form does this exam take?	UKCAT
Qualification gained	MBChB

Fascinating fact: You can fit a mini into the lifts in the medical school.

Leeds is the fastest-growing city in the UK outside London and is an exciting and vibrant city in which to train. The legendary Leeds MedSoc ensures all the medics have a great time with its superbly organized parties, balls, barbeques, trips and more besides!

The course at Leeds underwent a major overhaul several years ago. Clinically orientated teaching takes place from year 1 and hospital-based training begins as early as year 2. Staff and departments have been receptive to feedback, with student representatives sitting on the board for each module. This has generated a very student-friendly atmosphere, and a course that is continually being improved. There is a wide mix of students from around the UK as well as overseas and mature students. Medics can sometimes feel a little separated from the rest of the student population, as they are mostly based in the medical school, but most get a chance to mix in halls of residence and through sports clubs and societies.

Education

Applicants will need to sit the UKCAT (see Chapter 3). An excellent Medical Students' Representative Council (MSRC) has been instrumental in designing the new-style course and is in constant contact with the staff to ensure that it continues to run smoothly. The bulk of the course is based around modules (or 'integrated core units', as some choose to call them) which are focused on systems of the body. Students look at all the different aspects of this system – such as anatomy, physiology and biochemistry – then link this in with clinical practice. In this way an academic framework is created that is relevant to the different specialities within medicine, surgery and primary care. You also look at behavioural sciences, ethics, epidemiology and personal and professional skills, though not all at the same time! In the later years the focus is more on individual specialities and it is more clinically based. There is clinical teaching from the very start of year 1, with more clinical experience being incorporated as the course progresses. Leeds also offers a vast range of special study components (SSCs), where you can create your own projects or explore particular areas of interest which lie outside the core curriculum in more depth.

Teaching

Teaching at Leeds is well-integrated, with a mix of practical classes, online learning, small group work, tutorials, lectures and clinical sessions. The use of computer-based learning is core, with experiments, tutorials and practice test questions being placed on the intranet. Anatomy is still taught using full-body dissection of human cadavers in years 1 to 3, and you share a body with a group of 4 or 5 people in your year. Clinical teaching on the ward starts during year 2. Leeds has the largest teaching complex in Europe and ward-based teaching is split between the Leeds General Infirmary, St James' Hospital and Bradford Royal Infirmary.

Assessment

Assessments vary depending on the module. However, the major assessments are the integrated examinations at the end of the year, consisting of MCQs and EMQs that cover the year's work. There is a chance to do a preparatory formative exam, which helps you know what to expect and how much work you need to do for the real thing. SSCs also count toward a major part of the course and OSCEs, which assess clinical skills, occur in years 3, 4 and 5.

Intercalated degrees

Students have a choice as to whether or not they want to do an extra year to gain a BSc or a BA. The intercalated year can be taken after years 2, 3 or 4. The number of places available for intercalating has recently increased and a large number of scholarships are available. The range of degrees available is also expansive, from biomedical ethics to psychology, sports science and beyond.

Special study modules and electives

Self-selected components (SSCs) run throughout the course and the staff at Leeds have received awards for the range of SSCs offered. In year 1, the emphasis is on learning how to access medical literature, conduct a scientific investigation, and improve on computing and teamwork skills. In year 2, students undertake a literature review and also have the opportunity to do something a bit different such as training with the police. Year 3 offers students the opportunity to design their own project. This has resulted in many published articles for Leeds students (very useful on your CV!). There are three SSCs in year 4 and four in year 5, with the chance to travel abroad. The range is huge, with medical history, ethics, foreign languages, working with the police, developing teaching skills, giving sex education, research projects and going on clinical or community placements being just some of the projects on offer.

A 10-week elective is timetabled at the beginning of year 5, from the first week of August to the first week of October. Most students use this opportunity to experience a health service in another country, and find it a truly amazing experience. Where you go is entirely up to you, and the possibilities are endless!

Erasmus

There is no Erasmus scheme.

Facilities

Library   The medical school has its own library. This is well-stocked with the latest publications, core textbooks, a plethora of other medical literature and access to e-journals and the best medical databases online. The library is open every day of the week and stays open until midnight near exams. It is easy to use, the staff are always very helpful and you can always be sure to bump into some familiar faces – most people find it a great place to get some work done. Medical students also have access to all the other libraries in the university as well as hospital libraries.

Computers   There is excellent provision of computers throughout Leeds University. The 200 plus computers in the medical school have recently been updated to flat screens and medical students are also granted access to computer clusters in the local hospitals, and any other cluster within the university. An IT course is run at the beginning of year 1 to help those who need to update their computer literacy. There is also a 24-hour computer cluster on campus, and many of the other clusters are open until late.

Clinical skills   There are clinical skills laboratories at St James' Hospital, Leeds General Infirmary (LGI) and Bradford Royal Infirmary. These offer the opportunity to practise on the same equipment that will be used in the exams.

Welfare

Student support

There is a wide level of support at Leeds including the highly successful student-mentoring scheme, where you're adopted into a 'medical family' consisting of students in higher year groups: parents, siblings and all! The individual personal tutor scheme is also highly successful, with tutor group meals being a termly affair, and the counselling services are always on hand when things get a bit too much. The student-mentoring scheme (affectionately known as MUMS) means that every new medical student has two 'parents' from the year above to show them around, make sure they make it through the first week relatively unscathed and answer questions that you may not want to ask the staff. If you would prefer to speak to a member of staff, each student is also attached to a doctor who is a point of contact for personal and academic issues. Students in years 1 and 2 have the opportunity to meet with the academic deans to discuss their progress and highlight any fears or anxieties they may have. The MSRC also provides a direct link with staff: it can anonymously relay any problems you've encountered and is available to accompany you to any meetings that you might arrange with the staff, should you so wish. The Students' Union and the university also have excellent counselling services.

Accommodation

Most first-year students live in university accommodation, either halls or flats. These can be fairly costly, but standards are generally good and this can be a great way to meet non-medics. In the second year, many move out to back-to-back houses in Headingley, Hyde Park or Woodhouse. Rents starts at about £50 per week, but most pay a little more. Insurance is pricey and, like any student area, burglary can be a problem. The locals are mostly friendly, but can sometimes be a little anti-student, but your mates all live in the next street. There is help in finding accommodation available from the university Unipol scheme and there is always a whole bunch of other medics looking for housemates towards the end of the year.

Placements

The medical school is on campus but is also attached to the Leeds General Infirmary (LGI – one of the main teaching hospitals). The city centre is less than a 10-minute walk from the school, and free shuttle buses run from the LGI to St James' Hospital and to other hospitals that students may need to attend. Facilities in the teaching hospitals are of a high standard. The three main teaching hospitals are St James', LGI and Bradford Royal Infirmary. A lot of district general hospitals are also used, including York, Harrogate, Ilkley, Halifax, Scunthorpe, Otley, Hull, Huddersfield and Wakefield. A few third-year students even spend a term in the Yorkshire Dales! In years 4 and 5 attachments can be even further afield. All accommodation and transport is provided for residential attachments. Travel costs are variable and are to a certain degree supported by the university, although students may occasionally be expected to carry the cost. Free buses are provided to some placements. Associated district hospitals incorporate the majority of West and North Yorkshire with Sheffield medical school occupying South Yorkshire.

Location of clinical placement/ name of hospital	Distance away from medical school (miles)	Difficulty getting there on public transport*
Leeds General Infirmary, City centre	0	walking/cycling
St James' University Hospital	2.7	bus
Bradford Royal Infirmary	15	bus / car
Seacroft Hospital	7.2	bus
Wharfedale Hospital	12.9	car

* : walking/cycling distance;   : use public transport;   : need own car or (continued)
  : get up early – tricky to get to!

Sports and social

City life

The main city centre has all the shopping and nightlife your bank account can take, and is within a 10-minute walk from the main campus. Theatre, Opera North, museums and galleries cater for the culture vultures. Sport is big in Leeds, especially football, cricket, rugby union and rugby league.

Leeds nightlife is arguably unrivalled; there really is something to cater for everyone's taste! The usual student cheesey music is a-plenty with Creation and Evolution being huge nights. Halo, an old renovated church, seems to be the place to go for your dance, with Townhouse being an outlet for funky house. R'n'B also seems to be everywhere, at random club nights – particularly at the huge Majestik. There's a big Indie scene, with all the big bands coming to play in Leeds, either at the Cockpit, the Faversham, the Refectory, Joseph's Well or the Brundell Social club. And alternative nights aren't sparse either with the Cockpit putting on a few a week, bar Phono being a haven, with Wendy House and Star also being highly-rated. For jazz there are plenty of small bars, but Hi-Fi is a major attraction, with a decent live jazz night. In short, whatever you like you are spoilt for choice when it comes to a night out in Leeds!

It is also, quite possibly, the shopping capital of the north. The city centre boasts the first Harvey Nichols outside London, the ultra-trendy Corn Exchange and, with countless other shops, there is everything anyone could want. It is quite easy to get lost during the first couple of weeks! The people in Leeds are generally very friendly and happy to help, though they seem to be outnumbered by the students at the beginning of the year. The Yorkshire Dales are a short bus journey away and are a fantastic place to walk and get away from the hustle and bustle of life in the city. There are good road links and Leeds is on the fast rail network to London and Edinburgh, with good rail links to most places. Historic York is just a short journey away.

University life

The Students' Union has had a huge cash injection and comprises four bars, a nightclub, a new trendy café, a bistro and a supermarket. Leeds MedSoc is the largest and probably the most active society of the Union and organizes endless events, including two annual balls, bowling nights, pub-crawls, ice-skating, quizzes, ballet trips and lots of general drinking nights.

Sports life

Sports are huge at Leeds. After becoming a sports member for just £45 a year, you have pretty much unrestricted access to the huge amount of facilities at Leeds. It is free to book badminton, squash, and football courts/AstroTurfs. The huge multigym is only 50p a visit. The university has a huge number of teams and organizations from samurai jujitsu to aviation to good old-fashioned rugby! If you are too busy for uni sports the MSRC has huge number of medics' sports teams, which are organised to fit around the medic timetable. Medics' hockey is huge, mixed and attracts lots of non-medics too; best of all it doesn't take itself too seriously – you turn up as much or as little as you want, and it doesn't matter how good you are or even if you've played before! Medics' rugby is also massive, and is of a surprisingly high standard – they even beat the Leeds University first team last season. In addition there's medics' badminton, football, netball, cricket and – brand new – medics' lacrosse.

Societies

There is an infinite number of societies at Leeds University. From MedSIN (which raises awareness about international health) to WAMS (widening access to medical school), Rocksoc to Scottish Country Dancing and the Real Ale Appreciation Society to Theatre Group there is something to suit all tastes. A number of society fairs are held at the beginning of the year, from where you can sign up to whatever you fancy.

Great things about Leeds

- You get to learn the anatomy on real bodies, not just textbooks and videos (great for would-be surgeons).
- The city centre is right on your doorstep and everything you could want, from a multitude of shops to banks, bars and clubs, is all in one place.
- The Medical Students' Representative Council is highly-respected by the staff and so the course is very student-orientated.
- Proximity to the Yorkshire Dales – a city in the country!
- The staff go out of their way to make sure the transition from school life to medical school life is as easy and gentle as possible.

Bad things about Leeds

- Leeds University does not have a swimming pool.
- Medics always seem to have exams and holidays when the rest of the university hasn't, and vice versa.
- There is not enough parking on campus.
- Leeds has no major concert venue.
- Some medics struggle to make friends outside of the medical school.

Further information

Admissions Office
School of Medicine
University of Leeds
Leeds LS2 9JT
Tel: 0113 343 7194
Fax: 0113 233 4375
Email: ugadmissions@leeds.ac.uk
Web: http://www.leeds.ac.uk

Additional application information

Average A level requirements	• AAB
Average Scottish Higher requirements	• AAAAB plus two Advanced Highers
Make-up of interview panel	• Two staff members from university or affiliated hospitals or local GP plus one medical student
Months in which interviews are held	• January – March
Proportion of overseas students	• 16%
Proportion of mature students	• 5%
Proportion of graduate students	• 4%
Faculty's view of students taking a gap year	• Encouraged for those wishing to gain work experience, voluntary work or travel.
Proportion of students taking intercalated degrees	• 10%
Possibility of direct entrance to clinical phase	• Yes, but only for dentists wishing to gain a medical degree for maxillo-facial career.
Fees for overseas students	• £11,400 pa (years 1 and 2) £21,300 pa (years 3, 4 and 5)
Fees for graduates	• £3000
Ability to transfer to other medical schools If so, under what circumstances	• Not encouraged due to the integrated nature of the course.
Assistance for elective funding	• Yes, although applications with projects are more successful than those for clinical attachments.
Assistance for travel to attachments	• Shuttle buses and coaches are provided for some attachments but not others. In addition, students can apply through their LEA.
Access and hardship funds	• Many available through the university.

Weekly rent	• £50–95 (halls) • £50–75 (private)
Pint of lager	• £1.40 Union • £2.50 city centre pubs
Cinema	• £4.50
Nightclub	• £3–6

Leeds

Leicester

Key facts	Undergraduate	Graduate
Course length	5 years	4 years
Total number of medical undergraduates	1000	171
Applicants in 2006	2000	450
Interviews given in 2006	1400	250
Places available in 2006	175	64
Places available in 2007	175	64
Open days 2007	June	
Entrance requirements	AAB	2:1 in health science degree with at least 2 years' postgraduate work experience delivering health care to patients
Mandatory subjects	A in chemistry	
Male:female ratio	50:50	
Is an exam included in the selection process?	Yes	Yes
If yes, what form does this exam take?	UKCAT in 2007	UKCAT in 2007
Qualification gained	MBChB	MBChB

Fascinating fact: The university administration building used to be an asylum.

Leicester is a young medical school whose first students graduated in 1980. It is a friendly place, with teaching for phase I on the university campus in the Maurice Shock Building (MSB), around 15 minutes' walk from the city centre. Most halls are further out of town, in a lovely area of Leicester that boast the botanical gardens. The later phases of the course are largely based at the Clinical Sciences Building (CSB). This is part of Leicester Royal Infirmary and is also close to the city centre. The Students' Union on campus provides many good nights out, with a wide range of alternative nightlife and other events organised by the medical student society (LUSUMA) including balls, outings and the annual ski trip.

In 2003, the 5-year course in Leicester was joined by a new 4-year course in medicine for health science graduates. The 4-year accelerated course is the second of the Leicester Warwick Medical Schools programmes to offer graduates a specialized programme of study.

Approximately 10% of students on the 5-year course are mature students and there is a good representation of international students from a variety of countries.

Education

Applicants need to sit the UKCAT (see Chapter 3). Leicester's 5-year course is currently divided into 2 phases, each lasting 2½ years. Ahead of most other medical schools, Leicester has moved away from the traditional preclinical and clinical approach, in order to focus its curriculum on an integrated, interactive and proactive student-based learning approach. This is especially the case in the hospital-based part of the course.

Phase I is primarily taught at the medical school and its modular structure is based on tutorials, lectures and interactive group sessions. Students are introduced to both patients and cadavers in the first week of term, to ensure that students know from the outset how to effectively communicate with patients and their families and understand the importance of the interpersonal skills required as a doctor in addition to the academic acumen. Building on this, at the start of year 2, students are let loose on wards at one of the three major teaching hospitals in the city and are given excellent consultant-led opportunities to practise history-taking and examination techniques. Phase I students are heavily supported with many clinical teachers and learning aids, and are taught in an often imaginative and forward-thinking way.

Phase II is mainly clinical, with ward, clinic and theatre teaching in different specialities. The teaching in this phase very much depends on the consultant team each student is attached to. Phase II also includes an elective period, where students are encouraged to travel abroad in order to experience medicine in a different country, culture, or context. There have also been many students who have had successful electives within the UK in areas of medicine that are not covered by the undergraduate curriculum.

Progression from phase I to II is dependent upon passing a written and a practical examination.

The graduate course at Leicester has been incredibly successful, attracting students from all over the country, and indeed the world, to its 4-year programme. Students come from a variety of backgrounds including nursing, physiotherapy, radiography and psychology. Ages range from early twenties to early forties, with most students choosing to live in the city or county; however, there are an increasing number who cope with living further afield.

Phase I of the 4-year course is only 1½ years (as opposed to 2½ years in the 5-year course), but covers the same material. This makes the course intense but rewarding. Formal teaching time is around 25–30 hours per week plus your own self-directed learning time. The intensity of the timetable makes doing paid work difficult, although there is a long summer break between years 1 and 2.

Exams for both the year 4 and 5 courses take place primarily in January and June. Extra time is given to any student with specific educational needs, e.g. dyslexia. Phase II (the hospital-based phase) of both the 4- and 5-year courses has an identical format.

Teaching

During phase I, students are allocated to a group of eight for tutorial work. They remain with this group throughout the preclinical years. Each group is given its own cadaver to work on throughout the year in dissection and anatomy teaching. Tutorials are taken by academics in 4 groups of 8 students. Phase II teaching is on the wards, but it is backed by some lectures in the form of an academic half-day each week. Students are placed with a clinical partner of their own choice. Attendance is registered and contributes to passing each clinical attachment as well as the completion of case portfolios. There are thirteen 8-week blocks, which rotate through disciplines and include an elective. For each block, the pair of clinical students is attached to two or three consultant teams of different specialities.

Assessment

Module examinations are mainly written short-answer questions or assessed essays. There is a 15-station OSCPE (objective structured clinical and practical exam) examination at the end of semester two. Assessment in phase II includes patient portfolios (case studies) and clinical skills (histories and examinations); students also receive formative grading from their consultants on completion of each clinical attachment to help assess their progress. Finals have a clinical component and written examinations.

Intercalated degrees

Any student wishing to do an Honours year is encouraged to do so. Honours degrees can be science-based or clinical and there are a wide range of subjects to choose from, usually comprising either a research project within the faculty of medicine, or students may join the final year of a course within the faculty of medicine and biological sciences to pursue further study. Students have the option of intercalating after either year 3 or 4 of study, assuming their academic performance is good enough.

Special study modules and electives

All students have a 2-month elective module, which can be carried out in the UK or abroad, and takes place during year 4.

Two special study modules (SSM) are taken in phase I and one in phase II. It is compulsory to study one science SSM, although other subjects such as languages are available for the second in phase I. These allow the student to have an opportunity to pursue some of their specific interests that are not necessarily covered elsewhere in the curriculum.

Erasmus

Students currently take part in the Erasmus programme during the clinical phase of the course, with links to universities in Lausanne (Switzerland) Granada (Spain) and Homburg (Germany). Whilst there are many advantages to experiencing medicine in an overseas setting there are also disadvantages in that you do miss an entire block, which may cover an area of medicine or surgery that you won't cover again. Some working knowledge of the native language of the host is required when applying for Erasmus.

Leicester has recently entered the MedSIN/IFMSA exchange programme, which is organized by the MedSIN National Officer for Professional Exchanges. This allows clinical students to directly switch places with a foreign student for a 4-week period. The list of participating countries is globally vast. Interested students should consult the IFMSA website at www.ifmsa.org or the Leicester MedSIN organization.

All students have a 2-month elective module, which can be carried out in the UK or abroad, and takes place during March of year 4.

Facilities

Library   The main university library is on campus, near to the MSB, and is open until midnight Monday to Friday and until 6 PM on Saturdays and 9 PM on Sundays (times vary during vacations). There are also medical libraries at the three main teaching hospitals. The CSB library at the Leicester Royal Infirmary is the largest of these and is open 24 hours a day, making it popular around examination times! It is staffed between 9 AM and 10 PM on weekdays. The staffed hours are shorter on Saturday (9 AM–6 PM) and Sunday (2 PM–9 PM).

Computers   There are computer facilities for all university students on the main campus in the main library and the Charles Wilson and Ken Edwards buildings. The MSB has a computer room for medical students, which has recently been refitted with new computers. There are also PCs available at the clinical sciences libraries at all three University Hospitals of Leicester sites. Course work (case studies and essays) must be word-processed. The medical school is gradually introducing on line assessments in some modules.

Clinical skills   Clinical skills at Leicester begin during the first year of study. This initially takes the form of interviewing 'simulated patients' as well as practising physical examination skills on volunteers. These skills are examined at the end of year 1 in the form of OSCPEs. This progresses in year 2 to clinical placements one morning per week in one of the Leicester hospitals, where the skills learnt in year 1 are revised and put into practice.

Welfare

Student support

Student welfare takes a high priority at Leicester and is achieved through a number of structures, both within the medical school and in the wider university community. Within the medical school pastoral support is provided by personal tutors and the medics welfare team.

Each tutor group is allocated a personal tutor who is a nominated faculty member and plays a pastoral role. Overall, the faculty staff are very approachable and supportive. During phase II of the course each hospital has a student facilitator to deal with queries and problems. There is always a member of staff available (24 hours a day) if there are any major problems or emergencies.

The medics' welfare team was established several years ago and provides a comprehensive peer support structure for medics in all years. The team comprises a small group of medical students, appointed each year following interview, who provide a discreet pastoral support service to other medical students who might be experiencing difficulties, either personally or academically.

The team comprises members of varying ages and backgrounds, spanning both the 5-year standard entry and 4-year health science courses. They offer a range of services including drop-in clinics and also run a student mentoring scheme, which links medics who are having difficulty getting their head around one or more of the phase I academic modules with a student from the years above who is competent in the relevant subject(s).

In the wider University of Leicester community there are a structured range of services. These include a self-referral counselling service, services to support students with established or suspected disabilities, a centre specializing in developing study and presentations skills, a university welfare service, which provides a range of practical advice and support, including financial and housing guidance, and Nightline, which is run by students for students, providing support throughout the night (including telephone numbers for taxis and late-night food delivery!).

Most areas of the medical school and university have standard disabled access facilities, such as ramps and lifts. Anyone with specific requirements would be advised to check with the university before application.

Accommodation

University accommodation is available throughout the course, and some medical students stay in university accommodation beyond the first year. In the first year it is popular – and advisable – to live in catered halls, as there are loads of activities and great end-of-term balls and parties. Privately rented accommodation is inexpensive but variable in quality. It is best to shop around in advance for a good deal. A Union-run accommodation office can help you find places and there are many notices on the medical school noticeboards for house-shares.

Placements

Phase I is based on the university campus in the MSB, and phase II is based in the Robert Kilpatrick Building at the Leicester Royal Infirmary (LRI). The LRI is only a 10-minute walk from the MSB, and everything is in reasonable proximity. Teaching also takes place at the Leicester General and Glenfield General Hospitals, both of which are a short bus- or cycle-ride away for the more energetic. There is no student parking available at either the university or the LRI, but there is plenty of free parking at either Glenfield or the General. The medical school is currently undergoing an investment programme which will see a new multi-disciplinary medical sciences teaching building being built with an expected opening date in 2009. In addition, district general hospitals are used in Kettering, Northampton, Boston, Lincoln, Burton-on-Trent and Peterborough, where free accommodation is provided. GP attachments were traditionally in the Leicester area; however, due to the increasing numbers of students, placements further afield, such as Northampton, are increasingly being used.

Location of clinical placement/ name of hospital	Distance away from medical school (miles)	Difficulty getting there on public transport*
Leicester Royal Infirmary	0.5	
Leicester General Hospital	2.5	
Peterborough District Hospital	40	
Pilgrim Hospital, Boston	65	
Queens Hospital, Burton-on-Trent	34	

* : walking/cycling distance; : use public transport; : need own car or lift; : get up early – tricky to get to!

Sports and social

City life

The city centre is about a 45-minute walk from halls, or 10–15 minutes from the university campus. There is a regular bus service between halls, the town centre and the university during term time and a student bus pass is available to buy, giving discounted travel. Leicester has a good range of cinemas, a theatre, pubs, clubs, bars and shops, which reflect the city's diverse ethnicity. There are plenty of restaurants, and curry lovers in particular have a wide choice. There are popular clubs in town and late bars to suit all tastes. Many top bands come to Leicester on tour, visiting De Montfort Hall and De Montfort University. The Charlotte is also a renowned venue for smaller events and is frequented by several popular bands. Leicester has all the facilities of a city as well as some of the homeliness and friendliness of a smaller town.

The city is reasonably small, but has all the shops you could want. There is an excellent fruit, veg and fish market for fresh food (cheaper than the supermarkets). If you have your own transport, the Leicestershire countryside is attractive and makes a pleasant escape from the city. There is Championship football and world-class rugby on the doorstep. If you are lucky, on some of the wards at the LRI you can just about see into the rugby stadium!

University life

At the Students' Union there are club nights every Wednesday, Thursday, Friday and some Saturdays. There are also university events at local clubs – such as the exotically named Zanzibar every week. The Redfearn bar is open all day weekdays and food is available – it proves a popular place to relax after lectures or exams. Elements, which is found in the Union building, is open from 10 AM serving coffees and snacks. LUSUMA (the medics society) arranges a full social programme for the pre-session course named *Introweek*, and the largest social event of the year takes place during this week, the pyjama pub crawl. They also continue to arrange social events every term, such as Halloween parties, a medic's revue, a *Stars in their Eyes* show, and a summer and winter medics' ball. There are a large variety of university societies to choose from; you will be spoilt for choice and it is a great way to meet students from other courses. Many medical students are involved with university societies. The university provides safe transport for all students with its night minibuses, which take students from the campus to anywhere within the city limits. The buses run from approximately 6 PM in the winter (7 PM in the summer) until the Union closes at 2 AM. There is a minibus card available to buy which gets you a free ride, or each journey currently costs £1.

Sports life

Medical students have the opportunity to join university sporting teams (of which there are many) as well as the wide range of medics' sporting teams available. Thanks to team captains and the sporting secretaries, there have been vast improvements in recent years in the organization of the teams. Many teams receive sponsorship from local businesses. There are often sports days at home and away against other medical schools. The university has sports fields at Stoughton Road, two sports halls, two gyms, where there are circuits and aerobic classes, and an athletics track. There are plenty of swimming pools in town, or one near the university halls in Oadby. The medical school adheres (during phase I) to the non-scheduling of lessons on afternoon Wednesdays when matches take place. Due to timetabling commitments the 4 year course students are not released from teaching on Wednesday afternoons.

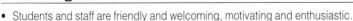

Great things about Leicester

- Students and staff are friendly and welcoming, motivating and enthusiastic.
- There are wide-ranging activities available for all organised by LUSUMA, the Union and other societies.
- Great improvement in Leicester's nightlife in recent years, with many new bars, clubs and restaurants for varying tastes.
- Leicester was ranked number one in *The Guardian* teaching league tables in 2003.
- Clear module objectives to assist with self-directed learning.

Bad things about Leicester

- The location of placements can present you with travel problems.
- Lack of temperature control in lecture theatres.
- Phase II students are spread about the region.
- Not near the sea. In fact, Leicester is about as far from it as you can be.
- No student car parking at the university and Leicester Royal Infirmary.

Further information

Dr Kevin West
Maurice Shock Medical Sciences Building
Leicester University
University Road
Leicester LE1 7RH
Tel: 0116 252 2969/2985/2966
Fax: 0116 252 3013
Email: med-admis@le.ac.uk
Web: http://www.le.ac.uk/sm/le/

Additional application information	
Average A level requirements	• AAB
Average Scottish Higher requirements	• AAB
Graduate entry requirements	• 2:1 in health science discipline
Make-up of interview panel	• One senior staff, one final year medical student
Months in which interviews are held	• November – February
Proportion of overseas students	• 5%
Proportion of mature students	• Not known
Proportion of graduate students	• Not known
Faculty's view of students taking a gap year	• Neutral
Proportion of students taking intercalated degrees	• 10%
Possibility of direct entrance to clinical phase	• No
Fees for overseas students	• Please contact university for details
Fees for graduates	• £3000
Ability to transfer to other medical schools If so, under what circumstances	• Transfers to other medical schools are not encouraged, but if necessary are allowed.

(Continued)

(*Continued*)

Assistance for elective funding	• Six small bursaries for electives per year. Contacts for other sources of potential funding also available.
Assistance for travel to attachments	• Small reimbursement for the Learning from Lives module at the beginning of phase II; otherwise no assistance.
Access and hardship funds	• Administered through the university welfare service.
Weekly rent	• £51–£90
Pint of lager	• £1.90–£2.20 (Student Union)
Cinema	• £4.50 with NUS card
Nightclub	• Free entry before 10.30pm weekdays. Thereafter £5–£7. Student nights in the week often only cost £2–£3

Liverpool

Key facts	Undergraduate	Graduate
Course length	5 years	4 years
Total number of medical undergraduates	1402	94
Applicants in 2006	2000	550
Interviews given in 2006	1043	90
Places available in 2006	292	32
Places available in 2007	292	32
Open days 2007	29 March	
Entrance requirements	AABB	2:1 degree in life/health sciences and BBB
Mandatory subjects	Biology and chemistry	Biology and chemistry
Male:female ratio	40:60	38:62
Is an exam included in the selection process?	No	No
If yes, what form does this exam take?		
Qualification gained	MBChB	MBChB

Fascinating fact: The Liverpool Medics Students Society is the oldest in the country. Its record for downing a yard of ale is only 12 seconds!

In 1996 Liverpool Medical School introduced a new curriculum, in accordance with GMC guidelines, and this is proving to be a success. August 2001 saw the first PBL (problem-based learning) students to graduate at Liverpool start on wards as doctors. The school has grown in size, with around 1200 undergraduates and the introduction of the new graduate-entry programme, but a strong medical students' society ensures there's always a friendly face around. The city is the European Capital of Culture for 2008 – a well-deserved honour – which has bought massive investment and is helping in continuing to transform this great city. In the words of Roger McGough, a local Liverpool poet: 'I used to have to defend the city, but now the city speaks for itself.'

Education ▌

Since the introduction of the PBL course, subjects are no longer taught in lecture theatres; instead, different areas of medicine are presented to students as case scenarios. Students discuss the issues and formulate learning objectives in small groups with tutor guidance, then go and research the topics for themselves. Community attachments start from the middle of year 1, and from the beginning of year 2 an increasing proportion of time is spent on hospital and community attachments. Studies follow the human lifecycle, from conception and birth through adulthood and into old age.

Teaching

The new course contains little in the way of formal teaching. In years 1 and 2, plenaries (lectures) are given that are designed to provide an overview only of each problem, in a newly built state-of-the-art lecture theatre (a plenary theatre?). Anatomy is visualized and self-taught with the aid of nearby anatomists, using models and prosections in a recently refurbished and improved multi-million-pound human anatomy resource centre. Clinical skills and communication skills are taught throughout the course.

From arriving in hospital, teaching is arranged during hospital placements with excellent standards of a variety of bedside and small group teaching in addition to ward rounds and clinics. The main teaching hospitals are well-respected centres of excellence at the cutting edge of modern research and practice.

The new graduate-entry course provides an accelerated course for graduates in which years 1 and 2 of the traditional course are merged into one.

Assessment

Assessment is continuous, designed so that everything you learn (including practical skills) will be recognized and recorded. Summative exams occur at the end of each year for the first four years, with no exams in the final year! The final year comprises five 8-week rotations, consisting of two self-selectives plus general practice, accident and emergency and the shadowing of a Foundation Year 1 doctor (an excellent chance to prepare students for the realities of the house job). Consultant assessment of performance takes place at the end of each of the rotations.

Intercalated degrees

It is possible to study for an intercalated degree at the end of year 4, with BSc, BA or masters degrees available dependent on the course taken. It is possible to transfer to undertake the degree and then return to complete the medical course at Liverpool. Limited funding is available to some students wishing to study for an intercalated year.

Special study modules and electives

There are 6 SSMs spread through years 1–4 of the course, covering a wide range of subjects: all bar one are 4 weeks in length. The fifth SSM in year 3 allows a more in-depth study of a topic, lasting one day a week for two-thirds of the year, providing the opportunity for students to arrange their own module. Topics from any speciality can be chosen, with a 2500-word essay for each module. Some students are able to get their work published in medical journals.

In addition, in the final year there are the two SAMPs – selective in advanced medical practice. These are 8-week placements, taken as part of the final year, spent in a speciality chosen by the student.

The elective takes place at the end of year 3, from June to the start of September. This is widely regarded as the most exciting prospect of most medical students' courses. You can study and practise medicine all over the world from Ashworth Prison to Zambia!

Erasmus

Two exchange schemes – Socrates and Erasmus – allow students to study at a participating European medical school for a period of 16 weeks during the final year. Current exchanges are set up with schools in France, Spain, Germany, Holland and Sweden. The scheme has recently been expanded to include Eastern European countries.

Facilities

Library　A short-loan system operates for the books most in demand. The library is open 24 hours a day on weekdays and closes at 5 PM at weekends (if you feel the need!). All hospitals in which students have placements have their own libraries, with varying borrowing arrangements. The books stocked are directly influenced by the demands of the students, so the latest books are always available – complemented by an increasing array of electronic resources and journals.

Computers　The university and hospitals have ample 24-hour computer facilities available for students, with free use of email and the internet. Free work-related printing is available for students at some of the hospitals.

Clinical skills　One of the real highlights of the new course has been the introduction of the clinical skills centre, where students are able to master a whole range of practical clinical skills, from taking blood and suturing wounds to advanced life support. There are weekly sessions in the first year, with an OSCE exam at the end of the year.

Welfare

Student support

Students generally mix well and there are good relations within and between year groups. There is a long-standing mentoring system set up by the LMSS (Liverpool Medical Students Society), so that each first-year student is given a second- or third-year 'tutor'. The role of the tutor is to introduce the fresher to the joys of all aspects of medical school life in Liverpool, which is particularly useful when exams come around and you need some handy revision tips! In recent years Liverpool has enjoyed a very constructive and student-friendly atmosphere within the faculty. In addition to facilities provided by LMSS, the Students' Union has the standard welfare and counselling services.

Accommodation

Most students only live in university accommodation for year 1. This is a good opportunity to meet other students. There is a wide variation in the standard of private accommodation, but there is plenty of choice. Most students rent through Liverpool Student Homes, which regulates the standard of accommodation that is available – thus decreasing the chance of getting a dodgy landlord!

Placements

Liverpool University was the original red-brick university. The campus dominates a large area adjacent to the city centre. The main University Hospital is adjacent to the university campus, and the medical school is well placed near to all the main university and hospital departments.

The medical school is part of a large teaching hospital, the Royal Liverpool University Hospital. In addition, the city boasts the largest specialist women's (LWH) and children's (Alder Hey) hospitals in the country, plus the Cardiothoracic Centre, University Hospital Aintree and the School of Tropical Medicine.

Students are also placed in local district general hospitals – all of which have high standards of teaching and are very popular with many students. In year 4, many students spend the year in Lancaster, Barrow, Chester or Birkenhead – this is very popular with some students, giving them a chance to move away from Liverpool for a year and experience the Lake District or Welsh countryside. General practice and community placements are spread throughout the course.

Location of clinical placement/ name of hospital	Distance away from medical school (miles)	Difficulty getting there on public transport*
Royal Liverpool Hospital	0	🚶
Alder Hey	3	🚶 🚌
Whiston	10	🚶 🚌
Chester	25	🚗
Barrow-in-Furness	101	✈

* 🚶: walking/cycling distance; 🚌 : use public transport; 🚗: need own car or lift; ✈: get up early – tricky to get to!

Sports and social 🏆

City life

Liverpool is a thriving multicultural city. It extends a warm welcome to students. It is a proud city, with its world-famous accent, sense of humour, two cathedrals, football teams and maritime history. It was once the biggest port in the British Empire. Having fallen on hard times in the 1970s and 1980s, Liverpool is now very much on the up and investment in the city has never been higher! Many students, from all courses, stay in the area after graduation.

The medical school and the student residential areas are well-placed for all the attractions and are adjacent to the many surprisingly beautiful parks within the city. Like many other cities there is crime about, but a common-sense approach will ensure that the good times aren't spoilt. Police statistics show that Liverpool is, in fact, one of the safest cities in the UK.

Liverpool has an excellent social life, with every taste catered for: excellent pubs, several cinemas, sports complexes and nightclubs of all hues. It has a great sporting tradition and is home of the Grand National steeplechase, two Premiership football clubs, and numerous other great sporting teams. It is also the birthplace of the little-known band The Beatles and the Cavern club is still packed with Beatle-maniacs. The city is only a short distance from Manchester, North Wales, Chester and the Lake District.

University life

LMSS is a major plus for studying medicine in Liverpool. It covers all aspects of medical student life, from interaction with the faculty to weekly meetings with guest speakers. There are regular balls, dinners and social parties, as well as the medics' own orchestra, choir, sports teams, play and the annual Smoking concert. The university also offers a wide range of societies. LMSS has its own website at http://www.lmssonline.co.uk/. There is also a very active and expanding branch of MedSIN.

Sports life

The medical society has football, rugby, hockey, netball, basketball, squash, badminton and cricket teams. Recent additions to the sports teams include Chinese martial arts and a celebrated tiddly-winks team! The university has all these, and more! The university sports hall, complete with swimming pool, gym and squash courts, has recently been renovated.

Great things about Liverpool

- The PBL course is self-directed, so you have to be self-motivated but this allows you to adapt your own learning to your own pace. During the early years this allows students to make time to pursue other interests – in effect, the course is on flexitime.
- Students have a real say in the course at Liverpool and course organisers are receptive to their suggestions.

- The course prepares students to work effectively as Foundation Year 1 doctors, with early patient contact and clinical skills training.
- A diverse syllabus allows all aspects of medicine and those affected by illness to be appreciated.
- The LMSS provides a strong backbone to all activities in Liverpool Medical School, from academic issues to social and welfare issues.

Bad things about Liverpool

- The necessary approach to course work at Liverpool can be very different from A level studies: PBL is not for people who want to be spoon-fed in lectures.
- Hospital placements can be some distance from Liverpool, and travelling by public transport can be time-consuming and expensive.
- The Medical Student Society President traditionally strips at the Freshers Initiation ceremony, which is never a pretty sight!
- The social life within the medical school can be so good that sometimes it is difficult to get to know students from other courses!
- The weather – it can be cold and wet, particularly in winter.

Further information

Admissions Officer
Faculty of Medicine
Cedar House
Ashton Street
Liverpool L69 3GE
Tel: 0151 795 4370
Fax: 0151 795 4324
Email: mbchb@liv.ac.uk
Web: http://www.liv.ac.uk

Additional application information	
Average A level requirements	• AABB
Average Scottish Higher requirements	• AAABB and two Advanced Highers in biology and chemistry
Make-up of interview panel	• Two interviewers
Months in which interviews are held	• November – March (undergraduate) • January – February (graduate)
Proportion of overseas students	• 8%
Proportion of mature students	• 4%

Proportion of graduate students	• 6%
Faculty's view of students taking a gap year	• Acceptable
Proportion of students taking intercalated degrees	• 10%
Possibility of direct entrance to clinical phase	• No
Fees for overseas students	• £17,300 pa
Fees for graduates	• Please contact university for details
Ability to transfer to other medical schools If so, under what circumstances	• Possible at the end of second year but happens infrequently.
Assistance for elective funding	• Elective travel bursaries are awarded by the School of Medical Education depending on destination and planned activity/ speciality.
Assistance for travel to attachments	• Only through LEA, nothing specific available.
Access and hardship funds	• Guild is supportive in applications.
Weekly rent	• £40 in the main student areas • £60 if you prefer the comfort of the increasingly popular purpose-built student flats
Pint of lager	• £1 (Raz) • £1.20 (AJ – on campus) • £2 Concert Square and Albert Docks
Cinema	• £4 at local Odeon and UGC plus an excellent art-house cinema FACT newly opened
Nightclub	• Numerous new clubs and bars in the city centre and docks which cater for all the tastes plus the old favourites like the Raz

Manchester and Keele

Key facts	Premedical	Undergraduate
Course length	6 years	5 years
Total number of medical undergraduates	20 pa	2100
Applicants in 2006	407	3076
Interviews given in 2006	42	1183
Places available in 2006	20	380
Places available in 2007	20	380
Open days 2007	Three – please contact university for details	Three – please contact university for details
Entrance requirements	ABB	AAB
Mandatory subjects	3 arts subjects or 2 and one science	Chemistry and second science
Male:female ratio	1:1.25	1:1.25
Is an exam included in the selection process?	Yes	Yes
If yes, what form does this exam take?	BMAT. UKCAT in 2007	UKCAT in 2007
Qualification gained	MBChB	MBChB

Fascinating fact: Manchester can claim to have started both the nuclear age and the computer revolution.

Medicine has been taught in Manchester since the early 19th century. In October 2004, a merger between UMIST and the Victoria University of Manchester created the University of Manchester, which is now Britain's largest single-site university. The merger also made it one of the world's top centres for biomedical research. The medical school is part of the University of Manchester and is the second largest in the UK. Manchester has a proud history of educating students. The city is home to a number of universities and colleges and boasts a terrific social life for students. Manchester is also home to one of the largest gay scenes in the UK. It is truly a city for everybody.

Manchester was one of the first medical schools in the UK to introduce a problem-based learning curriculum. The basic sciences are studied within a clinical framework of patient cases, which are used to direct learning each week. Students have some clinical contact from year 1, together with gaining a thorough introduction to what being a doctor is all about. In year 3 there is an intake of students from St Andrew's.

In addition, students may choose to undertake all of their training at Keele University. From 2007, Keele will found itself as an independent medical school.

Preston, a base hospital of the Lancashire Teaching Hospital NHS Trust, educates small groups of students in year 3 and above. This new base hospital is a permanent addition to the Manchester Medical Schools.

Education

Applicants need to sit the UKCAT (see Chapter 3). The course is 5 years long, with two preclinical years (phase I) followed by three clinical years (phase II), although the 'early experience' program has increased the clinical emphasis in phase I.

A premedical programme, lasting 1 year, is available for those who do not have the required science qualifications for entry into year 1. The programme is problem-based with patient case studies involving the relevant areas of physics, chemistry, biology and mathematics. See Chapter 4 for more information.

Students can apply to enrol on the European Studies Option during the first semester of year 1. Linguistic ability is required to A or AS level standard or equivalent in French, German or Spanish. During years 1 to 4, language skills will be enhanced by weekly tuition in the selected language. There is the option to study in a European country during one of the special study modules in years 3 or 4, and, in year 5, a 16-week placement will be undertaken at one of the partner universities in Europe.

Teaching

Phase I teaching involves group discussions, lectures and practical sessions, including basic clinical skills, early experience, computational skills and anatomy sessions using cadavers. These sessions are mandatory. The course is organized into four semesters in phase I, each with a theme: nutrition and metabolism; cardiorespiratory medicine; abilities and disabilities; and lifecycle. Students work in PBL groups to create and discuss weekly learning objectives, which are fulfilled in their own time with the aid of the above resources. Students change PBL groups every semester to make sure they meet new people. In semester 3, students benefit from additional neuroanatomy practical classes. The early experience programme allows phase I students to spend time meeting patients in both hospitals and GP centres, practise and learn new clinical and communication skills and learn how to record their experiences. Occupational health clearance is necessary to participate in early experience and early hepatitis B vaccinations are advised.

Years 3 and 4 (phase II) continue the case-based approach, but in a clinical setting. Four days per week are spent in one of the five teaching hospitals, and one day per week in general practice. Year 5 works on a four-block rotation system, whereby students will be on an elective, at a teaching hospital, a district general hospital or in the community at any one time. Because of the high attendance demands on final-year students, free hospital accommodation is provided during attachments, which allows students to shadow foundation doctors and gain practical experience to prepare them for their future jobs.

Assessment

In phase I, there are exams at the end of each of the four semesters. They comprise of two MCQ based exams, covering the semester contents (semester test) and general aspects of the course (progress test), and an OSCE (objective structured clinical examination). At the end of each semester, PBL groups are assessed and marked for communication skills and teamwork. For those studying the European option there are yearly exams. Students are also required to keep a portfolio of their work and interests developed whilst at Manchester – these are reviewed as part of the OSCE exam.

Assessment in phase II is twice a year and consists of a progress test and an OSCE. In the final year, students take one set of exams in May, comprising an OSCE, a patient management paper (PMP), and a final true/false question paper.

Intercalated degrees

Intercalated BSc and MSc courses are offered at the end of years 2 and 4. There is a wide range of bioscience subjects available to study, as well as more unusual subjects such as healthcare ethics and law, and history of medicine. The faculty encourages any student wishing to intercalate and some funding is available.

Special study modules and electives

In years 1 and 2 there is one 4-week special study module (SSM) per year, whereas in years 3 and 4 there are two per year. These modules can be on practically anything, but note that in the clinical years one of the SSMs must be in a district general hospital and one in the community.

In the final year there is an elective period, where students are encouraged to go abroad to appreciate medical education in a foreign healthcare setting. Students cover costs for electives, so often a great deal of organization and planning is needed. In addition, a report must be submitted upon returning to Manchester.

Erasmus

Socrates/Erasmus students are selected by the home university. Eligible Manchester students are also offered the chance to pursue the European option. Students who successfully complete this element of the course are awarded a degree that recognizes their medical training in the context of a foreign language and healthcare system.

Manchester University does not accept students moving outside an Erasmus agreement; these people must apply as a visiting EU student. Students should have a high level of English sufficient to follow courses alongside UK students. The Cambridge Certificate of Proficiency in English is recommended. Tuition fees are waived for incoming Erasmus students. Full-year students are guaranteed a place in university housing as long as they apply before the deadline.

Facilities

Library   The medical faculty library is well-equipped with the core textbooks. It is open during term time, weekdays only. The John Rylands University Library stocks most of the major journals. This library is open both in term time and during holidays. Hospital libraries vary in size and standard.

Computers   There are excellent computer facilities in the medical school and the John Rylands Library, with internet access, email and a number of computer-assisted learning programmes.

Clinical skills   More and more emphasis is being placed on the use of skills laboratories, and facilities in the clinical years of the course are constantly being improved. There has been a tremendous influx of cash into the skills laboratories over the last 2 years and there is a variety of mannequins for practising CPR, injections, blood taking, etc., and video resources on clinical skills.

Welfare

Student support

Faculty staff are approachable and student feedback is consistently encouraged. Elected student representatives sit on all major faculty committees, which gives students opportunity to raise issues close to their hearts. Good relationships between students and tutors are fostered through tutorials. Students are also allocated a member of staff and a mentor from the year above, who act as a pastoral tutor and social support, respectively. There are both faculty and Students' Union-based counselling services, which are highly regarded.

Accommodation

University accommodation is guaranteed for first-year students, and although most students choose to move into the private sector after this, some do stay. Halls may be catered or self-catering, and vary in price and standard. Most accommodation is within a short bus ride from the university and town centre.

Placements

In years 3 and 4, four days per week are spent at the base hospital and one day in the community. Royal Hope Hospital is served by the excellent Metrolink Tram service.

Location of clinical placement/ name of hospital	Distance away from medical school (miles)	Difficulty getting there on public transport
Manchester Royal Infirmary	0	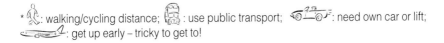
Royal Hope Hospital	6	
Wythenshawe Hospital	6	
Preston	39	
Keele	45	

* : walking/cycling distance; : use public transport; : need own car or lift; : get up early – tricky to get to!

Sports and social 🏆

City life

Manchester offers an endless choice of where to go and what to do. There is a wide variety of pubs, bars, clubs, stores, theatres and restaurants, each with a different character, theme or style. The city is truly multicultural and there is a good mix of home, overseas, mature, and postgraduate students, as well as a vibrant gay and lesbian scene. For those interested in music or comedy, Manchester is a fantastic place to live. As well as the local scene, most of the big-name tours include Manchester as a venue. However, should all the excitement get too much for you, the Peak District, Pennines, Lake District and North Wales are not far away for a little peace and tranquillity!

University life

The Medical Students Representative Council (MSRC) is the focus of medical school social life, organizing a number of medics' events throughout the year, including the infamous pyjama pub crawl and the annual winter ball. There are also year clubs, which organize trips, parties and one graduation ball for each year. The medics' dramatics society organizes an annual pantomime and a revue. Along with faculty events, a huge range of clubs and societies are run from Manchester Students' Union, which is opposite the medical school.

The campus has its own cultural attractions too: the internationally renowned Whitworth Art Gallery, Contact Theatre and Manchester Museum. Students can drop-in to gaze at a Hockney, marvel at mummies or see the best in contemporary theatre. Medical students normally take part in social gatherings in Rusholme – The Curry Mile – to introduce themselves and meet other medics for a PBL group curry.

Sports life

Being home to the most famous football team in the world is only the start for Manchester. Manchester boasts two Premiership football teams (City and United) and a top-flight rugby union team (Sale Sharks). Manchester City and Sale Sharks offer discount tickets for students.

Manchester's sports scene has seen huge benefits from the opening of many facilities built to cater for the 2002 Commonwealth Games, which has left a legacy of world-class sporting facilities, including an Olympic-sized swimming pool and national cycling, squash and netball centres.

Within the medical school, Manchester has a thriving sporting community. There are medics' rugby, hockey, tennis, netball, rowing and football teams, which actively encourage participation and socializing. The main university also has countless sports clubs, but medics tend to play for the medics' team if one exists in their sport. Most of the medics' sport teams have a not-to-be-missed annual tour.

Keele

In 2007, Keele will break away from Manchester and run independently with its very own medical course. New students entering from 2007 will receive a Keele medical degree after undergoing a very different course. More detail on this, including the medical student view of the course, will be provided in future editions of this publication.

Keele University is a campus university situated in North Staffordshire, just outside Stoke-on-Trent, the home of Robbie Williams. The area is referred to as 'The Potteries' by local inhabitants, reflecting its industrial background for the world-famous pottery production, including Wedgwood and Spode. In the past this was a major source of employment, but is now a common source of the locals' health problems. Until 2007, at the earliest, Keele can only consider applications from home and EU students.

Teaching

Students studying at Keele will undertake the Manchester medical course (except for subtle differences) and will graduate from Manchester. No premedical year option is currently available at Keele.

Year 1 and 2 students will spend the vast majority of their time on the Keele University campus. It is a large attractive campus university with restaurants, sports and social facilities, as well as library and academic buildings. Students are guaranteed accommodation on campus for their first year of study, which in 2005 ranged in cost from £53 to £86 per week, depending on facilities.

The clinical years at Keele will be spent predominantly at the University Hospital of North Staffordshire NHS Trust, only 3 miles away from Keele. This is a very busy hospital, offering the full range of clinical services, and is an excellent place to gain clinical experience.

Assessment

Generally, the structure of the course and the assessments are the same for both Keele and Manchester students. However, Keele has the advantage of being a new medical school, so the patients have not been exposed to our endless interrogation and are usually more than happy to help with our education.

Intercalated degrees

An intercalated degree leading to either a BSc or MSc can be taken at Keele and it may still be possible to intercalate in Manchester.

Facilities

The new clinical education centre (CEC), opened in September 2004, is available on the University of North Staffordshire NHS Trust Hospital site; it contains the new health library with up-to-date IT facilities, excellent clinical skills labs, and the usual seminar and lecture theatres. Students will also spend some time at Stafford and Shrewsbury District General Hospitals, both of which have received additional funding to expand their resources for medical students, including education and accommodation.

Welfare

Keele is conscious that a medical course can be challenging and has a similar pastoral system to Manchester. Many students decide to live off-campus, especially during their clinical training, living locally in Newcastle-under-Lyme or Stoke-on-Trent. The cost for private accommodation is around £35 plus per week, with utility bills on top.

Sports and Social

The area offers a variety of shops, takeaways, bars, nightclubs, and restaurants. There is also a gym 3-minutes' walk from the hospital. Due to the nature of the course students will spend time in the community during their GP and psychiatry placements; a car is very advantageous, but not essential as local public transport is adequate. Currently, students are provided with free accommodation in year 5, on campus and at the district general hospitals, depending on their placements.

Keele medical students have a number of committees to represent their views including the medical school committee, the intra-school committee, and the staff/student committee.

Great things about Manchester

- Enthusiasm for medicine is maintained by a course that emphasizes clinical problems from day 1.
- The faculty staff are very approachable and open to change, with plenty of opportunities to give feedback on both course and staff.
- The social life is excellent and there is generally lots going on at reasonable prices.
- The sheer size of the multi-faculty universities in Manchester, and the 2002 Commonwealth Games, have ensured top-level academic and sporting facilities.
- In the third year a load of new people arrive from St Andrew's, which spices things up a bit!

Bad things about Manchester

- Adjusting to self-directed learning can be difficult for some students who are used to being spoon-fed, although this is becoming the case at all UK schools with new courses.
- Differing interpretations of self-directed learning can often mean students perceive a lack of teaching.
- Some hospital placements are quite a distance away and can be difficult to reach on public transport.
- As with all major cities, Manchester does have a higher than average crime rate and insurance premiums can be high.
- Communication from the medical school can lacki in clarity, with students hearing about changes through rumour and speculation.

Further information

Manchester

Ms L M Harding
Admissions Officer
Faculty of Medicine
Stopford Building
University of Manchester
Oxford Road
Manchester M13 9PT
Tel: 0161 275 5025/5774 (undergraduate admissions)
Fax: 0161 275 5697
Email: ug.admissions@manchester.ac.uk
Web: http://www.manchester.ac.uk/medicine

Keele

Admissions and Recruitment Office
School of Medicine
The Covert
Keele University
Staffordshire ST5 5BG
Tel: 01782 583 632/583 642
Fax: 01782 583 903
Email: medicine@keele.ac.uk
Web: http://www.keele.ac.uk

Additional application information	
Average A level requirements	• ABB (premedical) AAB (undergraduate)
Average Scottish Higher requirements	• AAAAB
Make-up of interview panel	• Please contact university for details
Months in which interviews are held	• November – April
Proportion of overseas students	• 7%
Proportion of mature students	• 11%
Proportion of graduate students	• 10%
Faculty's view of students taking a gap year	• Gap year students considered equally
Proportion of students taking intercalated degrees	• 10%
Possibility of direct entrance to clinical phase	• No
Fees for overseas students	• Check current fees with university student services centre
Fees for graduates	• Check current fees with university student services centre
Ability to transfer to other medical schools If so, under what circumstances	• Students welcome to intercalate at other universities with equivalent learning opportunities.

Assistance for elective funding	• Prizes and bursaries available are updated annually on the Manchester Medical School website.
Assistance for travel to attachments	• GP placements are usually within 10 miles of your base hospital and information about public transport to each place is sent out with your placement pack.
Access and hardship funds	• As for electives
Weekly rent	• £60 approx
Pint of lager	• £2 upwards
Cinema	• £3–£5
Nightclub	• £5 upwards

Newcastle and Durham

Key facts	Undergraduate	Graduate
Course length	5 years	4 years
Total number of medical undergraduates	c. 1100	c. 40
Applicants in 2006	3000+	1000+
Interviews given in 2006	500	100
Places available in 2006	327	25
Places available in 2007	327	25
Open days 2007	Please see website for details	
Entrance requirements	AAA 2007 entry	2:1
Mandatory subjects	Chemistry or biology	
Male:female ratio	Not available	Not available
Is an exam included in the selection process?	Yes	Yes
If yes, what form does this exam take?	UKCAT 2007 entry	UKCAT 2007 entry
Qualification gained	MBBS	

Fascinating fact: Newcastle Medical School might have expanded with the creation of its link with Durham, but in fact the medical school started off in Durham. In a moment of insanity about 50 years ago, Durham actually gave it away to Newcastle, and has regretted it ever since.

Students who start at either Newcastle or Durham quickly develop an affection for their communities, whether it is vibrant Newcastle or the rapidly developing campus at Stockton. At both centres the large student presence makes for an excellent social life.

The medical school is well-established and highly regarded. The medical school is 5-minutes away from the main campus and has a diversity of national and international students from many different backgrounds. A new, state-of-the-art, 400-seat lecture theatre has just been completed. In addition to the traditional 5-year medical degree at Newcastle there is now the opportunity for graduates to apply for the accelerated 4-year course at Newcastle which is demanding but has the obvious advantage of being a fast track to qualification (see Chapter 4 for more information).

The medical school at Durham University is based at Queens Campus, Stockton, in brand new facilities set along the regenerated Tees riverside. Stockton students spend the first two years of their Newcastle medical degree being taught at this campus as members of Durham University, before being transferred and integrated with the much larger numbers of Newcastle students in years 3–5. Stockton is a small town with quite a new student population – as a result it doesn't always feel as student-friendly as Newcastle or Durham.

Education

The undergraduate medical course is split into two phases: phase I, which is mostly academic, lasts around 2 years, while phase II is predominantly clinical and lasts about 3 years. Approximately 220 places are available for students to enter phase I at Newcastle; however, the universities of Newcastle and Durham have paired to provide an additional 100 (approx.) phase I places with the University of Durham. After completing phase I, all students commence phase II with the University of Newcastle.

At Newcastle early patient contact comes from occasional hospital and GP visits in years 1 and 2, and the course attempts to break down the traditional preclinical/clinical divide. There are opportunities for extended contact with patients by way of the family and chronic illness patient studies.

The courses at Newcastle and Stockton are divided into two major phases based on the traditional preclinical/clinical model. In phase I (years 1 and 2) the course is case-led and systems-based, with an emphasis on the clinical approach from the start. There are several opportunities for early patient contact in the form of project work as well as hospital and GP visits. Communication skills are given a high priority from the very beginning. The systems covered in year 1 include cardiovascular respiratory and renal, gastrointestinal, endocrine medicine and metabolism. In year 2, clinical sciences and investigative medicine are taught, with immunology, haematology, neurology and musculoskeletal. Personal and professional development and medicine in the community are taught in years 1 and 2, in addition to the more traditional subjects.

At Stockton students do a 60-hour community placement in a local voluntary sector organization and are assessed on this in year 2. In addition, the Stockton students are required to maintain a personal and professional development portfolio over their two Stockton years and they undergo an interview on this before moving on to phase II. These aspects of the course reflect a greater emphasis on the social and cultural aspects of medicine at Stockton. A more traditional curriculum in Newcastle in years 1 and 2 presents the students with more emphasis on science-based subjects such as medical genetics.

The graduate-entry course aims to combine the essential elements of years 1 and 2 into one intense year, which it achieves by teaching core material over a 45-week year (rather than two years of 31 weeks), in which a problem-based learning method is predominantly used. Lots of support from tutors is available, with students being taught in groups of 8 to 10. This accelerated curriculum commenced for the first time in 2002, and feedback from the students has been very positive.

Teaching

The staff are generally approachable and supportive, and well liked by students. Phase I teaching is lecture based (40–50% of the time) for the Newcastle and Stockton students, except for the accelerated course students who have more structured tutorials and self-directed study. All students on phase I have small-group seminar work, practical sessions, clinical skills sessions and self-directed study. Anatomy in Newcastle is taught on prosected specimens to all students. Both universities protect Wednesday afternoons from teaching, except in the final year, to allow free time for inter-university sports.

Phase II sees the emphasis shift significantly to clinical experience. There is an introductory Foundations of Clinical Practice course, lasting 15 weeks, which introduces students systematically and thoroughly to clinical history-taking and examination. Students then embark on a series of essential junior rotations which takes them through to the end of year 3, spending time in reproductive and child health, chronic illness, rehabilitation, mental health, public health and infectious diseases. Throughout the year students spend one morning a week with a GP practice.

For their entire year 3 and final year, students are allocated to a 'base unit', which comprises a cluster of hospitals located within the sizeable northern region as follows:

- Teeside (Middlesbrough, Stockton, Bishop Auckland, Darlington, Hartlepool)
- Wear (Sunderland, Durham, South Tyneside)
- Tyne (Newcastle hospitals and the Queen Elizabeth Hospital in Gateshead)
- Northumbria (North Tyneside, Ashington, Hexham, and Carlisle)

Around 60% of students end up with their first or second choice of base units, and extenuating circumstances may guarantee a particular base unit. Free accommodation is only provided for placements in the west of the country.

Year 4 starts with another 16-week block, in clinical sciences and investigative medicine, based back at Newcastle. Teaching centres on lectures and group study using problem-based learning, and encompasses clinical pharmacology and therapeutics, and investigation and diagnosis of human disease. This is then followed by three 6-week student-selected components (SSCs).

At the beginning of the final year there is the 8-week elective period, followed senior rotations in the major clinical specialities: these are three 4-week-long senior rotations (women's health, child health, general practice, mental health), one 4-week period for preparation for practice, and 16 weeks of hospital-based practice. Students are again allocated to one of the regional base units. Final-year students spend 5 days a week in hospital and are expected to become part of the team to which they are attached, including being around during some evenings and even weekends. The emphasis is on taking responsibility for your self-directed learning, and therefore time is often left deliberately non-timetabled.

Students should consider carefully the various phase I options, as mature or local students might prefer the community spirit of Stockton but someone coming straight from school and wanting to be at the heart of the action might think Newcastle is more their scene. Either way, make the choice carefully because it might then determine your feelings about which base unit you want to be in for year 3.

Assessment

Phase I exams consist of a multiple-choice paper (MCQ), a data interpretation/problem-solving paper and a clinically-based objective structured clinical exam (OSCE). In phase I, exams are mid-year, and at the end of the year. About 6 weeks into year 1 there is a short formative exam, which gives students a chance to gauge how they're progressing. There are also several in-course assessments including essays, literature reviews, project work, presentations and posters and a student-selected component (SSC).

Phase II exams consist of data interpretation/problem-solving papers, MCQs and OSCEs. In-course assessment is by way of marks for the junior rotations and SSCs in year 4. Final exams at the end of year 5 consist of data interpretation/problem-solving, an OSCE and a long case or *OSLER*; this method of assessment is currently being reviewed.

In all exams there are viva voces for borderline or distinction students.

Intercalated degrees

Students can intercalate after either year 2 or year 4 on successful completion of these years on the first attempt. Normally this means a BSc in various science subjects (Newcastle) or health and human sciences (Durham). In addition, the options when intercalating at the end of year 4 include study for a research masters (MRes) or an MPhil. Research projects available in the intercalated year are wide-ranging, from clinical to laboratory-based work to topics in the social sciences.

Special study modules and electives

As mentioned above, SSCs are chosen in year 4 and can be followed anywhere across the northern region or even further afield for unique opportunities. Students with an interest in a particular subject can set up an SSC themselves with the university's approval either in the north, elsewhere in the UK or even abroad. The majority of students choose from the 300 modules on offer by the university, for example hospital-based, in the community and in investigative medicine.

Electives are entirely up to the individual to dream up and arrange, although the university has a database of information from previous student electives.

Erasmus

There is no formal Erasmus programme in the medical school, but options exist to do languages as SSCs.

Facilities

Library The Newcastle medical library (the Walton Library) is newly refurbished, situated within the medical school and well-stocked. It is open in the evenings during the week (more limited hours at weekends and outside term time). Students may also use the university library, which is close to the medical school (5-minutes' walk).

Durham students have full use of the Newcastle library facilities. There are more limited library facilities at Stockton, where emphasis is put on using web-based resources such as Medline in addition to textbook resources.

Computers   Much information is passed on to students via email and IT teaching is held as part of the course.

There are over 100 PCs in Newcastle Medical School, which are used not just by medics but also by dentists and all the courses based in the faculty of medical sciences. There is usually a computer available somewhere, except at the very busiest times, but there are numerous quieter clusters throughout the university available for use, including a 24-hour facility. Wireless connection points are also available at various computer rooms.

Stockton has 200 computers on campus, with a significant number being library-based. All facilities at the university in Durham itself are available to Stockton students as are the Newcastle University facilities.

Clinical skills   The clinical skills laboratories at Newcastle and Stockton are available for private revision sessions as well as for timetabled teaching sessions.

Welfare

Student support

All students are assigned a personal tutor for pastoral support, and faculty staff are friendly and approachable. Occasionally some tutors may be too busy to see their tutees, but there are other members of staff that students can approach. Both universities and Students' Unions have welfare officers and counselling services, including Nightline.

All first-year students are assigned a second-year 'parent' to guide them and many students find this useful to help them settle in and orientate themselves in the first year. Those at UDSC have peer families in Newcastle as well, to encourage integration of the courses.

Mature students have an increasing presence. Newcastle University has a mature students' officer for advice on issues such as finance and childcare. At Stockton, free kids' club places are available during half-term holidays. Stockton has developed strong links with schools and colleges of education in the local area, through a programme of open days and visits, and has promoted a widening access policy, the benefits of which can be seen in its non-traditional student intake. Its medical students have qualifications ranging from the usual three science A levels to first and second degrees in arts as well as sciences, and professional qualifications from spheres as diverse as law and nursing. Mature students are well-represented and their presence has contributed to a genuinely interactive style of teaching, with staff who are less didactic and more open to discussion than in many medical schools.

Accommodation

Newcastle first years are guaranteed accommodation in halls or self-catering flats, although not all are centrally located. The housing office provides help and advice to students renting in the private sector, as most do from year 2. Popular student areas for renting are Jesmond, Heaton and Fenham. As student numbers increase, Gosforth and Sandyford are becoming increasingly popular too. Renting is easy and low-cost in Newcastle compared to many other universities.

At Stockton, first-year students tend to live in halls, which are all within 5 minutes of the medical department. All offer an outstanding standard of accommodation because of the newness of the buildings and most rooms have internet access. In the second year, students tend to live out. Stockton has a lot of low-priced but reasonable quality accommodation close to the university.

Placements

The Newcastle campus is situated very close to the city centre and includes the Royal Victoria Infirmary. In years 1 and 2, students have about six visits to hospitals in the region, but all lecture-based teaching occurs at the medical school. At Stockton, the smaller numbers lead to good opportunities for integration with both other Stockton students and those from the rest of Durham University. In years 1 and 2, the majority of the teaching is based at the medical school, but some courses are taught in hospital teaching centres in the Tees and Durham area hospitals. Travel expenses for the students are not refunded by either university in phase I.

During phase II, clinical attachments may be much further afield. There is usually accommodation available in hospitals; reimbursement of travel expenses is limited. Some clinical attachments have been put under strain due to an expansion in numbers and student numbers can be high in certain clinics and rotations. As a result, students often find that the inconvenience of commuting to more distant attachments is outweighed by the fact that the smaller district general hospitals usually have fewer students than the central city teaching hospitals.

Location of clinical placement/ name of hospital (base unit)	Distance away from Newcastle medical school (miles)	Difficulty getting there on public transport*
Newcastle hospitals (Tyne)	4	🚶
Durham (Wear)	18	🚗 🚌
Sunderland (Wear)	16	🚗 🚌
Ashington (Northumbria)	18	🚗
Carlisle (Northumbria)*	50	🚗 🚌

* 🚶: walking/cycling distance; 🚌 : use public transport; 🚗: need own car or lift; 🚗: get up early – tricky to get to!

Sports and social 🏆

City life

Newcastle, the northernmost English university city, gives a warm welcome to its students. Newcastle is a very lively city within easy reach of the hills of Northumberland and the unspoilt northeast coast of England. In recent years, Newcastle was voted eighth best 'party town' in the world, with no shortage of bars and pubs, and an ever-increasing club scene. The medical school has good access to the city centre shops, theatre, cinema, museums, art galleries and music venues. More shops are to be found at the Metrocentre, just across the river Tyne in Gateshead. The locals are generally very friendly and eager for everyone to have a good time.

Stockton is nestled between the bustle of Middlesbrough and historic Durham, with easy access to both and to other cities in the north-east. It might not boast all the attractions of a traditional university city, but it has all the facilities you would expect of a big town, and has become student-friendly with new café-bars and clubs and an international summer art festival, as the Queens Campus has become more established. In Middlesbrough, pubs and clubs abound, and you can quickly get out to beautiful coast and moors of North Yorkshire. It is just as easy to visit the world heritage site of Durham Cathedral and lunch in one of the cosy cafés tucked away in Durham's narrow streets. In Stockton itself there is a shopping complex with a multiplex cinema and bowling alley just minutes from the campus, and there are many student bars and nightclubs throughout the town.

University life

MedSoc is a great melting pot of all the years in the medical school and provides an opportunity to meet up with friends every week. On a Friday night free beer is still currently available, with highlights including the Metro line pub crawl and a black-tie Christmas Ball. Stockton's MedSoc has been up and running for 3 years now and has quite a repertoire of events held throughout the year. The third years annually stage a medics' revue in May, which attracts quite a crowd and includes the participation of many members of the medical faculty! The Newcastle Medical and Dental Student Council runs the peer-parenting scheme and organizes events to support a wide range of charitable organizations.

Other organizations, such as MedSin, provide a campaigning link to international medical student organizations, and dedicated students forge links with the community working with local schools providing sex education for disadvantaged groups. 'Marrow' is a student branch of the Anthony Nolan Bone Marrow register and has considerable support in Newcastle. Regular student BMA meetings are held for those students politically minded.

A huge range of other clubs and societies are available through the Students' Unions of both universities.

Sports life

At Newcastle, medics' rugby, netball and hockey teams compete in leagues, and there are also football, volleyball, cricket, squash and other sports clubs for medics, and innumerable other university-run clubs. The university sports facilities are good following a £5.5m redevelopment of the Sports

Centre, with a brand new gym; it is close by and has facilities comparable to gyms twice its price. For the enthusiastic spectator there are Newcastle, Middlesbrough and Sunderland Football Clubs locally, as well as rugby, basketball, athletics, cross-country and more.

At Stockton there is a great deal of interest in sport at all levels, with rowing and canoeing being very popular, utilizing the nearby Tees Barrage canoeing facilities. Sport in Durham is taken seriously at college and university levels.

Great things about Newcastle

- The locals are friendly – adding to this vibrant, rapidly developing city where the atmosphere is never impersonal.
- Cost of living is relatively low.
- If you need a break from city life, it's easy to escape to the country or the coast.
- New pubs, clubs and restaurants spring up all the time, with the Quayside and Jesmond being student favourites and Friday nights at MedSoc are a weekly highlight.
- The course is constantly evaluated and modified through student feedback

Bad things about Newcastle

- There is some trepidation about how the increase in student numbers in recent years might affect course organization and the student body.
- Travelling around the region can be time-consuming without a car and expensive with one.
- Timetable planning is sometimes communicated to students late.
- The tutor system doesn't work for everyone and so the amount of pastoral support students receive is variable.
- The amount of time spent on non-traditional subjects, in the first two years, can be frustrating for those who are expecting a more scientific course.

Great things about Durham (Queens Campus)

- Brand new state-of-the-art facilities, with very committed staff.
- Small (190 medical students in the department in total).
- Most of the teaching is delivered by a wide range of clinicians who come from many different hospitals and primary care centres in the region.
- Access to both Durham and Newcastle University facilities, e.g. libraries.
- Patient-centred course with high emphasis on communication skills.

Bad things about Durham (Queens Campus)

- The library is noisy and lacks the comprehensive stock of a more established medical school library.
- The number of staff permanently in the medical school is very small.
- Stockton is a small town.
- The transition to Newcastle university in year 3 doesn't achieve good integration between the two groups and students believe this requires improvement.
- Durham University has much shorter terms than Newcastle but students have to cover the same amount of material in each semester, leading to quite a heavy and fast-paced workload.

Further information

The Medical School
University of Newcastle
Framlington Place
Newcastle Upon Tyne NE2 4HH
Tel: 0191 222 7005
Fax: 0191 222 6521
Email: medic.ugadmin@ncl.ac.uk
Web: http://www.ncl.ac.uk
        http://medical.faculty.ncl.ac.uk/

The Department of Medicine
University of Durham, Queen's Campus
University Boulevard
Thornaby
Stockton-on-Tees
TS17 6BH
Tel: 0191 334 2000
Web: http://www.dur.ac.uk

Additional application information	
Average A level requirements	• AAB
Average Scottish Higher requirements	• AAAAB
Graduate entry requirements	• 2:1 degree
Make-up of interview panel	• Two selectors
Months in which interviews are held	• November – March
Proportion of overseas students	• Quota 26
Proportion of mature students	• Not known
Proportion of graduate students	• Not known
Faculty's view of student taking a gap year	• Must use year constructively to gain experience
Proportion of students taking intercalated degrees	• Not known

Possibility of direct entrance to clinical phase	• No
Fees for overseas students	• Please see website for details
Fees for graduates	• Please see website for details
Ability to transfer to other medical schools. If so, under what circumstances	• Possible but needs exceptional circumstances.
Assistance for elective funding	• Yes, if in financial difficulty.
Assistance for travel to attachments	• Limited help – travel bursary for Tees, Northumbria and Wear base units.
Access and hardship funds	• Available, through university and the medical school.
Weekly rent	• £40–£60 or more
Pint of lager	• Between £1.30 at pubs/Union to £2 at Tiger Tiger on a Saturday night
Cinema	• £3.50–£5
Nightclub	• £1–£3 during the week, more at weekends

Nottingham

Key facts	Undergraduate
Course length	5 years
Total number of medical undergraduates	1155
Applicants in 2006	1900
Interviews given in 2006	395
Places available in 2006	246
Places available in 2007	246
Open days 2007	29 June, 30 June, 15 September
Entrance requirements	AAB
Mandatory subjects	Biology and chemistry
Male:female ratio	36:64
Is an exam included in the selection process?	Yes
If yes, what form does this exam take?	UKCAT
Qualification gained	BMedSci and BMBS

Fascinating fact: Emeritus Professor Sir Peter Mansfield designed the first MRI scanner at Nottingham. He has received the Noble Prize for his pioneering work.

Nottingham is a campus university, founded in 1881, with a community atmosphere in a vibrant student-dominated city. Medics and non-medics mix in year 1 in superb halls of residence on a beautiful campus built around a lake. The site is also next to stunning Wollaton Park, which has a manor house, deer and great open-air concerts. Off-campus accommodation is mostly located in the Lenton area between the campus and the city. This area is very student-orientated, so many of your friends will live within walking distance of you throughout the course. The medical school is a part of the massive Queen's Medical Centre (QMC) hospital at the city end of the university campus. The course is systems-based, with emphasis on the early introduction of clinical skills. Outside placements are accessible and the quality of teaching is high. All students do a BMedSci degree within the 5-year course, and there are opportunities to study abroad. The elective period follows finals, which is a great idea as it allows less worry and you have more knowledge. Most graduates choose to find their first job through the matching scheme and stay in the Nottingham area.

The graduate-entry medical (GEM) course is based in Derby for the first 18 months before joining the undergraduates for the clinical course at Nottingham.

Education

Nottingham offers a blend of traditional and modern-style courses and subjects are split into four themes: cell, person, community and doctor.

Years 1 and 2 are integrated clinically, with systems-based teaching arranged in four semesters. One morning every fortnight is spent seeing patients, either in general practice or in hospital; clinical skills are taught and examined in both years.

Year 3 is split into two halves: the first involves a research project leading to a BMedSci degree for everyone; the second marks the beginning of full-time clinical study and integration with the GEM students, with general medical and surgical attachments after a brief introductory course.

Years 4 and 5 are spent on clinical attachments in a variety of specialities, e.g. paediatrics, obstetrics and gynaecology and psychiatry, before returning to general medicine and surgery. Throughout the course there is significant and appropriate emphasis on personal and professional development, including communication skills, ethics and career advice.

The ISC (intra-school committee), which ensures students sit on all academic meetings, runs well in Nottingham medical school and ensures a high level of input and involvement of students in evaluation of teaching, development of the course and student support issues.

Teaching

Lectures form the basis of most year 1 and 2 courses. These are supplemented with a limited number of tutorials (about 10 students) and seminars (about 25 students). Anatomy is taught by group dissection (10 students) and clinical problem-solving in the newly renovated dissection laboratories. Practical classes are taught in large tele-linked laboratories. The GEM course has more problem-based learning (PBL) than the undergraduate course which still relies heavily on didactic teaching.

Assessment

The course is examined by continual assessment as well as final exams after the 5 years. Depending on your outlook, this either reduces or spreads the inevitable stress; however, they have recently changed the exam system – reducing the number of exams in the first 2 years from around 40 to 12. For the first 2 years, exams take place in January and June, often using MCQs, i.e. negatively marked true and false questions (these can be more challenging than they sound).

The BMedSci is assessed from all components of the first 3 years.

In the clinical years, logbook assessment and practical exams follow each attachment, with MCQ exams twice a year. In year 5, the finals are clinically orientated, involving medicine, surgery, ortho-paedics and clinical laboratory sciences. The final year was redesigned relatively recently to allow several practice attempts at finals before the real exam.

Intercalated degrees

Despite being a 5-year course, everyone does a research-based BMedSci (Hons) degree in year 3. Some find this research opportunity exhilarating and use their projects to publish scientific papers or present them at conferences. Others are bored rigid! Either way, it is certain that the ability to analyse research, and the experience of carrying it out, is an important skill. There is an element of chance in what you end up studying, but the vast majority of students are happy with their project in the end. The BMedSci is not likely to stand up as well as a BSc on future job applications but is better than no additional degree at all and students who leave the course after year 3 have the benefit of a degree qualification, although few students leave mid-course.

Special study modules and electives

There are two periods of 4-week SSMs. One is in year 4 and the other in the final year. The choices are varied and Nottingham currently offers 30 SSM placements abroad.

The 9-week elective is at the end of all clinical attachments and final exams in year 5. However, if you have failed any clinical examinations in the years 4 and 5, you may have to re-sit them in this period. Most people choose a mixture of work and play; a short report is expected from everyone.

Erasmus

Nottingham medical school no longer takes part in the Erasmus scheme. However, a limited number of students have had the opportunity to complete their BMedSci project overseas, many students study one of the SSMs abroad, and two students in year 4 spend 6 months completing their child health and obstetrics and gynaecology attachments at the University of Oslo.

Facilities

Library   The medical library is well-stocked with core texts and journals, but can become busy around exam times. It opens until 11.15 PM weekdays, and during the day at weekends for most of the year. There are other libraries around the campus with longer opening hours but few medical texts. There are libraries at outlying hospital sites that students can use.

Computers   IT facilities are good, with over 200 terminals in the medical school and computers available at all outlying sites (although some sites are better than others!). There is unlimited and free access to email, the internet, teaching CD-ROMs and computer-assisted learning packages for teaching and revision. The Networked Learning Environment (NLE) is a website to which all students have access. It contains lectures and other online resources for all years. It allows students to review lectures long after they were given – particularly useful before exams. There are also example exam papers, feedback from previous years, and a student area – so you can upload notes or ask questions! The main computer room is open 24 hours a day and wireless internet access is available across campus and at many bars and cafés throughout the city.

Clinical skills   There are a series of newly-built rooms dedicated to teaching clinical skills, such as examining patients. The laboratory is staffed and open out of hours. Resources have rapidly expanded to an excellent level. The rooms are used on a casual basis and have many self-teaching aids – suturing practice kits, models of eyes, ears, arms (for blood pressure), videos, etc.

Welfare

Student support

As a whole the university has a friendly and open feel. Student welfare is taken very seriously. In the medical school every student is allocated a tutor who can address academic or personal problems. Unfortunately, the amount of actual support given varies from tutor to tutor. There is a 'medic family' mentoring system in which first-years are allocated individual second-year 'medic parents'. Whether or not you meet regularly with your 'parent' depends on how well you get on; however, a high rate of adoption and incest leaves most people happy! The university and Students' Union have welfare, legal, financial, health and counselling services, along with an active Niteline (night-time counselling service) run by students.

Accommodation

Almost all first-years are housed in good-quality university accommodation; these are mostly catered halls, though some students opt for self-catering flats. There are 12 medium-sized halls on the main campus, each with its own bar. A further three large halls are found nearby on the recently built Jubilee campus, a pleasant campus with a library on a lake, although some students feel a little cut off from the main campus where most activities take place. Students in halls are not allowed cars on campus but everything is within walking distance and there are cheap taxis. Permits are available for people with disabilities or special cases. Students have to move all their things out of halls or into storage for every holiday, which can be frustrating.

In subsequent years you can apply to stay in halls, though most students move into private rented houses: 80% choose to live in Lenton, which is a relatively safe student area that is 20 minutes' walk from the campus and town. House-hunting begins very early after Christmas; most students organize it themselves without university vetting. The Union organizes house-hunting for first-years wanting to live out before their first term.

Placements

The teaching hospitals are all located within one rush-hour drive of Nottingham. For clinical visits in years 1 and 2 transport is provided. The smaller hospitals are generally friendlier (as they have more time to talk to you), but sometimes more work is expected from you. Students usually organize to share lifts, as some hospitals can be very difficult to travel to via public transport. Accommodation is provided free of charge in Lincoln; otherwise you are expected to travel daily. At Nottingham, students can state preferences for where their attachments are. It is unlikely that any student will have all their attachments in Nottingham itself, so a degree of travelling is inevitable.

Location of clinical placement/ name of hospital	Distance away from medical school (miles)	Difficulty getting there on public transport*
Nottingham City Hospital	5	
Derby Royal Infirmary	20	
Derby City General Hospital	25	
Kings Mill Hospital, Mansfield	30	
Lincoln Hospital	45	

* : walking/cycling distance; : use public transport; : need own car or lift; : get up early – tricky to get to!

Sports and social

City life

The city centre is attractive, compact and has good shopping facilities. Nottingham is renowned for its inexpensive and diverse bars, clubs, pubs, theatres, cinemas and restaurants. In terms of nightlife Nottingham is arguably the best city in the UK. As a student you are in the best position to take advantage and with the combined population of Nottingham and Nottingham Trent students, the town is certainly looking to attract student trade. The city centre is within walking distance of most off-campus accommodation, and a 10-minute bus ride (£1.20) from campus. Because of its central location, travel to most other cities is quick and easy. The Peak District and surrounding countryside provide a welcome escape where students can enjoy themselves, far away from anatomy revision.

University life

Student life is rich and varied, and there is plenty of time to enjoy it while doing a medical degree. The student medical society (MedSoc) provides a good range of social events, e.g. cocktail parties, balls and guest lectures. MedSIN is also very active in Nottingham, so it is easy to get involved in projects such as Sexpression, WaterAid, Heartstart and Marrow. Nottingham has one of the largest student RAGs in the country, called Karni. This raises about £230,000 for charity from activities in the first term.

The main distinguishing feature of Nottingham medics' social life is the extent to which medical students are mixed with the whole university population. On-campus entertainment revolves around hall life, and includes bars and themed parties. In later years the pub and club scenes of Lenton and the city dominate. After the first year, many medics live with their non-medic friends from halls. Lenton, the main student area, is well-equipped with cheapish pubs, launderettes, late-opening shops, take-aways, video rental shops and buses. Although the campus accommodation is excellent, the university could take more responsibility for off-campus housing. There are about 120 societies to join in the Union, including virtually all known sports, a large range of cultural/international societies and all mainstream religious and political movements, then the more obscure neighbours, James Bond and Mutantsoc! The university has an award-winning radio station, URN.

Sports life

Nottingham is one of the top five universities in the country for sport. It has a good-quality sports centre on campus comprised of squash and tennis courts, weights room, two large indoor halls, a sports injury clinic, a swimming pool with an adjustable bottom and over 20 football pitches. After a registration fee is paid, you can use almost all the facilities for £1 (except the pool). Medics' teams play against the hall teams; they are particularly strong in hockey, netball, rugby, tennis and football. Most sports and standards of ability are represented somewhere in the university. The clubs provide a focus for excellent social lives. Nottingham does of course have two universities and there are annual varsity games between the two. Trent Bridge and The City Ground are used and crowds can often top 4000 for these high-tension matches.

Great things about Nottingham

- You get a bonus degree (BMedSci) without having to do an extra year.
- Good social life for students, with variety, value and accessibility along with many active and friendly student societies.
- Beautiful campus, with good community spirit and healthy inter-hall rivalry.
- Integration of medics with non-medics in halls (especially in hall bars!) broadens social circles and reduces the cliqueyness that medics are sometimes accused of!
- After the first year all your hall friends remain within walking distance by moving to the student area (Lenton).

Bad things about Nottingham

- Because of the poor central Union bar and lack of a campus venue for top bands, there is little to attract medics back to campus after their first year.
- It is felt that the university attracts students from similar backgrounds, leading to a lack of diversity within the student population.
- House-hunting begins too early (January) and can be stressful.
- Schemes used to allocate students to BMedSci projects, PRHO jobs and other parts of the course are often felt to be unfair and students often feel like they have little control over their future – it's almost like a lottery!
- The medical school is notorious for not confirming where your next attachment is until the week before it starts, so keep a sharp eye on the Networked Learning Environment!

Further information

Admissions Officer
Faculty Office
Queen's Medical Centre
University of Nottingham
Nottingham NG7 2RD
Tel: 0115 970 9379
Fax: 0115 970 9922
Email: medschool@nottingham.ac.uk
Web: http://www.nottingham.ac.uk

Additional application information

Average A-level requirements	• AAB with grade As in biology and chemistry and a B in a third subject (excluding general studies)
Average Scottish Higher requirements	• AAB
Make-up of interview panel	• Consultants and academics
Months in which interviews are held	• November–March
Proportion of overseas students	• 10%
Proportion of mature students	• 2%

Proportion of graduate students	• 2%
Faculty's view of students taking a gap year	• Acceptable, provided it is used constructively
Proportion of students taking intercalated degrees	• 0%
Possibility of direct entrance to clinical phase	• No
Fees for overseas students	• £12,160 pa for years 1 and 2 in 2005. • Years 3, 4 and 5 will be set at the clinical rate applicable when student reaches year 3.
Fees for graduates	• £3000
Ability to transfer to other medical schools If so, under what circumstances	• Very rarely done but possible after year 3.
Assistance for elective funding	• Not directly, but students are invited to apply for elective prizes.
Assistance for travel to attachments	• No, students must apply to their LEA and the medical school will back the claim.
Access and hardship funds	• Yes, all cases dealt with individually and anonymously. Must be paid back in the future.
Weekly rent	• £105 per week (for 31 weeks) in fully catered hall; £50 per week (for 44 weeks) in self-catering halls; £40–£65 per week, excluding bills (private)
Pint of lager	• £1.45 in the Union bar; £2.30 in a city centre pub
Cinema	• £4 with NUS
Nightclub	• Free–£4 Monday to Friday

Oxford

Key Facts	Undergraduate	Graduate
Course length	6 years	4 years
Total number of medical undergraduates	900	120
Applicants in 2006	1076	250
Interviews given in 2006	425	90
Places available in 2006	150	30
Places available in 2007	150	30
Open days 2007	28-29 June, 14 September	Easter and summer
Entrance requirements	AAA	2:1 or better, GPA above 3.5 and 2 science A levels (including chemistry)
Mandatory subjects	Chemistry and one other science/maths	Bioscience or chemistry degree and A level chemistry
Male:female ratio	45:55	70:30 (2005 entry)
Is an exam included in the selection process?	Yes	Yes
If yes, what form does this exam take?	BMAT	UKCAT
Qualification gained	BM, BCh	BM, BCh

Fascinating fact: One lucky person every year at the clinical school will have the traditional honour of playing the rear end of a large pink elephant in the medical school pantomime!

Oxford is a unique place. If you wish to mix a sense of history with a centre renowned for cutting-edge research; have the choice of living in modern student accommodation or 15th-century, wood-panelled rooms; meet students of all backgrounds; have the double benefits of a small college and a large university and all with a traditional yet innovative medical course, then Oxford is for you!

As with most medical schools, the course has undergone some changes recently and the intake was increased in 2001. However, Oxford still retains the ethos of a small medical school, which is a real advantage. The addition of an accelerated course for bioscience graduates is another innovation.

Some may criticize the lack of clinical involvement during the first 3 years of the 6-year undergraduate course. However, the firm scientific basis of medicine strongly emphasized on the Oxford course is of vital importance clinically, and the acquisition of skills, such as the critical evaluation of papers and an understanding of research, is rightly given very high priority. In the early years a real effort is also made to highlight the clinical relevance of the 'basic science' being taught. Three years before significant patient contact may seem like a long time, but the knowledge and skills gained during the preclinical course will be of use for the rest of your career, and having an 'extra' science degree is no bad thing when applying for medical jobs.

The course demands the very highest level of academic ability and commitment. However, your college tutor, who selects you in the first place, has a vested interest in your success and, in most cases, works very hard on your behalf – no one is left to struggle. The short terms and long holidays also make the hard work survivable and enjoyable.

Education

The medical school is considered as a single 6-year course by the Quality Assurance Agency, but for practical purposes there remains a clear-cut division between the preclinical and clinical courses in Oxford. In the preclinical school, the first five terms are spent studying the basic medical sciences (anatomy, biochemistry, physiology, pharmacology, pathology and neuroscience). Some clinical contact is introduced through the Patient–Doctor Course by spending 2 to 3 afternoons a term with a GP tutor. The final four terms are spent working towards an Honours degree (BA in Biomedical Sciences). After finals, preclinical students 'stay on' for a clinical anatomy course. Application to the clinical school is competitive, and about 55–65% of the Oxford preclinical students stay on. Most of the rest go to London or Cambridge, and there is an influx of students – most from Cambridge and some from London medical schools.

The clinical course lasts 3 years and aims to deliver the best teaching of both scientific principles and clinical practice. It is in a good position to do so, because of the combination of its small size (about 150 per year, including the graduate-entry intake) and the very high quality of its academic and clinical staff. Year 4 starts with a 6-week introductory foundation (Patient–Doctor II) course, a fortnight of which is dedicated to teaching by the final-year students doing a Medical Education special study module, which is always greatly enjoyed. The remainder of year 4 consists of an 8-week laboratory medicine (pathology) course, general, medicine, and surgery rotations, a residential general practice attachment and a placement at a district general hospital. Courses on medical ethics and law, communication skills, complementary therapy, evidence-based medicine and basic life support are 'threaded' into the year.

Year 5 contains all the specialist rotations. Some of these rotations will be spent partially at a DGH outside Oxford; for example, Reading, Milton Keynes, Swindon, Northampton or Banbury, but most of the time is spent in Oxford itself. Year 6 focuses again on medicine and surgery. Students also undertake 'clinical options' and a DGH attachment before clinical finals in January. After this, there is a 10-week elective period – the chance to complete ALERT and ALS courses and several weeks of special study modules. All students complete a Preparation for Practice module comprising a taught course and a house officer shadowing attachment. There is a requirement to produce a portfolio during year 6, with reflective reports on the attachments or work completed, which is developed in conjunction with a supervisor, who students select individually. In addition, an extended essay is written. Throughout the clinical course there is a great deal of ward-based teaching, with both consultants and junior doctors (all of whom are keen to practise being teaching hospital consultants!).

The graduate-entry programme at Oxford is a 4-year course currently restricted to graduates in bioscience and chemistry. This is an intensive programme, with emphasis on academic science – both medical and clinical. Year 1 focuses on the basic sciences in a clinical context, with the introduction of essential clinical skills such as history-taking and physical examination. Teaching in year 2 begins to be integrated with first-year clinical students on the standard medical course. Emphasis here is on clinical teaching with a smaller science component. The final two years are fully integrated with the existing clinical course. Informal assessments are held at several points during the first year. Assessments are also held towards the end of each clinical attachment throughout the course. Formal university examinations take place at the end of the first and second years, and again towards the end of the final year.

Teaching

In the preclinical years, the basic medical sciences are taught by means of lectures and practicals, supplemented by college tutorials 2 to 3 times a week. In the clinical years, teaching practices vary between departments, with some lectures/seminars and some ward-based teaching. Some colleges provide clinical tutorials in addition to the central, medical school-based teaching.

Assessment

Currently, assessments are at the end of year 1 and before Easter in year 2, and consist of essay papers, short notes and problem-solving questions. The practicals are assessed continuously and practical books must be kept up to date.

In the clinical years, assessment is largely by OSCEs and the odd written paper. In year 4, assessment is largely formative; whilst in year 5, exams after each 8-week speciality rotation are pass/fail. The modular form of the specialist rotations means that there is no easy year 5, but the pressure at finals is much reduced.

In the final year, assessment consists of a written exam, a clinical exam, an extended essay and the satisfactory completion of a portfolio.

Intercalated degrees

All students spend the last terms of the preclinical phase working for an Honours degree in Biomedical Sciences (unless they are already graduates). The degree course has a large amount of flexibility, and students are encouraged to follow courses that interest them. It is a quirk of the Oxford system that the degree awarded is a BA (and, after a few years, it can be upgraded automatically to an MA), rather than a BSc!

Special study modules and electives

In year 4, SSMs can be taken in subjects such as philosophy, theology, chronic illness and foreign language, where students are free to explore their interests. The 14 weeks of SSMs in the final year are more clinical in nature than the modules of the first clinical year. There are over 60 options, ranging from the traditional (e.g. cardiology, anaesthetics, general practice) to the innovative (creativity in healthcare, medical publishing, medical anthropology or even a language), and can be either purely clinical or research, or a mixture of both. With the medical school's permission you may arrange your own SSM which can (on occasion) be undertaken outside Oxford and even abroad.

There is a 10-week elective in year 6 and most students go abroad. Some of the colleges can help financially. In addition, there are opportunities to undertake other placements abroad, for example during the paediatrics and obstetrics and gynaecology modules.

Erasmus

Whilst it is more challenging to arrange study abroad during the preclinical part of the course, there are plenty of travel opportunities during the clinical years. The year 5 placements in paediatrics and obstetrics and gynaecology can both be partly undertaken abroad. In addition, the 10-week elective scheme in the final year enables experience of medicine anywhere in the world. As well as these opportunities, it is possible to arrange an SSM in a foreign country (or partly abroad).

Facilities

Library   Oxford is very well-catered-for with respect to libraries. At preclinical level, the Radcliffe Science Library (RSL) and college libraries are the most useful and are well-used. College facilities vary, but are in general good to excellent. The RSL has an incredible number of books and journals, but rather limited opening hours out of term. The Cairns Library is located at the John Radcliffe Hospital, and is the library used during clinical years. It is very well-stocked and open 24 hours a day, 365 days a year.

Computers   The computing facilities are very good in colleges, departments, libraries and, at clinical level, in Osler House and the Cairns Library, where a large number of computers are reserved exclusively for medical students. Computer-assisted learning is gradually being introduced, and all lecture notes and resources for courses such as the laboratory medicine course are available electronically. The new Weblearn system is entirely computer-based, with up-to-date timetables, information about SSMs, and clinical school notices all being posted electronically.

Clinical skills   There are two large and recently renovated skills laboratories for teaching of medical and surgical skills. Two automated dummies are available for skills teaching.

Welfare 🏠

Student support

Oxford students are bright yet friendly and very social. There really is a niche for everyone. The collegiate system enables the pastoral care provided by tutors to work very effectively in the preclinical years. In clinical years, when links with the college are not as strong, the system does not work so well but is supplemented by good support, be it academic or pastoral, from the medical school. Colleges provide significant financial assistance, ranging from subsidized accommodation, meals and entertainment, to elective funding and hardship grants. Oxford University has welfare and counselling facilities, in addition to the provision by the medical school and colleges. In clinical years, an 'informal but structured' peer support system operates.

At preclinical and especially clinical levels medical students tend to know each other very well. Depending on your viewpoint, this can be an advantage or a disadvantage, but most seem to enjoy the camaraderie and banter, whether in the bar or the dissection room! One of the great things about Oxford is the collegiate system: this broadens your horizons and makes it very easy to make friends with non-medics. At the clinical level, Osler House Club (the Students' Union) provides a very relaxed way of meeting people and making friends.

Accommodation

Preclinical students will find their life completely integrated with that of students in other subjects and will live with them in college accommodation. Many of the college buildings are old and beautiful, but do bear in mind that sometimes the accommodation you will actually live in will either be 1950s or private lodgings. All the accommodation is of a reasonable to excellent standard.

Things are very different for clinical students, however. Very few live on college sites, as the majority of graduate accommodation is in nearby annexes. The exception is Green College, which was established for medical students and is still largely populated by them. Many prefer to live out during their clinical training, as it affords more independence than college can provide, and there is plenty of good-quality private accommodation in Oxford.

Placements

The early years are spent studying basic medical sciences in and around the centre of Oxford. This is amid the Oxford colleges, with their long traditions of study and learning. The clinical school is based at the John Radcliffe Hospital (JR), which is a large teaching hospital situated in Headington, 2 miles east of Oxford city centre and easily accessible by bus or bike. The Churchill Hospital is increasingly becoming a specialist centre for certain services, such as transplants, oncology, and diabetes and endocrinology. The Radcliffe Infirmary contains services for neurology, ENT, ophthalmology and plastic surgery. At the time of writing it was due to be closed down and relocated to the JR site within 2 years. The Nuffield Orthopaedic Hospital and the Warneford and Littlemore psychiatric hospitals are smaller centres used for specific modules of the course. All the hospitals are easily reached by bike, bus or car (although parking is almost impossible!). Although other hospitals in Banbury, Reading, Swindon, Northampton and Bath are used, the majority of a student's time will be spent in Oxford. Students are provided with free accommodation and travel expenses are reimbursed on residential placements outside Oxford.

There are also ample opportunities to travel (in addition to the elective): several of the specialities (such as paediatrics, and deliveries in obstetrics) can be studied in other parts of the country or world.

Location of clinical placement/ name of hospital	Distance away from medical school (miles)	Difficulty getting there on public transport*
Aylesbury	25	
Reading	27	
Swindon	30	
Northampton	42	
Milton Keynes	39	

* : walking/cycling distance; : use public transport; : need own car or lift; : get up early – tricky to get to!

Sports and social

City life

Oxford, the 'city of dreaming spires', is a small city with easy access to the rest of the country, and London in particular (only 50 minutes by train and 90 minutes by coach). Many preclinical students survive the first 3 years without needing to travel more than 5 minutes on foot from the centre of the city, but at clinical school you are forced to move a little further afield. The town centre has the usual core of shops, and you will find it sufficient for most needs. Having said that, Oxford can't compare with what many cities offer in terms of variety. Culturally there is a lot going on, particularly if you like theatre and music, but the club scene in Oxford is not comparable to that in the larger centres such as London or Manchester, so it may not suit the more dedicated punter! However, the clubs are getting better, and you can always get to and from London on buses leaving every 12–15 minutes, 24 hours a day.

University life

There are numerous university and college-based clubs and societies dedicated to ensuring that students get the most they can out of their time in Oxford. At preclinical level these often form a prominent part of most people's social life, with the medical society (MedSoc) supplementing this. The societies

Oxford

range from the sublime to the ridiculous, and you will find that talents you never realized you had are catered for.

The clinical school social life tends to revolve around Osler House, a 1920s house in the grounds of the John Radcliffe run for and by clinical students. There is a bar, a television room, computing facilities, pool table and a pleasant garden, with lunch served daily. The Osler Committee organizes many events – social, sporting and cultural. However, many clinical students also remain involved in other aspects of university life, be it at their college or elsewhere. The clinical school pantomime, *Tingewick*, deserves a special mention. This occurs every year and is a great chance for the students to get their own back at their consultants and anyone else who deserves parody.

Sports life

Oxford is famous for its rowing and rugby, but other sports are well-represented too. In particular, the collegiate structure means that there are both facilities and opportunities for involvement in sport at any level of ability. All the colleges have sports pitches and boathouses, and many can provide squash and tennis courts as well. Intercollegiate competitions (Cuppers) form one focus for the competitive energy, and the very committed can find themselves competing at the highest levels – the Varsity competitions. Even if you lack speed, strength, skill, accuracy or talent in general, you will still be able to find a team of your level and skill! In the collegiate events the clinical school is represented by the Osler–Green teams, who regularly manage to field competitive sides.

Great things about Oxford

- The collegiate system and relatively small size of the medical school means personalized teaching and allows you to meet students in a variety of subjects.
- The tutorial system – having one-to-one or two-to-one tuition, with the academic support that this offers. Consequently, very few students fall behind in their work.
- The influx of up to 50 new students from other medical schools in year 4 creates a fantastic opportunity to make new friends when you begin your clinical training.
- Excellent scientific and clinical teaching, together with a stimulating environment in a university with a first-class, worldwide reputation.
- Oxford is a beautiful city in which to work. Together with its traditions, this makes student life here a unique experience.

Bad things about Oxford

- The public perception of Oxford is behind the times and relies too much on stereotypes. These are inaccurate and unhelpful – don't be discouraged from applying!
- Some students at Oxford are incredibly hard-working, so the pressure can build up at times.
- The scientific nature of the course, particularly during the preclinical years, does not suit everyone.
- The nightlife in Oxford is limited, but London is nearby and easily reached.
- The scheme that matches graduates to their first job doesn't work well.

Further information

Oxford Colleges Admission Service (undergraduate admissions)
The University Offices
Wellington Square
Oxford OX1 2JD
Tel: 01865 288 000
Fax: 01865 270 208
Email: undergraduate.admissions@admin.ox.ac.uk
Web: http://www.medsci.ox.ac.uk/study

Clinical Medical School Offices
John Radcliffe Hospital
Headington
Oxford OX3 9DU
Web: http://www.medsci.ox.ac.uk

Additional application information

Average A level requirements	• AAA
Average Scottish Higher requirements	• AAAAA plus at least chemistry at Advanced Higher
Make-up of interview panel	• Undergraduate: Two interviews by those teaching the course, one of which will include a practising clinician • Graduate: Two or three (typically one clinician and one college tutor)
Months in which interviews are held	• December
Proportion of overseas students	• 3% (undergraduate) 2% (graduate)
Proportion of mature students	• Not known
Proportion of graduate students	• 1%
Faculty's view of students taking a gap year	• Generally supportive if used constructively
Proportion of students taking intercalated degrees	• 100% (the Honours degree is part of the course)

(*Continued*)

(*Continued*)

Possibility of direct entrance to clinical phase	• Yes (Honours graduates only) with preclinical qualification undertaken in the UK
Fees for overseas students	• £16,500 pa (preclincial) £23,500 pa (clinical)
Fees for graduates	• *c.* £7500 pa (2 preclinical years) • *c.* £2000 pa (3 clinical years)
Ability to transfer to other medical schools If so, under what circumstances	• Yes. Possible after completing the 3-year pre-clinical component of the course, but only to other schools (mainly Cambridge and some London medical schools) that run non-integrated courses.
Assistance for elective funding	• Yes – there are a variety of funds available. Each college has its own travel bursaries, as does the medical school itself.
Assistance for travel to attachments	• With placements out of Oxford, the medical school will reimburse travel costs in full (where accommodation is provided, only one return journey per week).
Access and hardship funds	• Administered through individual colleges, and always available, but vary in value and criteria for application. Usually very generous, worth finding out about from the colleges/websites before deciding which college to apply to.
Weekly rent	• From £65–£105 (varies with college)
Pint of lager	• £1.50 (college bars) upwards!
Cinema	• About £5 – there are great cinemas though, including great art-house ones
Nightclub	• Lots to choose from (contrary to popular belief, there are actually some decent ones); £5 entry for students with cheap(ish) drinks. There are always student promotions. Most colleges have 'entz' and 'bops', basically music (which is generally pretty good) and alcohol at very cheap prices.

Peninsula

Key facts	Undergraduate
Course length	5 years
Total number of medical undergraduates	804
Applicants in 2006	1946
Interviews given in 2006	699
Places available in 2006	215
Places available in 2007	215
Open days 2007	14 April (Exeter); 23 June (Plymouth)
Entrance requirements	ABB + 1 AS level (370-400 points)
Mandatory subjects	One science subject grade A
Male:female ratio	44:56
Is an exam included in the selection process?	Yes
If yes, what form does this exam take?	UKCAT for direct school leavers
	GAMSAT for non-direct school leavers
Qualification gained	BMBS

Fascinating fact: We are the southernmost medical school in the country. Some students have a chance to have placements with GPs on the Isles of Scilly!

Peninsula Medical School is the result of collaboration between the Universities of Exeter and Plymouth and NHS hospital trusts across the south-west. The three main bases of the medical school are Exeter, Plymouth and Truro and students are expected to spend some time at each site. It is a new and vibrant medical school that is passionate about medicine. The first undergraduate students started in 2002 and are now in their fourth year.

Plymouth, Exeter and Truro are very different cities and provide students with sometimes very contrasting experiences. All are pleasant to live in and the medicine seen on each site is very different, with different specialities and contrasting populations of patients. Exeter is fairly affluent and Plymouth significantly poorer. Truro is an interesting mixture of both.

The school has an exciting approach to medical training, with students having extensive exposure to primary and community medicine, the aim of which is to develop an understanding of patient care at all levels. Students are taught through self-directed learning in a supportive environment. The course is split into preclinical and clinical years and students are based at hospital sites from year 3. Practical clinical skills are taught from year 1 in brand new clinical skills suites across the south-west. SSMs are offered from year 1.

Education

The course at Peninsula is dynamic, with changes being made to improve it as the course develops. At the time of writing, the course was taught in three phases. Phase I is largely based at Exeter and Plymouth, with some clinical placements accompanied by lots of clinical skills teaching. Phase II is hospital-based in Exeter, Plymouth or Truro. Phase III is the 'apprentice PRHO' year, and consists of shadowing junior doctors in hospitals across the south-west, including Barnstaple and Torbay. Life sciences are a theme throughout all phases. Clinical and communication skills are timetabled from the first week of the course. Students also have clinical placements from the first week of the course.

In phase I, students learn about issues relating to different stages in the lifecycle of a human being. Each stage of human life, from conception to old age, is covered in a 2-week long case unit of which there are ten in year 1 and year 2. Emphasis in year 1 is placed on the normal functions of the body; in year 2 the emphasis is pathology. The lectures, clinical skills and placements during a case unit aim to supplement learning objectives for that case unit. For example, during the conception case unit, students research topics such as the menstrual cycle, reproductive system and fertility, while also learning how to carry out appropriate clinical examinations. Students will also visit a community clinical placement, which could be a local GP or a visit to a family planning clinic, and have a chance to discuss the issues arising from this visit in a small group session.

In phase II, students follow one of three 'pathways' each term, and have a 'trigger case' each week on which to base their learning, e.g. 'the confused drinker', 'shortness of breath' and 'the new baby'. Students are split into very small groups (twos or threes) and have several placements during each week, including a protected, timetabled 2-hour teaching sessions with the consultant in charge of each week.

Teaching

The course at Peninsula is based on problem-based learning (PBL), which involves students working in small groups to determine learning objectives, researching these objectives and sharing information obtained in subsequent sessions. In phase I these sessions are coordinated by a member of staff who acts as a facilitator and ensures that the sessions run smoothly. In phase II, students are supported in learning life sciences with extensive clinico-pathological conferences accompanied by structured supported learning sessions and have access to the full resources of the life sciences facilities. One day of each week in phase II is an academic day based at the hospital teaching centre, with lectures, small group work and clinical skills sessions.

Assessment

Students are assessed in four major areas – applied medical knowledge (AMK), clinical skills, special studies units (SSUs) and personal and professional development (PPD). Four times a year, all students sit a progress test (an MCQ exam which assesses AMK). The exam is not based directly on previous work – rather, it aims to assess progress across the board in all aspects of AMK and all year groups sit the same exam at the same time. This might mean that students in year 1 get very low marks, but are deemed satisfactory within their year group. By year 5 students are expected to get very high marks.

Judgements of PPD made by staff are collected together and form a portfolio, and this element is assessed by completing a reflective portfolio analysis written by the student. Assessment of clinical skills is carried out at the end of year 2 by an integrated structured clinical examination (ISCE – sometimes known as an OSCE). Students must pass all four major areas at the end of each year to progress into the next year of the course. Further to this, assessment in the clinical years includes weekly clinical reasoning assessments made by teaching consultants.

Intercalated degrees

Intercalated degrees are available for the highest performing students after the end of year 4. It is possible for students to choose between intercalating a traditional BSc degree or a non-traditional BA degree.

Special study modules and electives

Peninsula offers special study units (SSUs) from year 1 of the course. During phase I, these are mostly short, 3-week placements providing each student with the opportunity to research medical issues and topics of personal interest ranging from clinical (e.g. stroke management) or scientific (e.g. psychoneuroimmunology) to alternative medicine and community (e.g. shiatsu and yoga). In phase II, SSUs are mostly in specialist clinical settings, but also include themes such as 'doctors as managers' and medical humanities. Furthermore, SSUs in year 4 run across the year so that students may be attached to a research group for a whole year. During SSUs students are required to attend contact sessions with the SSU facilitators and to prepare a report and/or a presentation on their research topic.

Being a new medical school, no PMS students have undertaken an elective as yet. The elective is planned for the first part the final year. The first students to undertake electives are currently in the process of planning and will have the chance to travel, or to take an elective project based in the UK. The planning process and a final report will form part of the SSU assessment for year 5.

Erasmus

An Erasmus programme has not been established.

Facilities

Library   Students have access to the university libraries at Exeter and Plymouth, as well as hospital libraries across the south-west and various postgraduate centres and specialist libraries such as public health. There is not a separate 'Peninsula Medical School' library, although students are well supported by library staff at each site and have access to extensive internet resources. The medical school also has several life sciences centres across the sites and these have open-access facilities including books, databases and models, although resources cannot be removed from the allocated rooms. There is also extensive use of an online learning environment, known as Emily, where everything from timetables to anatomy texts can be found. In the past year, the lectures given to students have been streamed onto Emily and can be watched from the convenience of a home computer!

Computers   At all sites, including both universities and all three hospitals, students have 24-hour access to brand new, dedicated IT suites exclusively for the use of medical students. These suites are generously equipped and so far, there always seems to be a computer free to use at any time.

Email is used heavily to communicate with students. Teaching sessions are provided on the use of computers, and specialist support is also available.

Clinical skills   Students attend a clinical skills session in brand new, purpose-built clinical skills centres, based in each main hospital site. Teaching facilities include mock-wards and clinical kit such as defibrillation machines. Development of communication skills is also a key teaching theme which starts with 'initiating a consultation' and includes practising patient interviews with actors. Facilities for recording these 'patient' interviews onto DVDs are used so that students can have lasting, take-home records of how cringeworthy their first attempts at interviewing patients were!

Welfare

Student support

Students have access to pastoral tutors, who are one or two members of staff appointed to each phase and to each of the three main sites. This is a new system and staff are keen to provide appropriate support to students who need it during their time at the medical school.

As students of the universities of Exeter and Plymouth, PMS students have access to the student support services available in their locality. This includes the welfare and equal opportunities offices, student counselling centre, student advice centre, education unit and 'Nightline', a student support hotline. For students with families, support is also available from the student parent department and family centre.

One of the challenges for the medical school is providing comparable university-type student support for students based in Truro and other outlying hospital sites. However, the senior staff are working hard to remedy this and are developing support mechanisms, including buddying systems for staff and students.

Accommodation

Accommodation is provided for all year 1 students in Exeter and Plymouth and most clinical students in Truro. In Exeter, the accommodation is conveniently located near shops and is in walking distance of the campus, hospitals and many of the GP surgeries that students will visit for their placements. In Plymouth, accommodation is central to both the university and city centre. At Plymouth students are housed in a large new building, which is part of a planned development giving new arts space to the university and city.

Placements

While Peninsula is split across three main sites (Exeter, Plymouth and Truro), students are mostly based in Exeter and Plymouth for the first two years with community-based placements across the city. Clinical skills are also taught in the hospitals and in Plymouth a shuttle bus is provided to get the students from the university to the hospital.

In the subsequent years, students are moved around the south-west and usually have a year based in each of the three hospital sites of Exeter, Plymouth and Truro. These each have their own locality base at the main hospital bases of Royal Devon and Exeter (Exeter), Derriford Hospital (Plymouth) and the Royal Cornwall Hospital (Truro). Torbay Hospital and North Devon Hospital also take students on shorter-term placements. Other placements may be with the Primary Care Trusts, for instance in the smaller hospitals across the south-west, as well as the mental health care teams.

Location of clinical placement/ name of hospital	Distance away from medical school or university campus (miles)	Difficulty getting there on public transport*
Royal Devon and Exeter Hospital	0.5	
Derriford Hospital (Plymouth)	6	
Placements in Plymouth	0–4	
Placements in Plymouth/ Devon	0–50	
Placements across the south-west	up to 100	

* : walking/cycling distance; : use public transport; : need own car or lift; : get up early – tricky to get to!

Each student is attached to a GP practice for the year and has the chance to visit for a week at a time, three times across the year. In cases where commuting to GP placements each day is an issue, the medical school is in the process of negotiating appropriate accommodation for students and this is either fully paid for or a significant contribution is met by the medical school. Several students volunteer to go further afield, as placements include the seaside towns of Dartmouth and Torquay and moors towns such as Tavistock.

Sports and social

City life

Exeter is a city packed with a blend of modern and historical attractions for students. These range from popular nightspots in the city centre and on the waterfront to the magnificent Exeter Cathedral, cobbled alleyways and catacombs.

Plymouth is an interesting mixture of the traditional Devon appeal (think clotted cream teas) and modern edge. Part of the city centre is being redeveloped and will provide great new shopping and city centre venues. Many sailors and surfers live in Plymouth and it's not far from Dartmoor, which provides stunning scenery and the opportunity for fantastic outdoor pursuits. There are plenty of cinemas, good places for eating and drinking and the infamous Union Street for late-night going out.

Truro is a beautiful cathedral city, surrounded by amazing Cornish countryside. They say that nowhere in Cornwall is more than 16 miles from the sea – so the beach isn't far! Truro is full of good places to drink and eat, although the clubbing scene is rather limited and there is only one small cinema. Truro tends to also be a bit more expensive than the other cities, as there aren't as many students based there.

University life

Plymouth and Exeter provide rather different student experiences. In Plymouth, medical students are integrated into the student population – the halls in year 1 are mixed and many year 2 medics live with other non-medic students. By contrast, medical students in Exeter are mainly based on a separate campus from the other Exeter students and are hence less integrated into the wider university. The medical societies (MedSocs) on both sites have similar aims and provide similar events like going out, sometimes with charity fundraising, and themed evenings. There is also development of (less alcoholic) events that involve families, as there are a fair number of mature students with children. Highlights are the MedSoc balls: at the time of writing Exeter hosts the Christmas Ball and Plymouth the Summer Ball.

MedSIN groups in Exeter and Plymouth are rapidly growing and have started to attract attention from other student societies and students. MedSIN offers students the opportunity to run and participate in numerous different community projects such as Marrow, Sexpression and CPR in Schools.

Students also have the opportunity to set up new societies. Plymouth has a Student Union whereas Exeter has a Student Guild. Both do essentially the same job, although no doubt some argument could be made over who has the best socials!

Sports life

The British Universities Sports Association (BUSA) ranks the University of Exeter among the top 10 universities for sport in the country. Both the main campus and St. Luke's campus in Exeter have well-maintained sports halls that include a gym and swimming pool as well as basketball, badminton and squash courts. The Athletic Union in Exeter has over 40 sports clubs (including 7 different kinds of martial arts) ranging from archery to windsurfing. Water sports (sub-aqua, surfing) are extremely popular as there are regular trips on the weekends to the coast and nearby beaches. Intramural sport is popular: Exeter Medsoc enters teams for hockey, football and netball.

Plymouth University has its own sailing and diving centres, running courses at a small cost. The number of sports clubs is enormous – and if they don't have what you want you can set up your own club! There is also a university gym which is open to all students for a small annual fee. Intra-school sports competitions are bi-annual events.

Currently Plymouth and Exeter play each other twice a year on the football pitch (both girls and boys), with the hope that Truro may get a team together soon. PMS is proud to have achieved notable success with their rugby team, who take on local and medical school opposition most weekends. A mixed hockey team is also being developed.

Finally, it'd just be rude not to mention the surfing heaven that is Cornwall and North Devon – apparently, it's a natural high that can't be beaten!

Great things about Peninsula

- Students learn clinical skills from the first week.
- It's always only a short drive/train ride to the beach.
- Lots of patients are aware of the new medical school and are keen to help medical students to learn.
- Living costs in both Plymouth and Exeter are relatively inexpensive. Plymouth is particularly cheap.
- The brand new medical school buildings, with brand new facilities, exclusively available to medical students are excellent.

Bad things about Peninsula

- Limited student parking provided at medical school sites.
- After years 1 and 2 on both campuses, you are rotated around various Peninsula Medical School locations in Devon and Cornwall (Exeter, Plymouth, Truro, Barnstaple, Torbay). A downer if you're looking to settle down in one place!
- Peninsula doesn't have an assessment-based approach – this may not be good if you are not self-motivated.
- You may never get to meet other students in your year if they move to different campuses from you.
- You may move to a different site after phase I and away from your friends.

Further information

Undergraduate Admissions Office
Peninsula College of Medicine and Dentistry
John Bull Building
Tamar Science Park
Research Way
Plymouth PL6 8BU
Tel: 01752 247 444
Fax: 01752 517 842
Email: pmsenq@pms.ac.uk
Web: http://www.pms.ac.uk

Additional application information

Average A level requirements	• 320 points from three A levels including one science subject grade A, plus one further subject at AS level grade B
Average Scottish Higher requirements	• 320 points from three Advanced Highers including one science subject grade A, plus one further subject at Higher level grade B, or two Advanced Highers grade A including one science subject plus ABB at Higher level, or four grade As and one grade B at Higher level including one science subject grade A.
Make-up of interview panel	• Three: one clinician and two from the following: healthcare professionals, non clinical academics, lay community members
Months in which interviews are held	• November, December, March
Proportion of overseas students	• 7.5%
Proportion of mature students	• No information available
Proportion of graduate students	• 22%
Faculty's view of students taking a gap year	• Encouraged
Proportion of students taking intercalated degrees	• 7% of year 4 students

Possibility of direct entrance to clinical phase	• No
Fees for overseas students	• £12,000 pa (years 1 and 2) £19,500 pa (years 3, 4 and 5)
Fees for graduates	• £3000 pa
Ability to transfer to other medical schools If so, under what circumstances	• Difficult due to the very different course structure; but has been done successfully by a few students.
Assistance for elective funding	• Available
Assistance for travel to attachments	• Available - travel bursary provided to each student.
Access and hardship funds	• Available through main universities.
Weekly rent	• £55–£75, depending on locality
Pint of lager	• From £1
Cinema	• £5
Nightclub	• £5; can also be free

Royal Free and University College London

Key facts	Undergraduate
Course length	6 years (5 for graduates)
Total number of medical undergraduates	1700
Applicants in 2006	2215
Interviews given in 2006	800
Places available in 2006	330
Places available in 2007	330
Open days 2007	April
Entrance requirements	AAB + AS
Mandatory subjects	Chemistry at A2 plus biology at AS level
Male:female ratio	50:50
Is an exam included in the selection process?	Yes
If yes, what form does this exam take?	BMAT
Qualification gained	MBBS (BSc)

Fascinating fact: The main quad and the old laboratories on the quad side of Gower Street are haunted by three children – two girls and a boy. Each sighting is reported identically: they walk in a line, the same girl always at the front, followed by the other two, each with their hand on the child in front's shoulder as if the trailing two were blind.

One of the largest medical schools in the UK lies in an exciting, attractive and vibrant part of London. The Royal Free and University College London Medical School (RF&UCMS) is the combined product of two previously separate world-class institutions: Royal Free Hospital School of Medicine (Hampstead) and University College London Medical School (Bloomsbury). The schools are now completely integrated, and incorporate a number of world-famous institutions with excellent reputations for teaching and research. These include the Institute of Child Health (Great Ormond Street), the Institute of Neurology (the National Hospital for Neurology and Neurosurgery), the Institute of Laryngology and Otology (the Royal National Throat, Nose and Ear Hospital) and the Institute of Ophthalmology (Moorfields Eye Hospital). RF&UCMS offers an integrated systems-based course taught by respected academics and clinicians as well as some very friendly students.

RF&UCMS has three main campuses that students will frequent throughout their training:

- Archway – known affectionately as 'the Whit' to UCL students, this is the site of the Whittington Hospital;
- Bloomsbury – located in WC1, the Bloomsbury campus is the site of the UCL Hospital; as London's newest £420 million super-hospital, it offers the finest facilities available;
- Hampstead – charming, leafy Hampstead is home to the Royal Free Hospital and is a popular home site; offers pleasant shops, bars, restaurants, and walks on the Heath.

Education

The new curriculum started in 2000. It is a 6-year integrated systems-based course, including a mandatory intercalated BSc for non-graduates. Clinical experience starts from day one, and although full integration is close to completion, the preclinical/clinical divide has not entirely been abandoned.

Teaching

The systems-based medical degree programme integrates the basic medical sciences with clinical science and professional skills and competencies. The core curriculum is traditionally arranged into three distinct phases. Phase I (years 1 and 2) consists of sequential systems-based learning modules ('Science and Medicine'). Phase II (years 3 and 4) consists of a series of sequential clinical attachments ('Science and Medical Practice'), which builds on the systems-based modules of phase I. In year 3 there are eight clinical attachments, each comprising a core medicine and surgery teaching course half a day a week (including basic science), half a day of professional development (such as communication, ethics, law, etc.), and 1 week of pathology per two attachments. Year 4 contains nine clinical blocks. Each student undertakes clinical attachments at central London and district general hospitals during this year. In phase III ('Professional Development'- year 5) there are clinical attachments in general practice, accident and emergency, oncology and district general hospital medicine and surgery, as well as selective specialist clinical or research attachments and a period of elective study.

RF&UCMS prides itself on its Professional Development Spine (PDS). Integrated throughout all 5 years, the course comprises a series of themes including society and the individual, evaluation of evidence, law and ethics, sociology and communication skills. In recognition of the multidisciplinary nature of modern medicine, the course draws on UCL's wealth of pre-eminent legal, ethical and sociological minds to create a truly modern, rounded and complete medical course.

Assessment

Assessment in phase 1 of the course is mostly by multiple-choice questions, OSPEs (objective structured practical examination – practical and data interpretation assessments in a circuit of timed stations – otherwise known as OSCEs) and coursework. By phase II, students are heavily involved in clinical work, and the assessments change to reflect this with the introduction of EMQs, OSCEs and a logbook for the recording of clinical firm grades. The phase II, year 4 exams are technically final exams for the clinical specialities, but the main finals are in medicine, surgery and general practice at the end of phase III, year 5. These exams consist of 'long station' OSCEs, 'short station' OSCEs and written short answer papers.

Intercalated degrees

All non-graduate students are expected to complete an intercalated BSc. Most students intercalate between phases I and II, but students are welcome to opt to undertake a BSc later in the medical degree programme, especially if they wish to pursue a BSc programme designed for students with greater clinical experience. UCL probably provides the best intercalated BSc opportunities in Britain. Subjects range from medical ethics and law to forensic archaeology and space physiology and medicine. Competition for some BSc courses is tough, and some students may have to settle for their second choice.

Special study modules and electives

In addition to the core curriculum there are special study modules (SSMs), permitting the study of selected subjects in depth. Phase 1 SSMs tend to be non-medical and can include law, history of medicine, arts and modern languages (over 16 to choose from). A further two are undertaken in phase 3, and are clinical or research-oriented. RF&UCMS students have unparalleled opportunities, as many of the SSMs are offered at world-class institutions.

An elective period of 8 weeks is offered in the final year. The minimum time that must be spent in clinical practice is 6 weeks. The world is your oyster, although expect to do a lot of the leg-work yourself. Help finding placements abroad is scarce – contact opportunities are limited to your own, or those of friendly clinicians. A limited number of competitive bursaries exist but don't expect them to fall into your lap!

Erasmus

There are currently no opportunities for exchange under the Erasmus programme. Travel overseas is generally restricted to the elective period, although some people have been known to sneak off to Trinidad for their paediatric rotations.

Facilities

Library   All three campuses have large, well-stocked libraries with extensive collections of medical and clinical texts to suit students at all stages of their training. Each library subscribes to a large number of journals and photocopying facilities are available although not free. For students pursuing more specialized disciplines during their studies, the specialist centres listed in the introductory paragraph are all within walking distance of Gower Street. In addition, the British Library is a few minutes' walk from the medical school as are the School of Pharmacy and the London School of Hygiene and Tropical Medicine. Student members of the BMA have the extensive and elegant library and study facilities of BMA House just metres from Gower Street.

Computers   There are clusters of networked computers throughout all campus sites and in many residential halls. When they are not booked for formal teaching, students have free access on a first-come first-served basis. Most networked computers are Windows PCs, although there are some Apple computers. All students have free internet and email access, although the university have recently initiated an unpopular move to charge for printing above a certain quota. Wireless internet connection is available for students with wireless-enabled laptops. Students can also access the college server from home.

Clinical skills   There are clinical skills laboratories on all three campuses. They are run by some of the friendliest teachers you'll ever meet, the teaching is excellent, allowing you to perfect such techniques as inserting tubes into rubber penises to allow a patient to pass urine before being released to perform these important tasks on patients.

Welfare

Student support

All students are assigned a tutor in phase I, normally a basic scientist who oversees their personal and academic development and provide pastoral care. In phases II and III students are currently assigned personal tutors who are clinically qualified. In addition, the faculty tutorial team provide regular 'walk-in surgeries', and most academic staff at UCL have an open-door policy or clearly advertised hours when they are available to students.

Student feedback on course quality and teaching is actively sought through questionnaires, faculty education committees, and staff–student consultative committees. Comments are taken seriously and courses have been changed on the basis of constructive student feedback. Each course is generally well-organized with comprehensive lecture notes distributed early in each term.

Accommodation

Most first-year students stay at UCL or in University of London halls. Halls are generally acceptable, although of lower value-for-money than non-London halls. A second year in halls is occasionally available during the BSc or final year. The accommodation office at Senate House offers help and legal advice to London students. To find better-value accommodation, many students choose to travel into central London from places like Finsbury Park and Camden.

Placements

Most teaching in phase I occurs at the Bloomsbury site – except PDS teaching, which is split across the three home sites.

Most clinical teaching placements in phase II, year 3, and about half in phase II, year 4, are at UCH, Royal Free and Whittington Hospitals, all of which are in central London and are easily accessible by public transport. In the other half of phase II, year 4, and in almost all of phase III, year 5, placements are at more distant district general hospitals, which take anything from 30 minutes to a few hours to reach depending on your respective locations. It is generally possible to either select or swap district general hospitals most of the time to ensure you shouldn't have to travel an inordinate amount of time. In addition, accommodation is nearly always provided, given the travelling time, and where accommodation is unavailable, travel costs are reimbursed.

Location of clinical placement/ name of hospital	Distance away from medical school (miles)	Difficulty getting there on public transport*
UCH	0	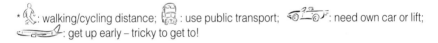
Royal Free	3.5	
Whittington	4	

* : walking/cycling distance; : use public transport; 🚗: need own car or lift; ✈: get up early – tricky to get to!

Sports and social 🏆

City life

UCL is surrounded by the greatest concentration of libraries, museums, archives and professional bodies in Europe! Soho and Covent Garden border its Bloomsbury campus and you just can't walk down a street in Central London without coming across a nightclub.

The Royal Free campus has both the cosmopolitan atmosphere of Hampstead and the open green parkland of Hampstead Heath. Nearby buzzing Camden offers live music, clubs and the super-cool Camden Lock market.

University life

RF&UCMS students are automatically members of University of London Union (ULU) and have access to all its facilities and services, including sports facilities, bars and cafés, clubs and societies, and welfare services. For the unique needs of the medical student there are also medical Student Union officers based on all three sites, which, together with the medical student community itself, form RUMS (Royal Free and University College Medical Students) – our own mini-union.

The family-like community of medical students here is encouraged from day 1, with freshers being assigned to a 'set' in which they may stay for social events and competitive sports. Throughout the year the RUMS officers organize various events including balls, theme nights and shows – kicking-off with the 14-day extravaganza that is 'The RUMS Freshers' Fortnight'. Additionally, RUMS runs over 30 clubs and societies and helps represent students over educational and welfare-related-issues.

Although ULU operate a variety of bars around its central sites, the medical school bar at Huntley Street is traditionally the habitat of choice for the RUMS student. With various themed nights and Wednesday night ('sports night'), it is rarely a place for quiet contemplation and reflection. The Royal Free has a new medical student bar and the Whittington has a curious little drinking hole under-ground that most students only discover by accident while trying to find the pathology lab in year 5.

Your motto should be 'work hard, play hard' and while the medical school will take care of providing the hard work, you get to take care of the play – and you couldn't want more choice. There are medics socie-ties as well as literally hundreds of clubs and societies at the Union to get involved in. RUMS has its own company of comics which produce the traditional medics revue comedy show. There are regular dra-matic and operatic productions as well as comedy and musical gigs at UCL's own Bloomsbury theatre. UCL has three museums and two arts collections, including works by Rembrandt, Turner, Constable and Dürer. The Slade Collection includes work by Augustus John and Percy Wyndham-Lewis. UCL's Petrie Museum is one of the greatest collections of Egyptian and Sudanese Archaeology in the world!

RAG week brings together the usual mixture of the insane and the civilized, all working for a good cause – you'll wind-up doing things you never thought you'd see yourself doing, and all in the name of charity.

However, one of the great things about being a RUMS student is that you're not confined to socializing within the medical school – you have all of UCL on your doorstep.

Sports life

Whether you're a honed and toned athletic masterpiece with your eyes on gold at Beijing in 2008 or a bit of a couch-fitness guru who likes the social and health benefits of doing sport, you have every opportunity of partaking in pretty much any sport at any level at RF&UCMS. RUMS has teams (1sts, 2nds, and 3rds, etc.) in most major sports which any RUMS student is eligible to try out for. Alterna-tively you can play for a ULU team. Both RUMS and ULU teams play on a local and national level. RUMS and UCL's home ground is based at Shenley, Hertfordshire. These 60-acres of hallowed turf are also the training venue for the mighty Watford FC!

UCL has a very strong tradition for water sports. Our oarsmen and women are based at the university boathouse at Chiswick. The United Hospital Bumps is a not-to-be-missed event taking place every summer on the Thames and is the inter-hospital rowing showdown for eights.

General sporting facilities at UCL are fantastic. Medical students have use of the swimming pool in John Astor House as well as the gym, squash courts and weights room. Bloomsbury campus now boasts the Somers Town Sports Centre and offers superb facilities very locally, including those for basketball, netball, hockey and football. UCL's Bloomsbury Fitness Centre contains an impressive gym complex and there is a further swimming pool as well as sauna and jacuzzi – for the lushes among you – based at ULU's Malet Street Buildings.

In addition, RUMS students are all encouraged to become members of the United Hospitals sports clubs.

Great things about RF&UCMS

- A top-ranking university with a worldwide reputation for research in basic medical sciences and clinical medicine. Opportunities to work alongside leaders in research. We are renowned for our teaching system, with small-group tutorials, a superbly equipped dissection suite and new teaching and learning facilities.
- The central London location places students very close to some of the finest theatres, concert halls and museums in the world.
- Get discounts on additional courses (evening/weekend) run by other faculties, such as in modern languages (good for electives) or fine art at UCL's Slade School.
- The new UCH is one of the most technologically advanced hospitals in the world, has works of art on its walls, 700 beds and the largest intensive care unit in Europe.
- Darth Vader and six Storm Troopers opened its paediatric unit in Autumn 2005! The Queen opened the rest.

Bad things about RF&UCMS

- RFUCMS requires applicants to sit the BMAT – sorry (see Chapter 3 and www.bmat.org.uk).
- The need to travel around London to get to different campuses (Bloomsbury, Archway, and Hampstead) is a bit of a drag.
- UCL is a big place. You can get that 'small fish, big pond' feeling at first – but then so is the NHS so at least you'll be prepared!
- Some DGH's are *very* far away (e.g. Bath or Devon!) and students must live-in. However, there are often students who are happy to swap with you.
- Tough retake policy.

Further information

Dr Brenda Cross
Medical Admissions
University College London
London WC1E 6BT
Tel: 020 7679 0841
Fax: 020 7679 5494
Email: medicaladmissions@ucl.ac.uk
Web: http://www.ucl.ac.uk/medicalschool

Students' Union: Medical Students' and Sites' Officer
25 Gordon Street
London WC1H 0AY
Tel: 020 7679 7949
Email: mss.officer@ucl.ac.uk
Web: http://www.uclu.org.uk

Additional application information

Average A level requirements	• AAB
Average Scottish Advanced Higher requirements	• AAB
Make-up of interview panel	• Three: two UCL staff (one clinical, one life sciences) and one other (student or teacher)
Months in which interviews are held	• November – March
Proportion of overseas students	• 7.5%
Proportion of mature students	• 15%
Proportion of graduate students	• 15%
Faculty's view of students taking a gap year	• Positive
Proportion of students taking intercalated degrees	• 100% (excluding graduates)
Possibility of direct entrance to clinical phase	• Yes – Oxbridge only
Fees for overseas students	• £21,320
Fees for graduates	• £3000
Ability to transfer to other medical schools	• Not normally, extenuating circumstances required, although students transfer into the school from Oxford and Cambridge after their year 3.
Assistance for elective funding	• Limited and very competitive.
Assistance for travel to attachments	• Travel outside of zone 2 is refunded. If accommodation is provided only one return journey is paid per week.
Access and hardship funds	• There is a large access fund available to all its (10,000) students throughout the year. Advisable to get your application in early.

(*Continued*)

(Continued)

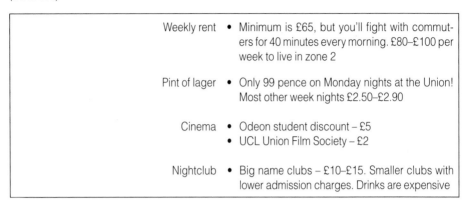

Weekly rent	•	Minimum is £65, but you'll fight with commuters for 40 minutes every morning. £80–£100 per week to live in zone 2
Pint of lager	•	Only 99 pence on Monday nights at the Union! Most other week nights £2.50–£2.90
Cinema	•	Odeon student discount – £5
	•	UCL Union Film Society – £2
Nightclub	•	Big name clubs – £10–£15. Smaller clubs with lower admission charges. Drinks are expensive

St Andrews

Key facts	Undergraduate
Course length	3 years (followed by 3 years at Manchester/Preston)
Total number of medical undergraduates	416
Applicants in 2006	1097
Interviews given in 2006	375
Places available in 2006	124
Places available in 2007	124
Open days 2007	See website for details
Entrance requirements	AAB
Mandatory subjects	Chemistry plus one other science. GCSE english at B or better
Male:female ratio	42:58
Is an exam included in the selection process?	No
If yes, what form does this exam take?	UKCAT from 2007
Qualification gained	BSc (Hons) in medicine; MBChB completed at Manchester Medical School

Fascinating fact: St Andrews may be a small town but it is home to around 22 different pubs – this is more per square mile than any other university town in Britain!

Established in the 15th century, St Andrews is the oldest university in Scotland. It is set in a small picturesque town on the east coast of Fife. In September 2004, the course was radically changed so that students graduate with a BSc (Medicine) at Honours level in 3 years – medical students gain direct entry into St Andrews University at the second-year level of a 4-year Honours degree programme for which the first year does not exist! During the 3 years, students are taught a systems-based curriculum, where important concepts are frequently revisited and consolidated. The faculty is small and students socialize with medics and non-medics alike.

On graduation from St Andrews, the vast majority of students have headed south for Manchester to complete their clinical studies (taking a further 3 years). The uniqueness of such a course provides a great opportunity for students to experience studying in both an ancient university town and a big vibrant city.

In September 2006, the Scottish Executive announced that 100 extra places would be made available for St Andrews' students to complete their medical training in Scottish medical schools. This is in part due to a review, which has sought to boost the medical workforce in Scotland by increasing the number of medical undergraduates completing their degrees in Scotland.

Education

St Andrews University is the oldest university in Scotland, which explains the traditions and customs that surround being a student here. However, as the university is always keen to keep up with the needs of a modern doctor in training, the course has been overhauled so that students are taught an integrated curriculum instead of the traditional pure preclinical sciences, like anatomy and physiology. Year 1 is spent learning about the foundations of medicine, in which cellular and molecular processes are emphasized as the starting point for disease, along with other biological sciences, leading to a good understanding of the structure and function of the body. The Honours programme begins over the next 2 years and takes the form of an integrated review of all the main body systems. The final semester consists of two modules. Applied medical science links the medical sciences through a series of clinical seminars and patient cases. The final Honours module is a significant student-selected component (SSC) of the course. This may take the form of a course of advanced study, a laboratory-based project or a library project.

Students graduate from St Andrews in Medical Sciences, and then progress to a clinical school for a further 3 years before graduating as a doctor. Students have previously been guaranteed a clinical place at the University of Manchester, the largest medical school in Europe, with outstanding clinical facilities and the two courses are very well integrated to allow a smooth transition. Students are based in one of Manchester's three big teaching hospitals, or at Preston campus. See the Manchester chapter for more information. In the future, there will be links with other Scottish medical schools to allow St Andrews' graduates to complete their clinical training in Scotland. Future applicants may wish to consult the chapters on Glasgow, Edinburgh, Dundee and Aberdeen (which will take 50, 30, 10 and 10 students, respectively).

Clinical relevance is emphasized throughout the St Andrews course in the form of a series of patients, which the students work on in small groups. The small class size for tutorials and dissection gives a great opportunity to develop good relationships between students and with staff. Some aspects of the course mimic the problem-based learning approach in operation at Manchester, and integration between the two schools has improved greatly over the last few years.

One of the benefits of the course structure at St Andrews is that students leave here with a degree, whether or not they continue medical studies.

Teaching

St Andrews aims to instil a comprehensive understanding of the workings of the human body, taking a traditional knowledge-based rather than problem-based approach. Throughout the course a wide range of teaching methods are used, including lectures, laboratory-based practicals, computer-based resources, small group tutorials and problem solving. The medical curriculum is delivered with the aid of the university's new web-based learning environment and students are taught how to use these extensive online resources at the start of their course. From here, students can access interactive timetables, and, most importantly, are given a set of detailed learning objectives. Unlike in some institutions, students have the increasingly rare opportunity to learn anatomy by careful regional dissection of the whole body. Scheduled classes occupy approximately 15 hours per week, with 6 additional hours set aside for guided study.

Assessment

The learning objectives are the basis of assessment, and students are encouraged to focus their learning in light of these learning objectives. Exams are varied and include a mixture of MCQs, short-answer questions, case studies and objective structured practical examinations. Mid-terms and practical work done throughout the year contribute a small amount towards the end of year mark.

Intercalated degrees

All students graduate from the University of St Andrews with a BSc in Medicine at Honours level.

Special study modules and electives

Different types of student selected components exist throughout the course, with a major component in the final semester that can take the form of a laboratory-based research project or taught module (e.g. reproductive biology, cancer biology, health psychology or ethics). There is also the opportunity to complete a library project based on current medical literature, on a topic of interest selected by the student.

The electives are taken at the clinical school you attend. Consult relevant chapters for more information.

Erasmus

There are no opportunities for Erasmus or study abroad at St Andrews.

Facilities

Library A small range of books is available, although many students buy the core texts because of the restricted availability of some titles. There is also a small negotiated discount for all first-year medics who buy their core texts at once. Books are available on short loan (4 hour/overnight/weekend slots for the most popular titles), 3-day and long loan. St Andrews' students are also allowed to borrow books from Dundee medical library. Opening hours are increased during exam periods and shortened over the vacations: currently, during term time, the library is open Monday–Friday 8:45 AM–midnight, Saturday 9:00 AM–5:00 PM and Sunday 1:00 PM–7:00 PM.

Computers   There are several computer rooms available, including a new 24-hour computer suite within the Bute Medical building itself and within halls of residence.

Clinical skills   Clinical skills training begins in year 1 and continues throughout the course. Access to the clinical skills laboratory is good and the staff are always helpful. There are strong links with the community and the opportunity to gain wider clinical experience through hospital visits, GP attachments, and a new primary care initiative in Fife known affectionately as the Levenmouth Project.

Welfare

Student support

Student support is an area of major strength at St Andrews. In such a small town, the medics are well integrated into the university, and you will have the chance to get to know everyone at the school and make friends outside the faculty. The dean and faculty are good and very supportive, and tend to get to know everyone by name quite quickly. The students' association provides welfare and counselling services, including a free confidential and anonymous Nightline service for students in need of advice. The locals tend to be student-friendly, if only because the university is the biggest local employer and students make up a third of the town's population. However, when the revelry surrounding some of the ancient traditions still upheld by the university gets a bit over the top (for example, during the infamous Raisin Weekend in November), town and gown relations can become a little strained.

Accommodation

All students are guaranteed a place in university accommodation in their first year, and there are often rooms available for further years, although these places are becoming increasingly scarce as the university expands. First year rooms are often shared, which helps you to make friends quickly, though there are double *en-suite* rooms available in the newer halls such as New Hall and the David Russell Apartments. The standard of flats is generally good. Students can opt to be catered or self-catered within university residences. Some halls are better than others, but none are bad. Other privately owned accommodation is available, facilitated by a housing office at the university. Rents average £60–100 a week, which is quite expensive compared to other university towns, though competition for the best flats is still fierce. Parking is difficult if you want to live in the town centre.

Placements

The medical school consists mainly of the Bute Medical Building, referred to by students as 'The Bute'. Some other buildings in St Andrews may be used, but they are all within walking distance of each other. St Andrews is very small for a university town, so there is no problem getting around.

The new curriculum allows students greater access to experience in hospitals and other local primary care facilities, with GP attachments and hospital visits becoming increasingly regular in year 2. Students visit a number of different clinics to see clinical teams at work and learn about public health medicine in practice. Thus, strong links are formed with the community from the very start of the course and students get to see the application of the knowledge and skills they have learned.

For clinical placements, see the entries for Manchester, Glasgow, Edinburgh, Dundee and Aberdeen.

Sports and social

City life

St Andrews is a beautiful coastal town, famed for its golf courses, with a population of around 18,000, one-third of whom are students. Being the oldest of Scotland's four ancient universities, it has more than its fair share of traditions and some of the oldest student societies. The students all live very near the centre of town, so it is never far to walk to meet a friend. There is a very good atmosphere among the students, with plenty of chances to mix with medics and non-medics, and enough things going on in the town, at the Union and with the societies, to keep you as busy as you want to be. Tourists and golf-followers can make the town bustle a bit too much at times, but you can often go celebrity spotting with some success!

The town has an excellent pub and café culture and there are easily enough pubs, restaurants, coffee shops, and cafes to keep most people happy. Ravers needing something more than the cheesy Union 'bop' every Friday will have to travel to Edinburgh or Dundee for some real action, along with equally die-hard shopaholics. Outdoor types have easy access to the Grampian Mountains, and the nearby sea and beaches can be good fun. There is no railway station at St Andrews; the nearest is Leuchars, which has regular bus services or taxis, which are about £8–10 one-way.

University life

You tend to make many firm friends within the school very quickly from having tutorials, practicals and lectures together. Outside of lectures, the Union is good – especially for freshers getting to know the place – and alcohol is reasonably cheap, but the club scene is lacking. There are twice weekly coaches to nightclubs in Dundee, 20-minutes away, which offer clubbers the chance to visit some of the busiest clubs in Scotland. The price for these buses is £5, which includes entrance to the club and a bus back to St Andrews. St Andrews' medical society is known as the Bute Medical Society, and has good socials, including a famed annual ball, pub crawls and 'cheese and wine' lectures from interesting medical speakers as well as a raucous revue. There many types of societies, from the very sensible to the downright silly (anyone for the Tunnocks' Caramel Wafer Appreciation Society?). Social life tends to focus around balls and events run by these societies – there is normally something each and every week, giving students plenty of opportunity to meet people both within and outside of the medical faculty, and to keep up with the 'work hard, play hard' adage that medics are famed for.

Sports life

Most sports are supported, especially hockey and rugby, and there is a medics' competition every year called the Hypertrophy. Medical school teams do not play every week, and keen players often get involved with their hall teams or the main university clubs. Inter-hall competitions are also popular. The facilities have been improved in recent years, such as the gym and Athletics Union. There is no university swimming pool though one is located within the town. It is, of course, golf heaven, with the Royal and Ancient offering excellent deals for students. Membership is around £100 a year, which includes the Old Course.

Great things about St Andrews

- Small year groups and good integration with non-medics and between medics in all 3 years.
- Traditional-style teaching gives students a grounding in basic medical sciences before clinical training.
- Excellent pastoral and education support, with most lecturers getting to know you on first name terms (can be a good or bad thing ...).
- Gives you the opportunity to study medicine in two different institutions.
- St Andrews has its own beach and there is dirt-cheap membership on the best golf courses in Scotland.

Bad things about St Andrews

- The traditional-style course can sometimes make you feel distanced from actual clinical medicine.
- Having to leave to pursue your clinical training – you can get very attached to the place!
- No nightclubs (if you discount the Union bop) nor many shops – you may have to travel to Dundee.
- It can get a bit cold and windy.
- Relatively small student numbers and the small size of the town can make it difficult to 'get away from it all'.

Further information

Admissions Application Centre
St Katharine's West
16 The Scores
St Andrews
Fife KY16 9AX
Tel: 01334 462150 (direct line)
    01334 476161 (switchboard)
Fax: 01334 463330
Email: admissions@st-andrews.ac.uk
Web: http://www.st-andrews.ac.uk

Additional application information

Average A level requirements	• AAB
Average Scottish Higher requirements	• AAAAB
Make-up of interview panel	• Two panel members – mix of teaching and honorary staff
Months in which interviews are held	• November – March
Proportion of overseas students	• 8.5%
Proportion of mature students	• 4%
Proportion of graduate students	• 4%
Faculty's view of students taking a gap year	• Positive, provided relevant to medical career
Proportion of students taking intercalated degrees	• N/A
Possibility of direct entrance to clinical phase	• No
Fees for overseas students	• £16,100
Fees for graduates	• £2700
Ability to transfer to other medical schools If so, under what circumstances	• Guaranteed transfer to Manchester/Preston for clinical training. You can apply to any other university for clinical training where curriculum complements that at St Andrews.
Assistance for elective funding	• N/A
Assistance for travel to attachments	• N/A
Access and hardship funds	• Financial department supplies a means-tested bursary – several different ones available.
Weekly rent	• £55–£100
Pint of lager	• £1.60–£2.30 (Union)
Cinema	• £3.65
Nightclub	• £3 (variable) at Union nightclub

St George's

Key facts	Foundation for medicine	Undergraduate	Graduate
Course length	1 year	5/6 years	4 years
Total number of medical undergraduates	18	1000	287
Applicants in 2006	149	2193	1368
Interviews given in 2006	50	850	310
Places available in 2006	20	202	70
Places available in 2007	20	188	84
Open days 2007	Last Wednesday of every month at 2PM (except July and September). Specific open days for graduate and foundation for medicine		
Entrance requirements	Mature non-graduate students who can demonstrate through work experience and personal development that they have the social and organizational skills and motivation needed to succeed in the study of medicine	AABB	2:2 degree in any discipline and GAMSAT
Mandatory subjects		Chemistry and biology	
Male:female ratio	40:60	40:60	40:60
Is an exam included in the selection process?	Yes	Yes	Yes
If yes, what form does this exam take?	UKCAT for 2008	UKCAT	GAMSAT
Qualification gained	Undergraduate Certificate but progression to 1st year MBBS	MBBS	MBBS

Fascinating fact: Probably one of the few medical schools that can boast having a dead cow by the name of Blossom in its library (who helped Jenner pioneer vaccination).

St George's, University of London (SGUL) is the former St George's Hospital Medical School – same lovely medical school, just with a trendy new logo. It's located in the heart of Tooting, in South London, 5-minutes' walk from Tooting Broadway underground station. It genuinely is a very welcoming school, with plenty of atmosphere and a wide variety of clinical experience available. St George's Hospital itself is one of the largest teaching hospitals in Europe, situated in a heavily-populated part of London with pressing health needs. The school offers two medical degree programmes: an established 5-year course and a 4-year graduate-entry programme. Together with medical students, St George's also trains students in other allied health professions. While the courses are run separately, the Students' Union runs events available to all. Staff, students and the SU are friendly and welcoming, which creates a strong feeling of community within the hospital. It is this, in particular, that makes SGUL a great place to study. Most will thoroughly enjoy the atmosphere, and will, at the very least, appreciate what is has to offer.

Education

Teaching

On the 5-year course, teaching begins with the common foundation module in the first term, shared by all first-year allied health professional courses. Subsequent teaching is divided into two core cycles. In cycle 1 (years 1 and 2) students study system modules integrated with some clinical experience and undertake two SSMs. In cycle 2 (years 3–5) students gain clinical experience in hospitals and general practice covering a wide range of disciplines. Structured clinical teaching is provided in all clinical attachments, in addition to lecture programmes at St George's. Students go on to complete three more SSMs in core cycle 2, the last of which is the 10-week elective. Clinical skills are taught from the first year by older students and dedicated clinical teaching fellows, with an intensive period at the beginning of year 3 before starting clinical attachments.

On the 4-year course, the first two years are spent in problem-based learning (PBL) across six modules, which together cover basic and clinical science. Within these modules, objectives are listed under four different themes: basic clinical science, community and population medicine, patient and doctor, and personal and professional development. Most learning is self-directed, with some lectures and seminars provided. The final 2 years are spent gaining clinical experience with general clinical attachments (GCAs) and specialities. SSMs are also a requirement for this course.

In keeping with modern curricula, there is an emphasis on communications skills from an early stage; this comprehensive teaching offers an invaluable opportunity to meet patients and practise history-taking before entering the clinical years, and covers challenging areas, such as breaking bad news, before facing the real situation.

Assessment

On the 5-year course, exams are termly for the first 2 years, contributing to the end-of-year synoptic exams. Each year must be passed for progression. The third-year exam contributes 20% of the final MBBS qualification. Three exams taken in year 4 from topics covered in the preceding clinical firms provide 10% each towards written finals, which come at the end of year 4. Electives and clinical finals are in the final year. Written assessments take the forms of: MCQs (negatively marked multiple-choice questions), EMIs (extended matching items, essentially lists from which the correct answer is chosen), SAQs (short-answer questions) and, in major exams, essays. Practical skills are assessed with OSPEs or 'spotters', which are predominantly anatomy-based and OSCEs, which test clinical skills using actors as patients.

On the 4-year course, exams are after every module in the first 2 years (every 4 to 7 weeks): these are formative in the year 1 and summative in year 2. The only requirement in year 1 is to pass the SSM. Exams are similar in format to the 5-year course with MCQs, EMIs and SAQs. In year 2, the 'mini-case' is introduced, where clinical scenarios are given out progressively during the exam, requiring investigation and diagnosis of a problem from initial presentation onwards. Year 2 also sees the introduction of OSCEs to assess clinical skills, history-taking and ethics. Year 3 is assessed at the end of the year with written papers and OSCEs, with electives and final exams taken alongside 5-year course students.

Intercalated degrees

An intercalated BSc can be taken after years 2, 3 or 4 on the 5-year course. The later the degree is taken, the more clinical in nature it can be. Study may be at St George's, other London colleges/ medical schools or further afield if you wish. A wide range of courses is available – choices are not restricted to medical or science subjects. Intercalation is currently not offered to 4-year medicine students.

Special study modules and electives

SSMs provide an opportunity to study an area of personal/specialist interest. On the 5-year course, the first two (in year 2) are taken at St George's, after which the choice is open, with the option to study abroad. Many students take the first three at St George's and use the fourth as a 'mini-elective' before the main 10-week elective, which is the final SSM. The 4-year course is more prescriptive: the first SSM is an obstetrics family attachment requiring an essay; the second a research project culminating in a poster presentation; the third a clinical mini-elective; and the fourth is the main elective.

All electives last over two months, and only require signing off by the host institution and a 1500-word report.

Erasmus

The IFMSA exchange scheme (handled by the MedSIN group) has recently been introduced to St George's, allowing medical students to swap places for a few weeks. The exchange scheme involves over 100 countries, so possibilities are immense. The 4-year course offers the opportunity for some people to swap for a term with students from Flinders University in Australia, which runs a similar course. Places are allocated by lottery.

Facilities

Library The library has just undergone a multi-million pound refurbishment and is open 7 days a week. Facilities are extensive, with approximately 40,000 books, 800 journals on current subscription, and a total of 77,000 journals available. Other facilities include inter-library loans, photocopying, a large history and archive collection and an audiovisual room with a large variety of video material. Students also have access to the library at the University of London for anything that cannot be found at St George's.

Computers   There is an excellent range of computing facilities available, with networked database, CD re-writers, ZIP, USB-key and interactive media. This can get busy at peak times, but queues are usually short-lived; this is further minimized by the provision of free wireless access in the library and bar for laptop users. The library has an electronic catalogue which can also be used to renew and reserve books, and is accessible over the internet. Over 100 workstations for network access, Word and Excel are available, with a few computers set aside with scanning facilities and Photoshop. Colour and monochrome laser printing are operated using the library copier cards. There is also a 24-hour access computer room with approximately 30 terminals and printing facilities. Good online teaching facilities are available, especially for anatomy. Key topics pages for problem-based learning cover the basic knowledge for the 4-year, and increasingly 5-year, courses.

Clinical skills   The facilities have hugely improved in recent years, with an incredible range of realistic models for students to practise on before being faced with real patients. The rooms housing these gadgets are open 9 AM–5 PM Monday to Friday, so students can walk in any time. In addition, the clinical skills facilitator is usually on hand to offer guidance on techniques. It is a very valuable resource which students are encouraged to take advantage of.

Welfare 🏠

Student support

Students at St George's tend to be friendly and easy-going. There is a strong spirit and students support each other. All freshers are assigned a 'mother' or 'father' student to look after them in their first year. There is normally no problem in borrowing lecture notes and getting useful advice. The school has counselling services on-site, and students can use all ULU (University of London Union) facilities. Relationships between the two medicine courses are good and students from all courses are involved with every aspect of St. George's life.

The medical school is part of the main teaching hospital but occupies its own distinct area. There are six floors containing the library, computer rooms, lecture theatres, clinical laboratories, Students' Union, NatWest Bank, school shop, a bookshop, a coffee shop and offices. The Students' Union, on the second floor, comprises the student bar, Students' Union offices, coffee facilities, games room, music room and snooker room. Many students and staff go there to relax for lunch and coffee breaks, and many of the extra-curricular activities are held there.

Accommodation

All first years are offered accommodation in halls, costing only £62 a week – which represents superb value. These are self-catered and about 10 minutes from the medical school. The rooms are a little small, and baths, toilets and kitchen facilities may have to be shared between six or eight people.

A small onsite computer room is provided, and wireless networking with direct access to the school network is in place.

Tooting itself is filled with eager landlords waiting to accommodate local medical students, and rents in the area are more favourable than in many other parts of London. The average rent per week is about £70 to £80. Watch out for estate-agent managed properties, where the landlord may be difficult to track down, and 'hidden' fees (e.g. contract renewal) may appear.

Placements

From year 3, students are placed at a variety of other hospitals for speciality training. Approximately half of the training takes place at St George's, and some placements allow a choice of where you go. Travel expenses may be reimbursed, depending on distance, with accommodation provided for more distant attachments. Travel to hospitals other than St George's may take from 30 minutes to 2 hours by public transport. The distance to attachments increases in the final year, as you reach the end of your training, with the furthest being Darlington, although many students enjoy the contrast.

Location of clinical placement/ name of hospital	Distance away from medical school (miles)	Difficulty getting there on public transport*
Bolingbroke	2	🚶 🚌
Springfield	0.5	🚶
St. Helier's	4.5	🚶 🚌 🚗
Kingston	6.5	🚌 🚗
Epsom	10	🚌 🚗

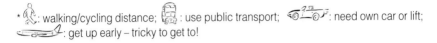

* 🚶: walking/cycling distance; 🚌 : use public transport; 🚗: need own car or lift; ✈: get up early – tricky to get to!

Sports and social

University life

St George's bar is one of the biggest and cheapest in the country, and is the scene of many a great night for many students. Discos are frequent, comedy nights and bands are well-attended, and much fun is had by all. There is big-screen TV with satellite, films, and main football, international cricket, and rugby matches, etc. There is a wide range of societies and clubs to join, from conventional sports to a parachuting club and a hill-walking society. Other societies include religious, cultural, LGBT, language, performing groups, our revue which frequently performs at the Edinburgh festival and many more. The Students' Union is supportive of new clubs and societies and students are also welcome to join those at ULU.

St George's is now the only free-standing medical school in the UK. All of the students here are studying healthcare subjects or biomedical science. There is a great feeling of camaraderie in the college: you will get to know most people in your year and others. There is much mixing between year groups and with students of other disciplines, which can be an immense benefit whenever you have questions about the course, etc. This is partly because there are so many social events organized by the Students' Union. The medical school itself encourages students and staff to take as positive an attitude to their extra-curricular interests as it does to studying.

Sports life

St George's currently owns a sports ground at Cobham, Surrey, but is looking to move to newer premises in nearby Tolworth. The rowing teams use the boathouse at Chiswick, where many other London colleges row. The Robert Lowe Sports Centre is on the hospital site and offers extremely cheap student membership, with six squash courts and three general fitness rooms with exercise bikes, treadmills, rowing machines and step machines. There is also a weights room and a large sports hall for team sports, such as five-a-side football, badminton, volleyball, netball and basketball. There are regular circuit training and aerobic lessons.

Great things about St George's

- It's a close-knit community, with many easy-going, fun-loving people for company.
- Location, location, location! The medical school is part of one of the biggest teaching hospitals in Europe, giving easy access to loads of weird and wonderful pathologies.
- If you do have to travel to a distant site, expenses are reimbursed or accommodation provided.
- Much support from both staff and students to help you along your way.
- Freshers' month lasts a month-and-a-bit. Yes, that's right – St George's offers 5 weeks of continuous freshers' events, from the St. George's Ball to a three-legged pub crawl. Numerous discos and non-alcoholic events also feature.

Bad things about St George's

- Although a London medical school, St George's is hardly central London. Tooting to Leicester Square is a mere 30 minutes on the tube and 50 minutes on the night bus (you'll learn to nap through it).
- Lack of students studying anything apart from health sciences can limit the conversation!
- The small size can mean that if you don't get on with someone you're unlikely to be able to avoid them!
- Parking at or even near the hospital can be difficult and expensive (no charge at halls – 15-minute walk).
- St George's cannot offer all students an intercalated BSc, although most who wish to study a BSc can normally do so.

Further information

St George's, University of London
Cranmer Terrace
London SW17 ORE
Tel: 020 8725 5201
Fax: 020 8725 2734
Email: medicine@sgul.ac.uk
Web: http://www.sgul.ac.uk

Additional application information	
Average A level requirements	• AAB
Average Scottish Higher requirements	• Advanced Highers required – AABB
Make-up of interview panel	• Three interviewers and a senior medical student
Months in which interviews are held	• November – March (undergraduate course) • March – April (graduate course) • February (foundation for medicine)
Proportion of overseas students	• 7.5%
Proportion of mature students	• 50%
Proportion of graduate students	• 0% on 5 year MBBS (graduates not accepted on the 5 year course from 2007 – graduates should apply for the graduate entry programme only)
Faculty's view of students taking a gap year	• Encouraged
Proportion of students taking intercalated degrees	• 60%
Possibility of direct entrance to clinical phase	• Yes, but very limited (undergraduate) • No (graduate)
Fees for overseas students	• £14,175 pa (years 1 and 2) • £24,875 pa (years 3, 4 and 5)
Fees for graduates	• £3000
Ability to transfer to other medical schools	• Yes – for clinical years (3, 4 and 5)

Assistance for elective funding	• Some, limited. Although good resources and help with applications to other funding bodies available.
Assistance for travel to attachments	• Most are close, public transport predominates; limited funding provided for more distant attachments.
Access and hardship funds	• Hardship funds (for home and international students) available on application • St George's bursaries
Weekly rent	• £65–£75 (self-catered halls) • £75–£90 (rooms in Tooting)
Pint of lager	• £1.80
Cinema	• £5 (Wimbledon)
Nightclub	• £3 at St George's if in costume • £5–£7 student nights in Wimbledon and Kingston

Sheffield

Key facts	Premedical	Undergraduate
Course length	6 years	5 years
Total number of medical undergraduates	18	c. 1300
Applicants in 2006	362	2904
Interviews given in 2006	54	837
Places available in 2006	18	241
Places available in 2007	18	241
Open days 2007	Please see website for details	
Entrance requirements	AAB	AAB
Mandatory subjects		Chemistry and another science
Male:female ratio	1:1.4	1:1.7
Is an exam included in the selection process?	Yes	Yes
If yes, what form does this exam take?	UKCAT	UKCAT
Qualification gained	MBChB	

Fascinating Fact: Professor Anthony Weetman, the Dean, is an internationally renowned thyroid expert.

Sheffield is one of the eight largest cities outside of London, with a population of around 500,000 people. It is reputedly one of the best cities in Britain (see *The Virgin Alternative Guide to British Universities*): a city built on seven hills, like Rome, and almost as scenic! Roughly a third of the city lies within the Peak District National Park, making it England's greenest city.

Sheffield University has a large undergraduate population (18,000+); including Hallam University there are approximately 40,000 students in the city. Sheffield University is rated among the top in the country and took the title of Times University of the Year 2001.

With the largest Students' Union in the UK, and a city that is compact, accessible, friendly, safe and cheap, it is easy to see why so many students love Sheffield.

According to results published in August 2005 by the Royal Bank of Scotland's Student Living Index, it has the lowest student living costs in the UK, compared with the other 21 main university towns and cities that were surveyed.

The medical school attracts students from all walks of life and there is a good mixture of backgrounds. There are approximately 250 students in each year, made up of around 20% mature students and 6% international students. The medical school is situated adjacent to the Royal Hallamshire Hospital (RHH), which is a 5-minute walk from the Students' Union and a 15-minute walk from the city centre and halls of residence.

The early years of teaching take place at the medical school, the biomedical sciences building and the excellent Union cinema! In the clinical years, lecture blocks and clinical skills teaching take place at the Northern General Hospital (NGH), which is situated on the other side of town (about 20 minutes away by car/bus). Ward-based teaching on placements takes place in Sheffield and in the various district generals hospitals (DGHs).

Education

The course uses a systems-based teaching scheme, which has been running since 1994 and which is under regular review (the latest update was in 2003). The curriculum is a hybrid of the traditional science-based course and the newer problem-based approach. There tends to be one set of exams at the end of each year, with some student-selected componenets (SSCs) and integrated learning activities (ILAs).

The course is divided into 6 phases. Phase Ia and Ib are the first 2 years and consist of systems-based lectures, anatomy dissection, a research project, medicine and society, and SSCs.

Clinical skills such as history-taking from actual patients are introduced from year 1 onwards and there is an intensive clinical experience (ICE) for 3 weeks in year 1.

Phase II lasts for 6 months and introduces clinical medicine; it comprises of two 10-week clinical attachments, SSCs and lectures introducing basic clinical sciences. Phase III runs from January to December and is split into IIIa and IIIb. The year is broken into rotations of 9 or 10 weeks, during which students are attached to the various specialities. During this period students also undertake a 7-week student-selected component (SSC) and the elective, both of which provide an opportunity to study medicine outside of Sheffield.

Phase IV starts with a 4-week SSC and a 10-week clinical attachment, and ends with 2 weeks shadowing a foundation house officer before you sit your final exam to attain the MBChB.

Teaching

In the first two preclinical years, lectures, tutorials, practical sessions and self-study form the basis of the teaching. The emphasis is on grasping key scientific concepts and applying these to clinical scenarios. On-line formative assessments, lectures and tutorials supplement the teaching and are found on the e-learning environment (Minerva).

Practical sessions give you the chance to get 'hands on' experience. Sheffield is one of the few medical schools left that offer anatomy dissection. This is invaluable in understanding how we fit together and gives budding surgeons their first opportunity behind a knife! Physiology and histology teaching are supplemented by lab sessions; these help in understanding the mechanics of how things work.

The following 3 years consist mainly of ward-based attachments, interspersed with lectures and small-group tutorials. By this stage, self-directed learning and development are encouraged, to produce doctors who are committed to life-long learning.

Teaching is monitored externally and by the students themselves. An elected year representative is extensively involved with the academic staff and is the first port of call in times of poorly organized teaching. Formal teaching sessions are rarely cancelled. Ward teaching is variable, largely depending on the clinician doing the teaching.

Assessment

Assessment of students is mainly by the end-of-year exams, which comprise written multiple-choice paper, short note, and practical multi-station spotter exams. The practical exam consists of dissection specimens to test anatomy, physiology, biochemistry and histology. There is also some continuous assessment, including projects and practical write-ups. Formative assessments also exist to help you monitor your own progress, but these don't count towards the end-of-year exams.

In the later years, objective structure clinical exams (OSCEs) are introduced as well as written papers, and are used to examine clinical skills.

Intercalated degrees

The option of spending an extra year studying for a Batchelor of Medical Science (BMedSci) is open to anyone who has passed all their phase I and II exams. Funding is available for most places, which are generally research- and/or laboratory-based. There is little competition for places and students can 'design' their own degree. The school publishes a list of projects open to BMedSci students, and staff are very keen to recruit students. However, owing to Sheffield's unique course format, which runs January to January, students wishing to study away from Sheffield will have to apply to the medical school for special permission to leave midway for the BSc/BMedSci, which is usually no problem (typically Honours degrees run September to September).

Special study modules and electives

SSCs allow students to further their development in a chosen area, which can be outside of the core curriculum. Overall, two-thirds of SSCs must be directly related to medicine but in the latter stages of the programme, a third may be in any subject area. Many students choose to undertake some research or take an audit.

There is a 7-week option, 7-week elective (which takes place in summer of year 4) and a 4-week option that run throughout the course. You are allowed to spend a maximum of 15 weeks outside of the Sheffield University-linked NHS trusts to pursue an area of medical interest.

Erasmus

Sheffield does not participate in the Erasmus scheme as the course is completely integrated and does not allow sufficient flexibility. Students who nevertheless are keen to experience medicine in a different country are encouraged to do so through the elective or SSC option.

Facilities

Library   Libraries are situated around the university and in all hospitals used for teaching. The two main medical libraries have been refurbished and the Royal Hallamshire Hospital library has recently extended its opening hours to include weekends. They contain all the major publications, journals, and access to Medline.

Computers   There are 25 open-access IT rooms in the university, offering over 900 terminals, 32 of which are located in the medical school. Opening times vary although one site is open 24 hours a day.

Clinical skills   There are two main clinical skills centres. Clinical skills teaching such as blood-taking are taught here. The staff are really helpful and supportive, and individual sessions can be booked.

Welfare

Student support

Year 1 students are eased into the course fairly gently and there are usually plenty of people around to help you with problems. Most lecturers are willing to help solve academic problems, and the undergraduate deans are very approachable.

A buddy scheme has been initiated whereby a couple of students in year 2 act as 'parents' for a couple of students in the year below. The point of this is not as it may first seem, as an extension of the nanny state! Instead it serves to provide a source of information for first years in case they are unwilling to approach academic staff.

The university and the Students' Union offer a very wide range of support services, all of which are available to medical students.

Accommodation

Within the next couple of years a new purpose built, state-of-the-art community for students is being developed. It will feature a mix of catered and self-catered accommodation and a new central building, which will include a full range of catering, retail, recreational and welfare facilities.

Currently all first-years are guaranteed accommodation, the standard is good, in a nice part of town and within easy walking distance of the university.

Placements

Year 1 students shadow a patient suffering from a chronic illness, to assess the impact of disease on daily living. This is known as the community attachment scheme (CAS), and takes a different approach to most of the medical course because it emphasizes the social effects of disease, rather than how to treat it. Throughout the clinical phase there are peripheral attachments in hospitals throughout South Yorkshire and Humberside (up to 50 miles away). There is also a 10-week attachment at a GP practice in or around Sheffield, to which students commute.

On-call rooms are available in Sheffield, with more permanent (free) accommodation in district general hospitals.

Location of clinical placement/ name of hospital	Distance away from medical school (miles)	Difficulty getting there on public transport*
Royal Hallamshire Hospital, Sheffield	20 metres (!)	
Rotherham DGH	11	
Chesterfield and North Derbyshire Royal Hospital	16	
Doncaster Royal Infirmary	27	
Hull Royal Infirmary	68	

* 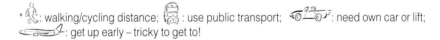: walking/cycling distance; : use public transport; : need own car or lift; : get up early – tricky to get to!

Sports and social

City life

The city centre is compact and not terribly well-formed, but has a good collection of small shops and restaurants. Division Street has lots of trendy student shops and many trendy bars. Eccleshall Road boasts many trendy cafés and shops and is situated in the more scenic part of Sheffield, not far from the centre. (Real shopaholics go to the huge purpose-built out-of-town Meadowhall Centre, accessible by bus, train and tram, with every high-street store under the sun.)

Sheffield is famous for having the most bars and pubs in one city outside London. There are an ever-increasing number of new nightclubs, café-bars, and live music venues. With so many clubs there is a student night nearly every day of the week, with cheap entry, drinks promotions and a free bus to and from the venue. There are two theatres and five cinemas which all have student discounts for those after a bit of culture: the Cineworld cinema contains the biggest screen in Europe, appropriately called The Full Monty.

The crowning glory of Sheffield is the Peak District. This attracts many active outdoor types (especially climbers) to the university, as well as those who like to relax over a pint in a nice country pub. Just 10 minutes' drive from the university you can walk, cycle, climb, admire the stunning scenery and forget about medicine. The locals are generally cheery and it is very easy to settle in at Sheffield quickly.

University life

Sheffield University Union is considered to be one of the best in the country, and has just been refurbished again. If you are looking to be part of a medical clique, Sheffield may not be for you. Medics are very much part of the university as a whole and the city has such a small, friendly feel to it that settling in is quick and easy.

The MedSoc organizes regular social events; the annual November Ball (be prepared to save up for it) and the legendary medics' revue are particularly well-supported. The infamous annual fancy-dress three-legged pub crawl draws in huge crowds of medics and non-medics alike – in 2006 a new record was set with over 1200 people registering! The society is open to new ideas for clubs and societies and forms the largest student society at both Sheffield and Sheffield Hallam University!

The Students' Union organizes cheap and cheerful events every night of the week. Tuesday club is widely and credibly regarded as the best night of its kind in the country. It has consistently championed the finest live artists and DJs in hip hop, drum 'n' bass, electronica and beyond. There is a huge variety of clubs and societies available to join: anyone fancy the Warhammer Assassins' Guild or Star Trek the Whistling Society?

The Union also runs a programme called Give it a Go which gives you a chance to try out a mind-blowing range of different activities. Whether you are sporty, musical, creative, adventurous, want to improve your IT skills, enhance your CV or go on a day trip, you'll find something to suit you.

In addition, people from all religious denominations are catered for through their respective religious societies. Prayer rooms are located in the medical school and the Union. The Christian Medical Fellowship holds weekly meetings, socials and a weekend away.

Sports facilities

The city of Sheffield has inherited a large range of world-class sports facilities after hosting the World Student Games, including the Olympic swimming pool at Pondsforge and Don Valley athletics stadium. There are two major football clubs as well as rugby, ice hockey and basketball teams competing at international level, national athletics events, speedway and not to forget the city's Crucible Theatre is the venue for the World Snooker Championships.

Sheffield Ski Village, Europe's biggest artificial ski-slope resort, offers snowboarding, as well as skiing. For walking, rock-climbing and many other sports from hang-gliding to horse riding, the Peak District is right on the city's doorstep.

The university's facilities are excellent; the Goodwin Sports Centre has just completed a major £6 million re-fit. The facilities are all accessible and a medics membership rate is available in the clinical years. The medical school has numerous sports teams that range from hockey, rugby and football to golf, squash and tennis. These teams compete with other medical schools and within the university intra-mural leagues.

Great things about Sheffield Medical School

- The course allows individuals to learn things at their own pace. Lecturers are accessible and are usually happy to help with any problems.
- There are still dissection and hands-on practicals, instead of prosections, which are beginning to turn up at all new medical curriculums. Definitely a dying breed.
- There are endless clubs for all music tastes, bars and coffee shops for the trend setters, and just about every type of entertainment under the sun.
- Student accommodation is in the nicer parts of town, within easy (and safe) walking distance of the university and all local amenities. Sheffield was voted the safest student city in the UK, in 2001.
- Medical students are part of the university as a whole and not just the medical school. This enables them to make use of all the facilities available, and to escape from medicine when they want to.

Bad things about Sheffield Medical School

- Students complain of a lack of organization within the school, this relates to the continually changing curriculum.
- You can feel anonymous in the medical school.
- Self-directed learning is hard if you are a poor self-motivator and leave things to the last minute; with formal assessment only at the end of the year, it's easy to fall behind.
- Some of the peripheral attachments are to slightly less than glamorous towns – Grimsby, Rotherham, Scunthorpe, Barnsley, etc.
- Hills – good practice if you're training for Everest!

Further information

Medical School Admissions Office
University of Sheffield
Beech Hill Road
Sheffield S10 2RX
Tel: 0114 271 3349 (medical school reception)
0114 271 3727 (medical admissions)
Fax: 0114 271 3960
Email: medadmissions@sheffield.ac.uk
Web: http://www.shef.ac.uk

Additional application information

Average A level requirements	• AAB (in two sciences, one of which must be chemistry)
Average Scottish Higher requirements	• AAAAB and Advanced Higher at grades AB in chemistry and another science subject
Make-up of interview panel	• Three: medically qualified senior staff, biomedical scientist and medical student or lay person
Months in which interviews are held	• Mid November – mid March
Proportion of overseas students	• 5.3%
Proportion of mature students	• 17.4%
Proportion of graduate students	• Not known
Faculty's view of students taking a gap year	• Acceptable
Proportion of students taking intercalated degrees	• 3.5%
Possibility of direct entrance to clinical phase	• No
Fees for overseas students	• £10,800 (preclinical) • £19,900 (clinical) (2006 figures)
Fees for graduates	• £3000 pa
Ability to transfer to other medical schools If so, under what circumstances	• Yes, if other medical school consents.
Assistance for elective funding	• Yes, bursaries and loans available.
Assistance for travel to attachments	• Yes
Access and hardship funds	• Available
Weekly rent	• £65–£110 (halls) • £38–£60 (private)
Pint of lager	• £1.50 Union bar • £2.40 city centre
Cinema	• £2.50–£4.50
Nightclub	• £5–£10

Southampton

Key facts	Premedical*	Undergraduate	Graduate
Course length	1 year	5 years	4 years
Total number of medical undergraduates	30	1092	124
Applicants in 2006	397	3320	1337
Interviews given in 2006	140	160 across both programmes	
Places available in 2006	30	206	40
Places available in 2007	30	206	40
Open days 2007	26 June and 8 September		
Entrance requirements	200 UCAS points. Selection based on academic and non-academic criteria plus UKCAT	AAB – selection based on academic and non-academic criteria plus UKCAT	2:1 or above in any discipline plus pass at A level chemistry. Selection based on academic and non-academic criteria
Mandatory subjects	Biology/human biology and chemistry	Chemistry	Chemistry
Male:female ratio	43:57	33:67	35:65
Is an exam included in the selection process?	Yes	Yes	No
If yes, what form does this exam take?	UKCAT	UKCAT	
Qualification gained	BM Medicine		

*Six-year widening access programme with Year 0 – This programme offers a guaranteed place on the BM5 programme (conditional upon satisfactory completion of the Year 0).

Fascinating Fact: Granada TV's *Young Doctors* was filmed in Southampton!

The medical school at Southampton University is progressive and student-friendly. It is a young medical school, with a well-developed modern course. Southampton pioneered the new integrated curriculum now in operation in most UK medical schools. As such, it has had more experience than most schools at adapting to and refining the new ways of learning medicine. In the first two years, a significant amount of time is set apart for inter-professional learning, a programme which involves working with other health science fields such as nursing, midwifery and rehabilitation sciences. Much emphasis is therefore placed on teamwork and communication, both with colleagues and patients. The medical school's international research strengths lie in: cancer sciences; clinical neurosciences; human genetics; developmental origins of disease; infection/inflammation and repair; and community clinical sciences.

Southampton offers a foundation year for students who come from a background where access to medical education might previously have been denied, which teaches the relevant sciences at a level that allows the smooth transition to year 1 of the 5-year programme. There is also a 4-year graduate-entry programme, open to science and arts graduates.

Southampton Medical School was awarded the maximum 24 points by the Quality Assurance Agency.

Southampton has just about everything city life has to offer, but on a scale which is easy to cope with and, of course, it's by the sea!

Education

The fully-integrated course has an increasing clinical component throughout the 5 years. During the first 2 years, each term deals with the basic science and clinical aspects of a major organ system, and includes clinical sessions in general practice and in the labour ward. Year 3 is the first full-time clinical year, and students work in the Southampton area. Exams at the end of this year integrate basic science and clinical knowledge, a feature that is valued by students. Year 4 comprises clinical experience in the minor specialities, plus a research project. This educational innovation enables students to study an area of their choice for 8 months, finishing with a dissertation and presentation. Most are fascinated by their project, but some are not and feel they forget a lot of the first 3 years' teaching, returning to their final year with blunted clinical skills. However, these are soon refreshed, and the value of learning research skills should not be underestimated. Final-year students are spread throughout the Wessex region in large teaching hospitals and smaller district general hospitals. Southampton has complied with GMC recommendations to limit the amount of factual knowledge that is required, and as a result the examinations are not structured to make you regurgitate thousands of facts but to test your ability to solve clinical problems, i.e. to be a good doctor!

The accelerated graduate-entry programme began in 2004, with an initial cohort of 40 students, open to both arts and science graduates. The course structure is slightly different to that of the 5-year programme, with greater emphasis placed on group learning, using cases and problems, clinical exposure at the Royal Hampshire County Hospital, Winchester, and self-directed learning. However, as the curriculum is also arranged by organ systems, there is the opportunity to attend some lectures alongside year 5 students at Southampton General Hospital. In years 3 and 4, students also join BM5 students on clinical attachments in the Wessex area. The first group of graduate entrants commented very favourably on the enthusiasm of the staff at Winchester, and the quality of the teaching there. As the course is in its infancy, formative assessments have yet to be written, which means that students need to demonstrate greater responsibility for their learning.

Teaching

In the early years students spend most of their time on the main university campus with other, non-medical students, learning in lectures, tutorials and laboratory practicals. Southampton has also been introducing computer-based learning into the curriculum, which has worked particularly well in anatomy and pathology teaching. Dissection is not taught at Southampton – students work with prosected cadavers instead.

Assessment

The major exams are at the end of years 1 and 3 and throughout the final year.

Intercalated degrees

Between 10% and 20% of students take the opportunity to spend an extra year between years 3 and 4 to study for a BSc, usually in Biomedical Science. Only a few students do this because of the extra expense and because all students spend time in research during year 4. Currently, students who already have undergraduate research experience may skip the fourth-year project and take an accelerated course, qualifying 6 months earlier, although this privilege is being phased out with the advent of the new, 4-year graduate-entry programme.

Special study modules and electives

At the end of year 3 students have an 8-week elective, during which they may decide to spend time working in a hospital abroad.

There are special study modules during years 2 and 3, where students may choose to study a particular area in depth, and in year 5 there is a 5-week block when students choose which speciality to gain additional experience in.

Erasmus

The medical school has no Erasmus programme, but you always have your elective.

Facilities

Library Students have access to the Biomedical Sciences Library on the main campus and the Health Sciences Library at the General Hospital. Library facilities are good, although the most popular books are always in demand and students often find it more convenient to buy core texts. Some texts are freely accessible online.

Computers   The computer facilities are very good and are updated regularly. Workstations are available all over the campus, at the General Hospital and in some halls of residence. Access, however, is not always 24 hours.

Clinical skills   The clinical skills lab is an excellent facility and is used in the Medicine in Practice course in years 1 and 2, as well as in some of the clinical attachments in years 3 and 4. It is also used for revision during the final year.

Welfare

Student support

Most people are struck by the friendliness of the staff and students at the medical school when they visit. A scheme has recently been set up whereby students run mini-tutorials for newer students in order to pass on the most relevant information – which books to buy, which books not to buy, which consultants have the nice, big yachts requiring crew for trips round the Channel Isles … all the really important stuff! Also, upon arrival at the introductory toga party, all freshers become part of a 'super-family', which allows for fantastic cross-year integration. Southampton University has a counselling service, and the Students' Union runs welfare services.

Accommodation

Students are offered a place in halls of residence for their first year only. There are a range of options, from a small self-catering room with no sink, to a large *en-suite* room with breakfast and evening meal. Which option you choose depends largely on your bank balance! A limited number of places is available in halls for subsequent years, but most people move into private rented houses in the Highfield and Portswood areas. Most halls are within a mile of the medical school and are well served by the excellent university bus service – Uni-Link. A year's Uni-Link bus pass is included in the accommodation fees. Most halls have a bar/games room and very active social committees. Inter-mural sporting events are also very popular.

Placements

The main university campus is in the Highfield/Bassett area of Southampton and is close to most of the halls of residence. The General Hospital, where most of years 3 and 4 are spent, as well as 1 or 2 days a week in years 1 and 2, is about 1-mile away in Shirley. The university bus service connects all sites.

Clinical attachments are normally in local Southampton hospitals during year 3 and are further afield in the final year (e.g. Basingstoke, Bournemouth, Dorchester and Poole). In these final-year placements there are fewer students per hospital and, consequently, more individual attention; students give excellent feedback from these placements. Weekday accommodation is provided on peripheral attachments, although travel expenses for return travel to Southampton at weekends is not.

Location of clinical placement/ name of hospital	Distance away from medical school (miles)	Difficulty getting there on public transport*
Southampton General	2	
Portsmouth	20	
Isle of Wight	10 (including a ferry!)	
Salisbury	24	
Guildford	60	

*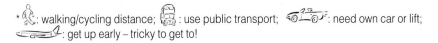: walking/cycling distance; : use public transport; : need own car or lift; : get up early – tricky to get to!

Sports and social

City life

Southampton has been widely rebuilt, having been heavily bombed during the Second World War. The town centre is therefore modern, but slightly characterless given the distinct lack of historical architecture. However, the harbour areas, which come alive during Boat Show week, are stunning and are what provides Southampton with its distinct nautical feel. Despite the small size of the city, shopping facilities are superb. There are a number of decent restaurants to fit all budgets and plenty of pubs. Serious nightclubbers though might be somewhat disappointed, with most clubs closing at 2 AM after playing a night of ubiquitous cheese. Trendy bars are also a bit thin on the ground, although a number of new ones have just opened up. In terms of live music, Southampton's scene bubbles. Whilst not always attracting the biggest bands, Southampton nonetheless offers up new and exciting jazz, classical and rock music in varying-sized venues including the Guildhall. Recently, The Bravery, James Blunt and Goldie Lookin' Chain have played there to packed houses. Just outside the city, the New Forest proves popular with nature lovers, cyclists, and pub-lunchers, and the Solent and the Isle of Wight are popular with sailors. The proximity to Bournemouth beach is a bonus for when the sun shines, a phenomenon that occurs with much regularity! Bournemouth is only 40 minutes away by car, and is set to become a Mecca for surfers when the artificial surf break is finished in 2007. London is also close enough for a day/night out by car, coach, or train.

University life

The Students' Union runs every club under the sun, including political, religious, arts and sports societies. The Union building hosts weekly nightclub events, bands, and comedians: for example, the Fresher's Ball this year welcomed the legendary Trev' and Simon! The university campus is modern, leafy, and well-appointed and is about 2 miles outside the city centre. The on-site theatre and concert hall host lots of non-mainstream acts and performances, and is a major arts hub for the whole of Southampton. The medical school itself, housed in the concrete bunker that is the Boldrewood Biomedical Sciences building, is renowned for its strong social life and camaraderie. The annual medics ball, which is the most popular in the university, is held in the Guildhall and the extravagant Christmas revue never fails to entertain with its eyebrow-raising take on medical school life. There are a number of very active health-related societies – Stop AIDS, Friends of MSF and MedSIN, all of which run informative events. Also, a lot of students get involved with medics sport, which is generally taken slightly less seriously than sport at university level.

Sports life

The University of Southampton has excellent water-sports teams. The facilities are accessible to everyone, from those who have never sailed/rowed/canoed in their lives to those who wish to compete at an international level. Southampton has teams in most sports, many of which are successful in national competitions. The new Jubilee Sports Centre provides some of the best sporting facilities on the south coast, with a fantastic swimming pool, well-equipped gym and squash and basketball courts. Yearly membership is a very reasonable £65.

Great things about Southampton

- Excellent course, which is well liked by students and recognized nationally for its quality.
- Good patient/doctor-to-student ratio on attachments.
- Students are part of the main university, not just the medical school.
- Staff are very student-friendly and approachable and there is a great support network if you experience problems.
- It's on the south coast, therefore relatively warm – and it's by the sea!

Bad things about Southampton

- As it's one of the newest medical schools, some of the older consultants tend to be sceptical about any 'newfangled' ways of doing things, although this is changing.
- Too many distractions – university social life, medical school social life, good lectures, beautiful countryside.
- The city's nightlife isn't what it could be, but again this is slowly changing.
- Having the elective after just 1 year of clinical work makes you less useful in a hospital abroad.
- Some of the fifth-year attachments can leave you feeling isolated and far removed from Southampton during the week (e.g. Isle of Wight), but this doesn't last too long – a maximum of 8 weeks.

Further information

Admissions Office
University of Southampton
Biomedical Sciences Building
Bassett Crescent Building
Bassett Crescent East
Southampton SO15 7FX
Tel: 02380 594 408

Fax: 02380 594 159
Email: prospenq@soton.ac.uk
   bmadmissions@soton.ac.uk
Web: http://www.som.soton.ac.uk/

Additional application information

Average A level requirements	• AAB
Average Scottish Higher requirements	• AAAAB
Graduate entry requirements	• 2:1 or above in any discipline
Make-up of interview panel	• Two members of Medical Selection Committee (where appropriate)
Months in which interviews are held	• February – April (premedical) • January – April (undergraduate and graduate)
Proportion of overseas students	• 9.5%
Proportion of mature students	• 5%
Proportion of graduate students	• 7%
Faculty's view of students taking a gap year	• Encouraged if used constructively
Proportion of students taking intercalated degrees	• 18% per intake
Possibility of direct entrance to clinical phase	• No
Fees for overseas students	• £11,300 pa (years 1 and 2) £20,400 pa (years 3, 4 and 5)
Fees for graduates	• £3000
Ability to transfer to other medical schools If so, under what circumstances	• If the other medical school consents.
Assistance for elective funding	• Some bursaries are available.

Assistance for travel to attachments	• For those without a car efforts are made to arrange attachments within the city limits if possible. Some though will have to be on attachment to hospitals in the region, but usually at least one person will have access to a car. Reimbursement for travel is provided.
Access and hardship funds	• Through the central university
Weekly rent	• £60–£90
Pint of lager	• £1.70 Union • £2.15 city centre pubs • 50 pence certain places and nights
Cinema	• £4.50
Nightclub	• Several, prices vary

Warwick

Key facts	Graduate course
Course length	4 years
Total number of medical undergraduates	660
Applicants in 2006	c .900
Selection Centre Places in 2006	c. 300
Places available in 2006	164
Places available in 2007	164
Open days 2007	Please see website for details
Entrance requirements	Biological science related degree
Mandatory subjects	Cell biology, genetics, molecular biology, biochemistry
Male:female ratio	1:2 years 2-4, but closer to 1:1 in year 1
Is an exam included in the selection process?	Yes
If yes, what form does this exam take?	MSAT and selection centre
Qualification gained	MBChB

Fascinating fact: The University of Warwick is consistently ranked in the top ten of UK universities. Interestingly, the estate in which the university is situated once belonged to Henry II, and covers four medieval farmsteads!

The Universities of Warwick and Leicester joined up in 2000 to offer an accelerated 4-year medical degree course to graduates in biomedical sciences. The course started with 67 students and the first intake began studying in 2000. Now in its fifth year, any early problems have been ironed out, resulting in a well-run and organized curriculum delivered by enthusiastic teachers. As a relatively new medical school there has been much investment in student facilities, with brand new buildings and learning resources. A new university hospital has been built in Coventry, completed in 2006. As was always planned, Leicester relinquished much of its hand in the course and Warwick Medical School was formally established as a faculty of the University of Warwick in January 2003, gaining full independence in June 2006. It has recently been expanded to accommodate the rapidly growing courses for other healthcare professionals. This gives the medical school a great feeling of innovation and an atmosphere of cutting edge healthcare research, all within a friendly environment.

Education

The medical course, open to graduates of biomedical sciences, is 4 years long and is spilt into two phases. Phase I lasts 1.5 years and is delivered partly at the medical school building at Warwick University and partly at the new clinical sciences building at Walsgrave Hospital. This phase covers the basic medical sciences as well as the psychosocial aspects of medicine. Communication and clinical skills are introduced early in the curriculum and supplement preclinical learning. An introductory clinical skills course (ICC) begins at the end of semester 1, and includes weekly hospital placements. Working as part of a healthcare team is emphasized and the innovative module, Health in the community, introduces this to students.

Phase II last 2.5 years and is predominately clinical. It is divided into 13 eight-week blocks that are split into junior and senior rotations based in the local hospitals. Students in phase II work in pairs and are attached to two consultant teams in different specialities.

Teaching

Phase I of the course is run over three semesters. Most learning in this phase occurs through a balance of lectures and group work. Students are placed in groups of 10 for group work and stay in this set until the end of phase I. Each module session lasts for approximately 3 hours and involves a mixture of lectures and group work. The lectures offer an overview of the topic, which is then developed further in group work by working through cases or discussion of issues. Anatomy is integrated in each of the modules and is supplemented with dissection sessions at Leicester, in which each group has their own cadaver. Clinical skills are taught at the beginning of the course in semester 1 and then further developed by weekly placements in hospitals in semesters 2 and 3. Developing interviewing skills in consultation (DISC) is a strand of the course that helps to develop communication skills and is first taught using highly convincing simulated patients played by actors. Following this you spend four sessions in general practice.

Phase II is clinical and mainly taught in hospital, with community teaching where appropriate. Weekly academic half days supplement ward learning and include student case presentations.

Assessment

Assessment in phase I of the course is varied, with a mixture of short-answer questions, multiple-choice questions, essays and case studies. The musculoskeletal module also includes a viva voce exam. Students are graded as excellent, satisfactory, borderline satisfactory or unsatisfactory. Clinical skills are assessed at the end of semester 1 with a 12-station objective structured clinical examination (OSCE) testing a variety of skills gained during the year. The introductory clinical course is assessed in November of semester 3 by attendance, patient portfolios and a clinical exam. Also in phase I is the integrated medical sciences assessment (IMSA). This is an MCQ exam that takes place at the end of each semester. It covers all modules taught up to the point of the exam and tests integration of knowledge with clinical practice. At the end of phase I there is an over-arching IMSA: a 3-hour paper that tests learning objectives from all modules taken in phase I. A 7500-word dissertation to be written on a clinical topic of your choice is also a component of phase I. Indications are that assessment in phase I will change in the near future.

Phase II assessments contain a mixture of clinical and written exams. Eight-week rotations require students to produce written portfolios for each block, with a total of 36 portfolios to be completed overall. The main clinical assessments are the intermediate clinical assessment (ICE) in year 3 and the clinical finals in year 4.

Intercalated degrees

All students are graduates and intercalated degrees are not offered.

Special study modules and electives

One SSM is taken in phase I. Topics include advanced anatomical studies, pre-hospital trauma medicine, sleep medicine, current research topics in medicine and a variety of languages, as well as other skills, including counselling and sign language. In the senior rotation of phase II, compulsory SSMs ensure exposure to emergency medicine and alternative therapeutics.

The elective is taken in year 3 of the course. Students can choose to go worldwide and, like other medical students, are required to complete a report about their experience.

Facilities

Library   Warwick has a huge library on the central campus with an increasingly well-stocked medical section. WMS also benefits from a Biomed Grid, with library and group work facilities tailored specifically to medical and biological science students. Many resources are available electronically and all hospitals have clinical libraries. The clinical sciences building at the University Hospital in Coventry in particular has excellent facilities. However, lecture notes and module handbooks contain the majority of information required for self-directed learning.

Computers   Computer facilities are excellent within the medical school, with 24-hour access. There are also many clusters located around the Warwick campus. Again all hospitals have IT facilities, most with 24-hour access.

Clinical skills   The medical school is equipped with three clinical skills rooms that contain all the required resources needed for practising and developing clinical skills. Seminar rooms also contain a range of equipment from full body skeletons to blood pressure instruments (sphygmomanometers). There is also a resource room containing many anatomical models, books and DVDs/videos that aid learning. All of the main teaching hospitals have well-resourced clinical skills centres that are staffed by friendly teachers that all students can use.

Welfare

Student support

Students can access the main university counselling and welfare services, as well as those available through the Students' Union. A personal tutor scheme operates in the school and inter-year relations are good, so there is always someone you can ask advice from about the course. The faculty take pride in their approachable staff, and students are encouraged to take advantage of this. First-year students are allocated a student mentor in the year above to provide informal support and information about life at the medical school.

Accommodation

Accommodation in university halls is not guaranteed but may be available. Most prospective first-year students are accommodated in nearby university housing in the Earlsdon, Canley and Tile Hill parts of Coventry, with some in Leamington Spa. All student accommodation is a bus or car ride away from the main university campus.

In the second year, most students choose to live in private accommodation in Leamington Spa, Kenilworth or one of the areas of Coventry adjacent to the university.

Placements

The medical school building is located on Gibbet Hill, a quiet part of the campus, a short walk away from the main centre. Most phase I teaching occurs here and in local hospitals. The main teaching hospitals are outlined in the table below.

Location of clinical placement/ name of hospital	Distance away from medical school (miles)	Difficulty getting there on public transport*
University Hospital Coventry and Warwickshire	5	walking/cycling; need own car or lift
George Eliot Hospital, Nuneaton	20	need own car or lift
Warwick Hospital	8	walking/cycling; need own car or lift
Alexandra Hospital, Redditch	30	need own car or lift
Hospital of St Cross, Rugby*	20	need own car or lift

*: walking/cycling distance; : use public transport; : need own car or lift; : get up early – tricky to get to!

Phase II teaching is at the main teaching hospitals and hospitals in Rugby and Redditch. Accommodation can be provided at hospitals should you require it. GP placements are located all over the

Midlands. It is worth noting that public transport to clinical placements is limited and a car (or a friend with one!) is almost essential. With this in mind, the school does try to place students as near to their home as possible and special circumstances are catered for.

Sports and social

City life

Warwick University may be in Warwickshire, but it is really a part of Coventry. Much of the centre was unimaginatively rebuilt after the Second World War but dramatic new renovation is ongoing. It has everything you might expect of a medium-sized city: theatre, museums, good shopping, restaurants and excellent travel links. Nearby Leamington Spa offers a wealth of fine dining, shopping and culture, and Birmingham is within easy reach for a tantalising change of scenery. A short journey in any direction can get you into pretty countryside, and places to visit in Warwickshire include Kenilworth Castle, Warwick and Warwick Castle and Stratford-upon-Avon.

University life

In spite of its relative youth, Warwick has a thriving MedSoc, which runs regular events for medics. Freshers' week 2006 was a huge success and included 'mums and dads, doctors and nurses' and the freshers' ball. It also saw the return of the now legendary WMS medics revue, extended to two performances by popular demand. There is a wide range of medical student run societies including Sexpression, Basic Life Support, MedSIN, and the Surgical Society. Students at Warwick can take advantage of a wide range of facilities on campus. A very large Students' Union provides a wide range of entertainment: bands, balls and student theatre are all regular events. A large and busy arts centre hosts many touring theatre and dance companies, as well as big name music acts of all genres. There are loads of student societies with every possible activity imaginable. Banks, shops, and a post office are all part of the campus.

Sports life

There is a huge sports centre at Warwick, offering a plethora of sporting facilities including an athletics track, swimming pool, climbing wall and playing fields. All the main sports are catered for, as well as many smaller ones, with facilities open to all. Medical students have their own teams in football, rugby, netball and hockey. There is also a popular medics' squash ladder.

Great things about Warwick

- A well-run and well-organized course with excellent new facilities and resources available 24-hours. All lectures and course material are placed on the web, giving students easy access.
- A brand new state-of-the-art teaching hospital has been built, with a fantastic new clinical sciences building. Upgraded clinical skills facilities at all the hospitals used for teaching also means students are never short of things to do whilst on placements.
- Significant clinical content from early on in the course and clinical application of learning is constantly emphasized. In clinical years, a pair of students is allocated to a pair of consultants keep-

ing staff student ratios low. This allows students to fully integrate into each attachment and feel as though they are part of the firm.

- Friendly staff in all parts of the medical school are always willing to help. You can even get post delivered to the medical school and the porter will sign for it!
- Warwick campus has a great range of student facilities with a nationally renowned arts centre that attracts top names. The surrounding Warwickshire countryside is beautiful and is easily accessible to escape to when revision is looming. Birmingham is only a 20-minute car or train journey away and is great for a night out and shopping.

Bad things about Warwick

- Access to clinical placements is difficult without a car (or a friend with a car).
- At the end of a long day, it is often a tiring journey home if you live off campus.
- Car parking during the day both on campus and in hospitals is expensive and limited.
- The main centre for shopping is Coventry: whilst having all that you need, it is not the most attractive of city centres. However, die-hard shopaholics have easy access to the new Bullring in Birmingham which is only a 20-minute train journey from Leamington Spa.
- As the medical school is not based on the main campus and the workload makes socializing with non-medics difficult, you can feel a bit isolated from the rest of the university.

Further information

Student Recruitment and Admissions Office
University House
University of Warwick
Coventry
CV4 8UW
Tel: 024 7652 8101 (medical admissions)
Email: pgteam4@warwick.ac.uk
Web: http://www2.warwick.ac.uk/fac/med/

Additional application information	
Average A level requirements	• N/A
Average Scottish Higher requirements	• N/A
Make-up of interview panel	• N/A
Months in which interviews are held	• February – March
Proportion of overseas students	• 7.5%
Proportion of mature students	• 100%
Proportion of graduate students	• 100%

(Continued)

(Continued)

Faculty's view of students taking a gap year	• N/A
Proportion of students taking intercalated degrees	• 0%
Possibility of direct entrance to clinical phase	• Yes – limited circumstances
Fees for overseas students	• £10,000 (year 1) £20,000 (years 2, 3 and 4)
Fees for graduates	• Likely to be £3000
Ability to transfer to other medical schools If so, under what circumstances	• Yes, requests are dealt with on an individual basis. Reasons can be financial, personal or health related.
Assistance for elective funding	• There is at present no financial assistance for electives by way of scholarships or bursaries but students may take a loan from the school, which has to be paid back at graduation.
Assistance for travel to attachments	• Travel to clinical attachments is covered by NHS bursary in years 2, 3 and 4 for English and Welsh students. Scottish students do not receive an NHS bursary but can claim from start of course for travel to clinical placements.
Access and hardship funds	• There is access to the Access to Learning Fund (ALF) as hardship funds no longer exist at any HE institution. Students are required to see the University Student Financial Adviser to state their case before a decision is made.
Weekly rent	• £45–£55 (halls) • £55 (private)
Pint of lager	• £1.20 Union bar • £1.70 city pub
Cinema	• £2.80 with NUS card
Nightclub	• Free–£10

Appendices

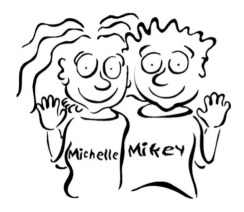

Mikey and Michelle's quick compare table

Mikey and Michelle's quick compare table

University	No of applicants (2006)	No of places (2006)	% Interviewed (2006)	Entrance req.	Mandatory subjects	M:F	% Intercalated year	% Mature	% Overseas	Graduate course
Aberdeen	1582	175	73	ABB	Chemistry	1:1-2	20	12	8	No
Barts	2500	268	52	AAB	Chemistry and biology	40:60	40	20	9	Yes
Belfast	734	180	4	AAA + A at AS Level	Chemistry, biology to at least AS Level	40:60	7	No info	7	No
Birmingham	2000	350	60	AAB (340 - 360)	Chemistry and either biology, physics or maths	2:3	31	5.5	8	Yes
Brighton & Sussex	1884	128	35	(320 - 340)	Chemistry and biology	37:63	0	25	0	No
Bristol	1885	217	35	AAB	Chemistry	1:2	30	6	5	Yes
Cambridge	1619	280	17	AAA	Chemistry	50:50	100	No info	No info	Yes
Derby	1200	90	21	2:2 Bachelors degree	N/A	43:57	N/A	100	N/A	N/A
Dundee	1433	154	36	ABB	Chemistry	42:58	17	N/A	8	No
East Anglia	966	130	47	AAB	Biology A2	40:60	N/A	50	0	No
Edinburgh	2330	218	2	AAB + B at 4th AS subject	Chemistry and either biology, physics or maths at least AS Level	36:64	40	5	7.5	No
Glasgow	1693	241	59	AAB	Chemistry	36:64	30	No Info	7.5	No
GKT	4443	372	29	AAB + AS (B)	Chemistry and biology	35:65	Not known	Not known	Not known	Yes
Hull & York	1690	130	47	AAB	Chemistry and biology	40:60	0	20	0	No
Imperial	2600	326	33	AAB (B in Chemistry)	Chemistry and biology	44:56	100	2.5	7	No

(Continued)

Mikey and Michelle's quick compare table. *(Continued)*

University	No of applicants (2006)	No of places (2006)	% Interviewed (2006)	Entrance req.	Manditory subjects	M:F	% Intercalated year	% Mature	% Overseas	Graduate course
Leeds	2606	238	40	AAB	Chemistry	35:65	54	2	5	No
Leicester	2450	239	67	AAB	Chemistry	50:50	10	No info	No info	Yes
Liverpool	1850	283	49	AAB	Chemistry and biology	35:65	10	4	5	Yes
Manchester/ Keele/Preston	2964	340	34	AAB (340)	Chemistry and one other science	1:1.22	5	17	6	No
Newcastle/ Durham	2640	315	25	AAB	Chemistry and biology		9	10	10	Yes
Nottingham	2500	246	31	AAB (As in chemistry and biology)	Chemistry and biology	33:67	N/A	4	10	Yes
Oxford	1187	150	36	AAA	Chemistry	45:55	100	0-4	4	Yes
Peninsula	1517	167	42	(370 – 400)	One science	44:56	0	25	0	No
Royal Free & UCL	2500	330	35	AAB	Chemistry and biology	46:54	100	15	8	No
St Andrews	737	124	30	AAB	Chemistry and either biology, physics or maths	45:55	10	4	16	No
St George's	1730	187	41	AAB + B at AS Level	Chemistry and biology	40:60	60	80	7.5	Yes
Sheffield	3251	238	31	ABB	Chemistry and another science	1:1.4	10	26	8	No
Southampton	2392	200	mature & o/s only	AAB	Chemistry	39:61	4	25	12	Yes
Wales	1569	298	46	ABB (370)	Chemistry and biology	1:2	13	6	7	No
Warwick	1100	164	29	2:1 Biological sciences degree	N/A	2:3	N/A	100	3	N/A

Glossary

Medicine is full of jargon and abbreviations. Estimates suggest that students' vocabularies double over the course of a 5-year medical degree. Unfortunately, it is such a part of life for medical students and doctors that they sometimes forget to speak in plain language to the general public. The following is a very brief list of words pertaining to medical education that you are likely to come across in this guide, and perhaps in medical school prospectuses. Our apologies for any jargon we have used in the guide that is not listed here!

Advanced life support (ALS): Generally refers to courses that aim to teach the theory and practical skills to effectively manage cardiorespiratory arrest, peri-arrest situations and special circumstances until transfer to a critical care area is possible.

Anatomy: The study of the structure of the body. While this used to be taught by dissection, prosections (pre-dissected specimens) are more commonly used nowadays.

Attachment: The term given to clinical placements. The student is placed under the supervision and guidance of a hospital consultant and his/her team (firm) or a GP for a period in the course.

Bachelor of Medicine/Bachelor of Surgery (MBBS/BMBS): Degree awarded on qualification from medical school. Some schools still retain the traditional MBChB, which substitutes Latin terminology for the English MBBS/BMBS.

Biochemistry: The study of the structure and functioning of the body at the molecular level.

BioMedical Admissions Test (BMAT): Test introduced in order to assess whether students who have graduated in the biomedical field have reached a suitable level to undertake a degree in medicine.

Blood-borne virus (BBV): A term used to describe a whole host of viruses which are passed via the blood. Includes hepatitis B, hepatitis C and HIV.

British Medical Association (BMA): The doctors' professional association and trade union, providing representation and services for doctors and medical students.

BSc (Honours): see *Intercalated degrees*.

Clerking: Taking a history from and examining a patient on admission. A very useful learning experience if you are the first person to see the patient.

Computer-assisted learning (CAL): Computer programmes are sometimes used to teach a topic in a more interactive format than a lecture/tutorial, and let the student set his/her own learning pace. They may also give the opportunity for self-assessment on a topic.

Computer Tomography (CT): A form of 3D X-rays.

Consultant: The senior specialist doctor, usually based in a hospital.

Core curriculum: Under GMC directives the medical course is split into a core curriculum (in which all students must cover the same key topics to a high standard) and special study modules (in which the student can go in his/her own direction and study an area of interest in more depth) which may not be covered by all students.

Department for Education and Skills (DfES): The English government department responsible for policy connected to all educational institutions in the United Kingdom. Has equivalents in the devolved nations.

Department of Health (DH): English government department responsible for delivering the National Health Service. Has equivalents in the devolved nations.

District general hospital (DGH): A regional hospital which treats a broad spectrum of patients but refers more specialist cases to a teaching hospital. Medical students are taught by NHS staff, not university-employed consultants and registrars.

Elective: A period (usually 6 to 12 weeks in the latter years of the course) when students can choose an area of interest to study independently outside their medical school, either in the UK or, more often, abroad.

Endocrinology: The study of the hormonal function of the body.

Epidemiology: The study of the pattern and causes of diseases in society.

Extended matching questions (EMQ): Popular examination technique which comprises a form of multiple-selection questions.

Foundation House Officer: New term, introduced by the Modernising Medical Careers (MMC) reforms, which describes doctors who are undertaking their first 2 years of work following graduation from medical school. Foundation House Officers 1 and 2 complete the 2-year foundation programme.

Foundation Programme: New 2-year training and education programme taken up immediately after graduation from medical school; to be introduced in August 2005 for all UK graduates.

Firm: see *Attachment*.

Fitness to practice: Generic term used to describe a doctor's suitability to work. It covers issues including health status, professionalism, behaviour and attitudes to patients and colleagues. Guidance can be viewed on the General Medical Council website. Students need to be fit to practice in order to graduate from medical school.

Formative assessments/exams: Exams or assessments that will not officially contribute to your year mark. They are, however, compulsory and are an excellent indicator of your progress.

Foundation programme (FP): The first 2 years of the new postgraduate training for doctors in the UK which aims to build the generic skills of newly qualified doctors. The programme was introduced in 2004 as a result of the Modernising Medical Careers (MMC) reforms.

General Medical Council (GMC): All medical degree courses must be approved by the GMC. It is the medical profession's self-regulatory body, which ensures professional standards are maintained and patients are protected. Doctors must be registered with the GMC to practise in the UK.

Graduate Australian Medical Admissions Test (GAMAT): Admissions test used by some medical schools to assess graduates' suitability to study medicine.

Graduate entry programme (GEP): A fast-track medical course, lasting 4 years rather than the standard 5 or 6, open to applicants with a previous degree (usually in a biological science).

Honours year: see *Intercalated degrees*.

Hippocratic oath: An early verse written by Hippocrates, which outlines the basic duties and functions of a physician. This oath was traditionally sworn by all new doctors; however, it has been replaced by other more up-to-date duties laid down by the World Health Organization (WHO).

International Federation of Medical Students Association (IFMSA): The student-equivalent of the world medical association which aims to improve health at an international level for all the worlds citizens. MedSIN is a national member of this group; many medical schools have MedSIN branches.

Integrated courses: Integration is the merging of several disciplines into one (hopefully more meaningful) course. Integration may be partial, within a single year or phase (for example combining anatomy, physiology and biochemistry to teach body systems, combining respiratory, cardiovascular, reproduction, etc.), or it may be full, across all years, starting clinical teaching with basic medical sciences from the outset.

Intercalated degrees: Most schools offer students the opportunity to take an extra year (or two) in the middle of the course to study a subject of interest, leading to a BSc(Hons) or equivalent at the end. Some schools only offer this to high achievers, while others have an intercalated BSc(Hons) built into the course for everyone.

MBBS: The degree awarded to medical school graduates. This varies slightly between schools, for example MBChB, MBBChir, but all are equivalent.

Medical Students Committee (MSC): UK committee of elected representatives that looks after the interests of all UK medical students.

Medical microbiology: The study of microorganisms and the diseases they cause.

MedLine: A widely used and comprehensive computer database of articles published in medical journals.

Medical society (MedSoc): A group within medical schools which is responsible for organizing social events and support for medical students locally.

Modernising Medical Careers (MMC): Government policy to reform the early years of postgraduate training of doctors, introduced in 2004. The new structure consists of the 2-year foundation programme followed by speciality training to become a consultant or GP.

Multiple-choice questions (MCQs): A popular form of assessment used in undergraduate and postgraduate medical education comprising a list of answers (1 to 4) and one question which links to one of those answers.

Objective structured clinical examination (OSCE): A form of assessment where the students are set several tasks: taking histories; examining patients; or performing tests/procedures to complete in front of the examiner within a set time. The student is marked according to a standardized marking scheme. Every student is thus assessed identically, ensuring fairness and comparability of results between individuals.

Pathology: The study of disease processes and their effect on the structure and function of the body.

Peripheral attachments: Placements in hospitals/general practices outside the university area and normally outside the university town.

Pharmacology: The study of the action of drugs and their application.

Physiology: The study of the functioning of body systems and tissues.

Postgraduate medical education and training board: The government board responsible for continuing education once you have received full registration with the GMC. It oversees all the exams and diplomas offered through the Royal Colleges.

Premedical year: Students without the necessary science entrance qualifications can apply to do a premedical year, which takes them to a sufficient level of scientific knowledge to join the medical course the following academic year (not offered at all schools).

Pre-registration house officer (PRHO): A newly qualified doctor working in the first year after graduation. House officers, while able to call themselves doctors and prescribe drugs, are provisionally registered by the GMC until they have completed this year satisfactorily. After this they achieve full registration.

Problem-based learning (PBL): Students learn from researching and solving a relevant (usually clinical) scenario, rather than being given all the information passively. Small group problem-solving tutorials, facilitated by members of staff, take the place of lectures. Facilitators are usually present to ensure harmonious and structured work.

Prosections: Pre-dissected cadaver specimens of the human body used to teach anatomy. These have replaced actual dissection by students themselves in many schools.

Provisional registration: Conditional registration with the GMC after graduation from medical school. Full registration is granted at the end of the F1 year once competencies have been achieved.

Registrar: A doctor who is undergoing specialist training (usually for between 3 and 9 years) before becoming a consultant or general practitioner. The next step up the ladder after SHO.

Self-directed learning: Learning under the student's own initiative from lists of objectives, rather than didactic teaching (such as lectures).

Senior House Officer (SHO): A junior hospital doctor who has completed his/her year as foundation house officer.

Student selected modules/Student selected components/Student selected studies (SSM/SSC/ SSS): Periods of the course when students study areas of interest outside the core curriculum. These may be taught, or may be independent research projects.

Tution fee: Student contribution to the cost of undertaking a university degree which is payable for each year of study.

Top-up tuition fees: Differential fee charged by the university for courses within their institution, payable from 2006 entry. The amount of fee levied may depend on the type of degree studied, but for medicine in 2006, it was £3000.

Teaching hospitals: Normally the main hospital(s) in the university town or city. Services provided are part of the NHS, but the senior clinical staff will often be employed by the university and hold medical academic posts. Teaching hospitals usually handle specialist cases, which can be referred to them from DGHs across the region. Many such hospitals will have regional centres for particular specialities or centres of excellence, such as cardiology, plastic surgery, neonatal intensive care, etc.

Viva: An oral examination (sometimes referred to as a viva voce).

United Kingdom Clinical Aptitude Test (UKCAT): A new psychometric test introduced in to the UK which aims to examine an applicant's suitability to study medicine and practice as a clinician.

Universities and Colleges Admissions Service (UCAS): Central body responsible for receiving applications to any medical school in the country.

Abbreviations

BMA:	British Medical Association
BMAT:	Biomedical Admissions Test
CAL:	Computer-assisted learning
CSYS:	Certificate of sixth-year study (Scottish students)
DGH:	District general hospital
GAMSAT:	Graduate Australian Medical Services Admissions Test
GMC:	General Medical Council
MCQs:	Multiple-choice questions
MSC	BMA's UK Medical Students Committee
OSCE:	Objective structured clinical examination
PBL:	Problem-based learning
SSM:	Special study module
UCAS:	Universities and Colleges Admissions Service

Further information

British Medical Association

The British Medical Association (BMA) is both the doctors' professional organization and their trade union, protecting the professional and personal interests of its members. It is the voice of the medical profession in the UK and represents the profession internationally. Members and staff are in constant touch with ministers, government departments, Members of Parliament and other influential bodies, conveying to them the profession's views on healthcare and health policy. Most medical students and practising doctors are members.

The BMA's head office is in London, and there are national offices in Scotland, Northern Ireland and Wales. There are an additional 15 regional offices throughout the UK. The BMA is a medical publisher in its own right, but also includes the BMJ Publishing Group. The BMJ Publishing Group is a major medical and scientific publisher and publishes the weekly *British Medical Journal* and the monthly *Student BMJ*.

Student BMJ   The *Student BMJ* is an international journal specifically for medical students. It is published monthly and includes articles on education, medical careers, student life, science and news. Many of the articles and papers are written by medical students. Individuals or schools and libraries can subscribe to the journal.

For more information or a sample copy contact:

Student BMJ
BMJ Publishing Group   Tel: 020 7383 6402
BMA House   Fax: 020 7383 6270
Tavistock Square   Email: bmjsubs@dial.pipex.com
London WC1H 9JR   Web: http://www.studentbmj.com

BMA Medical Students Committee (MSC)

The Medical Students Committee (MSC) represents students within the Association and also to important outside bodies, such as the Departments of Education and Health and the General Medical Council. Through the committee, the BMA campaigns on many issues, such as student finances and debt, reforms of the medical degree syllabus and health and safety. Following devolution, the BMA has established MSCs in Northern Ireland, Scotland and Wales. There are student representatives and BMA committees in every medical school, and the BMA runs many local events and talks for students. The vast majority of medical students join the BMA.

Medical students who are members of the BMA receive a variety of benefits, including a free subscription to *Student BMJ*, free guidance notes, a free copy of *Clinical Evidence*, library and information services and book discounts, to name but a few. General information, guidance, and student chat board can be found on the BMA's Medical Students Committee website.

British Medical Association	Tel: 020 7387 4499
BMA House	Fax: 020 7383 6494
Tavistock Square	Email: students@bma.org.uk
London WC1H 9JP	Web: http://www.bma.org.uk/students

The remainder of this chapter is divided into sections relating to education, finance and welfare corresponding to the different subcommittees within the MSC. Information in the other organizations' section relates to other medical student organisations that have a member that sits on the MSC.

Education

Universities and Colleges Admissions Service (UCAS)

Universities and Colleges	
Admissions Service	
Rose Hill	
New Barn Lane	
Cheltenham	Tel: 01242 222 444
Gloucestershire GL52 3LZ	Web: http://www.ucas.com

- *UCAS Handbook and Application Pack*: essential reading and material for applicants to university courses.

Department for Education and Skills

England

Tel: 0870 000 2288
Email: info@dfes.gsi.gov.uk
Web: http://www.dfes.gov.uk

Castle View House, Runcorn	Caxton House, London
Castle View House	Caxton House
East Lane	Tothill Street
Runcorn WA7 2GJ	London SW1H 9FN

Moorfoot, Sheffield
Moorfoot
Sheffield S1 4PQ

Sanctuary Buildings, London
Sanctuary Buildings
Great Smith Street
London SW1P 3BT

Mowden Hall, Darlington
Mowden Hall
Staindrop Road
Darlington DL3 9BG

Scotland

There are many publications about higher education and funding for Scottish students available on the web or from:

The Stationery Office Bookshop
71 Lothian Road
Edinburgh EH3 9AZ

Tel: 0131 228 4181
Fax: 0131 622 7017
Web: http://www.scotland.gov.uk

Scottish Executive Education Department
Victoria Quay
Edinburgh EH6 6QQ

Tel: 0131 556 8400
Fax: 0131 244 8240

Wales

Tel: 0800 731 9133
Web: http://www.dfes.gov.uk
Email: info@dfes.gsi.gov.uk

Northern Ireland

Department of Education
 Northern Ireland
Rathgael House
43 Balloo Road
Bangor BT19 7PR
County Down

Tel: 028 9127 9279
Fax: 028 9127 9100

Finance

Financial information

As mentioned in Chapter 5 the money4medstudents.org website is superb. Developed by the Royal Medical Benevolent Fund, the BMA Medical Students Committee and the National Association of

Student Money Advisors, it provides practical, unbiased information and advice to help you develop the financial knowledge and skills to enjoy your time at medical school but qualify with a manageable level of student debt. It includes budget planners, an advice clinic, specific information about each medical school and tips on how to borrow money sensibly. Go to www.money4medstudents.org.

Financial arrangements and support vary depending on which country you intend studying in. Some support is provided by the Departments of Education and Skills, and some from the Department of Health.

The Educational Grants Advisory Service provides information about student support systems in the UK and can help identify additional sources of funding.

Family Welfare Association
501–505 Kingsland Road
London E8 4AU

Tel: 0207 254 6251 (opening hours: Mondays, Wednesdays, and Fridays 10 AM–12 noon and 2 PM–4 PM)
Email: egas.enquiry@fwa.org.uk
Web: http://www.egas-online.org.uk

Relevant contact information for each nation is below.

England

For information and guides on student support ring the Department for Education and Skills (DfES).

Helpline: 0800 731 9133
Web: http://www.dfes.gov.uk

Financial Help for Health Care Students, a booklet by the Department of Health, explains NHS funding in more detail. Order one or download from the website:

Department of Health
PO Box 777
London SE1 6XH

Tel: 0845 60 60 655
Email: doh@prologistics.co.uk
Web: http://www.doh.gov.uk/hcsmain.htm

You can obtain bursary information from:

Student Grants Unit
Hesketh House
200–220 Broadway
Fleetwood
Lancashire FY7 8SS

Tel: 0845 358 6655
Fax: 01253 774 490
Email: nhs-sgu@ukonline.co.uk
http://www.nhsstudentgrants.co.uk

Scotland

Student Awards Agency for Scotland
3 Redheughs Rigg
South Gyle
Edinburgh EH12 9HH

Tel: 0845 111 1711
Web: http://www.student-support-saas.gov.uk

Wales

Further and Higher Education Division of the National Assembly for Wales
Tel: 02920 825 831
Web: http://www.learning.wales.gov.uk

You can obtain bursary information from:

NHS Wales Student Awards Unit
2nd Floor
Golate House
101 St Mary's St
Cardiff CF 10 1DX

Tel: 02920 261 495

Northern Ireland

Information for students from Northern Ireland can be obtained from the Department for Employment and Learning:

Also try:

The Department of Health
Social Services and Public Safety
Human Resources Directorate

Tel: 02890 524746
Web: http://www.dhsspsni.gov.uk
Web: http://www.delni.gov.uk

In addition, the following Government sites may be helpful:

English domiciled students studying in UK (pre NHS bursary years)

http://studentfinance.direct.gov.uk/index.htm

NHS tuition fee and grant page for English domiciled students studying in the UK, and non-UK EU domiciled students studying in England, in years 5 and onwards (standard course) and years 2–4 (graduate entry course)

http://www.nhsstudentgrants.co.uk

Welsh domiciled students studying in the UK

http://www.studentfinancewales.co.uk

Non-UK EU students studying in England and Wales	http://www.dfes.gov.uk/studentsupport/eustudents/index.shtml
Scottish domiciled students studying in UK and non-UK EU students studying in Scotland	http://www.saas.gov.uk
Northern Irish domiciled students studying in the UK	http://www.delni.gov.uk/index.cfm/area/information/page/StudentFinance
DfES marketing site! For international (non-EU students)	http://www.dfes.gov.uk/international-students
Isle of Man domiciled studying in UK	http://www.gov.im/education/support/grants.xml
Jersey domiciled studying in UK	http://www.gov.je/ESC/Culture+and+Lifelong+Learning/Careers+and+work+related+learning/Student+Finance/default.htm
	http://www.gov.je/NR/rdonlyres/12D04D0F-8DC3-401B-BCA2-87EC77184EE4/0/StudentFinance.pdf
Guernsey domiciled studying in UK	http://www2.gov.gg/ccm/navigation/education/education-dept-info/grants-awards

Charities

Copies of the following books should be available in the reference section of most public libraries:

- *The Charities Digest* – published by the Family Welfare Association
- *Money to Study* – published by UKOSA/NUS/EGAS
- *The Educational Grants Directory* – published by the Directory of Social Change
- *Directory of Grant-Making Trusts* – published by Charities Aid Foundation/Biblios

The British Medical Association Charities Office (see BMA address) has information about awards and grants for mature and second degree medical students.

Welfare

National Union of Students (NUS)

For general information on issues relating to students:

National Union of Students
Nelson Mandela House
Holloway Road
London N7 6LJ

Tel: 020 7272 8900
Fax: 020 7263 5713
Email: nusuk@nus.org.uk
Web: http://www.nusonline.co.uk

Gay and Lesbian Association of Doctors and Dentists (GLADD)

GLADD was formed in 1995. It has an active student section and provides professional support and educational and social meetings, both locally and nationally. GLADD campaigns vigorously within the health service and in the country at large on issues of equality relating to the lesbian, gay, and bisexual community.

Email: gladd@dircon.co.uk
Web: http://www.gladd.dircon.co.uk

SKILL

National Bureau for Students with Disabilities is a registered national charity, which promotes opportunities for disabled people in further and higher education, training and employment. Skill operates a freephone information service that provides expert information on studying and training – from applying to university or college through to obtaining a Disabled Students Allowance and getting adjustments in exams. Skill also works with policy-makers, tutors and disabled student advisers to ensure that disabled students are empowered to achieve their potential.

Information Service	Tel: 0800 328 5050 (voice) 0800 068 2422 (text)
Email	info@skill.org.uk
Web	www.skill.org.uk

Other organisations

Junior Association for the Study of Medical Education

JASME	Tel: 0131 225 9111
c/o ASME	Fax: 0131 225 9444
12 Queen Street	Web: www.jasme.org.uk
Edinburgh EH2 1JE	Email: info@jasme.org.uk

Medical Students International Network (MedSIN)

Founded in 1997, MedSIN is an independent, student-run organization which aims to facilitate medical students' involvement in humanitarian and educational activities at local, national and international levels. MedSIN groups in medical schools carry out sex-education projects, international exchanges, bone marrow registration drives, seminars on topical issues and much more. Through its membership of the International Federation of Medical Students' Associations (IFMSA), MedSIN also provides opportunities to go on projects all over the world, from Angola to Zimbabwe. The IFMSA was founded in 1951 and promotes international co-operation on professional training and the achievement of humanitarian ideals. To get in touch or find out more, visit the MedSIN website: http://www.medsin.org.

Other useful information

Armed forces: cadet recruitment

Army
Royal Army Medical Corps
Recruiting Office
Regimental Headquarters
Army Medical Services
Slim Road
Camberley
Surrey GU14 4NP

Tel: 01276 412 730
Fax: 01276 412 731
Email: ramc.recruiting@army.mod.uk.net

RAF
Medical and Dental Liaison Officer
Directorate of Recruiting and Selection
(Royal Air Force)
PO Box 100
Cranwell
Sleaford
Lincolnshire NG34 8GZ

Tel: 01400 261 201 ext 6811
Fax: 01400 262 220
Email: mdlo@royalairforce.net

Royal Navy
Med Pers (N)2
Room 133
Victory Building
HM Naval Base
Portsmouth PO1 3LS

Tel: 02392 727 818
Fax: 02392 727 805

Further reading

Learning Medicine by Peter Richards (formerly Dean of St Mary's Medical School) and Simon Stockill, published by BMJ Publishing Group and updated regularly. Now in its 16th edition, this title is available through Hammicks BMA Bookshop, Manchester. Tel. 0161 276 9704, email orders@hammicksbma. com, website www.bmjbookshop.com. Price £13.95 (discount available for BMA members). http:// www.bmjbookshop.com.

Medical Specialities: the way forward (2005), available free of charge from the Science and Education Department to BMA members or at £10 to non-members. Tel 020 7383 6164, email: info. science@bma.org.uk. Also available through Hammicks BMA Bookshop, Manchester. Tel. 0161 276 9704, email orders@hammicksbma.com, website www.bmjbookshop.com.

Becoming a doctor: entry in 2007 (2006), available from the BMA website http://www.bma.org.uk/ ap.nsf/Content/becomingadoctor2007.

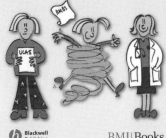
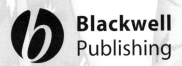